A groundbreaking exploration into PTSD and severe mental illness, encompassing psychotic, severe mood, and borderline personality disorders. This exceptional book equips readers with a meticulous, hands-on guide to assessing and treating these complex conditions. From comprehensive etiological knowledge to evidence-based cognitive restructuring treatment, this book is rich with empirical support. Authored by distinguished clinical researchers in PTSD and psychosis, this work stands as a testament to their expertise. An indispensable resource for clinicians, this is a definitive must-have for anyone working with people with severe mental illness.

—**Tania Lecomte, PhD,** Professor of Psychology, University of Montréal, Montréal, Québec, Canada; Director of The Canadian Network for Research in Schizophrenia and Psychoses

In this important volume, Drs. Mueser and Gottlieb provide us with a sensitive and skillful guide to assessing and treating PTSD in individuals with serious mental illness. Their years of clinical experience, combined with their considerable research, shine through in every chapter. Thank you for this important resource and for so ably helping some of the most vulnerable trauma survivors in our care systems.

—**J. Gayle Beck, PhD,** Emerita Professor of Psychology and former Chair of Excellence, University of Memphis, Memphis, TN, United States

Treatment of Posttraumatic Stress Disorder in Serious Mental Illness

Kim T. Mueser & Jennifer D. Gottlieb

Treatment of Posttraumatic Stress Disorder in Serious Mental Illness

The Cognitive Restructuring Program

Foreword by Douglas Turkington

AMERICAN PSYCHOLOGICAL ASSOCIATION

Published by
American Psychological Association
750 First Street, NE
Washington, DC 20002
https://www.apa.org

Order Department
https://www.apa.org/pubs/books
order@apa.org

Typeset in Meridien and Ortodoxa by Lumina Datamatics, India

Printer: Sheridan Books, Chelsea, MI
Cover Designer: Gwen J. Grafft, Minneapolis, MN

Library of Congress Cataloging-in-Publication Data

Names: Mueser, Kim T., editor. | Gottlieb, Jennifer D., editor. | American Psychological Association, issuing body.
Title: Treatment of posttraumatic stress disorder in serious mental illness : the cognitive restructuring program / edited by Kim T. Mueser and Jennifer D. Gottlieb
Description: Washington, DC : American Psychological Association, [2025] | Includes bibliographical references and index.
Identifiers: LCCN 2024013490 (print) | LCCN 2024013491 (ebook) | ISBN 9781433841651 (paperback) | ISBN 9781433841668 (ebook)
Subjects: MESH: Stress Disorders, Post-Traumatic—complications | Stress Disorders, Post-Traumatic—therapy | Psychological Trauma—complications | Cognitive Restructuring—methods | BISAC: PSYCHOLOGY / Clinical Psychology | PSYCHOLOGY / Psychopathology / Post-Traumatic Stress Disorder (PTSD)
Classification: LCC RC552.P67 (print) | LCC RC552.P67 (ebook) | NLM WM 172.5 | DDC 616.85/21—dc23/eng/20240806
LC record available at https://lccn.loc.gov/2024013490
LC ebook record available at https://lccn.loc.gov/2024013491

https://doi.org/10.1037/0000423-000

Printed in the United States of America

10 9 8 7 6 5 4 3 2 1

To my colleague and friend, Stanley D. Rosenberg, whose shared passion for reducing the effects of trauma on the lives of others made this work possible.
—KIM T. MUESER

To Jed, for always bringing out my best. To my family, and my friends who are like family, for all of their support and love along the way. And in memory of David Schuldberg, PhD, for his encouragement to become the psychologist that I am today.
—JENNIFER D. GOTTLIEB

CONTENTS

FOREWORD

It is a great honor to be invited by two of the greatest thinkers and exponents of cognitive behavioral therapy (CBT) for severe mental disorders to write this Foreword. I have had the fortune to work with Kim (and latterly Jen) for many years since the Cognitive Therapy of Psychosis Academy was first formed by Aaron T. Beck in the 1990s. I have personally worked in the field since 1988 and have been involved in most developments in CBT for severe mental disorders (specifically psychosis) since that time, publishing 13 books and manuals and 240 peer-reviewed publications. I worked with Aaron T. Beck as he and his team developed recovery-oriented CBT as a viable treatment for disabling negative symptoms of schizophrenia by changing defeatist beliefs. David Kingdon and I first described traumatic psychosis as the largest subgroup of "the schizophrenias" in 2008. Tony Morrison and colleagues clarified the role of trauma further, and therapies began to be developed and piloted. Initially, the Ehlers and Clark approach was piloted to begin to work with the cognitions linked to trauma-related emotional "hot spots" linked to the psychosis. Subsequently, prolonged exposure and then eye movement desensitization and reprocessing were piloted and shown to be safe and promising. The field has been integrated and has made a giant leap forward in the volume that you are about to read.

Kim Mueser's interests have closely (and perhaps slightly eerily!) paralleled my own, including developing cognitive techniques to enhance family psychoeducation, treatment of comorbid substance use, recovery from severe mental disorders, and more recently trauma within psychosis. I have followed Kim's work closely over the years and recognize in him a kindred spirit and a true pioneer in the field.

Jennifer Gottlieb is younger than Kim and I and has both the energy and determination to further describe, develop, and test the rapidly developing field of treating trauma in severe mental disorders. Jen has been involved in the development of rating scales and running randomized controlled trials of new interventions for trauma in severe mental disorders. Jen has also pioneered the implementation of CBT for psychosis across North America and the use of online treatment options.

To have both authors work together to complete this volume on CBT for trauma in severe mental disorders is an exciting prospect for the reader.

Why do we need this book at this point in time?

Well, the role of trauma in the causation and maintenance of severe mental disorders is being increasingly recognized. Services are increasingly attempting to be "trauma focused." However, classification systems have not yet caught up with clinical practice. Every clinician—whether in community treatment teams, rehabilitation, or acute inpatient services—recognizes clients with (complex) posttraumatic stress disorder (PTSD), emotional instability, self-harm, psychosis, and a history of unprocessed trauma. There is also the emergence of a group of dissociative psychoses with trauma and dissociative identity disorder. These clients often make only placebo-level response to medication but have the potential to recover with integrated psychological treatment regimes. But the process of therapy has never been adequately described until Kim and Jen wrote this book. Thank you very much!

One of the key points is the breadth of the book. A clear approach to using cognitive restructuring to treat PTSD within the schizophrenias, bipolar disorder, treatment-resistant depression, and borderline personality disorder is presented. The clarion call is made by the authors to ask about and diagnose/formulate the presence of trauma and PTSD in serious mental illness as it is so treatable and so frequently camouflaged by voices, delusions, and negative symptoms. Aaron T. Beck would have been delighted to note that the good outcomes with cognitive restructuring are mediated by changes in trauma-related cognitions. The low dropout rate with Cognitive Restructuring is impressive as many clients with severe mental illness struggle to accept the techniques of prolonged exposure. Specific modifications are described to work with comorbidities, including substance use. The intervention is meticulously presented and is cost-effective, being delivered to clients with severe PTSD and serious mental illness with 12 to 16 sessions being given over 3 to 6 months. One of the great delights of this volume is to be introduced to Kim and Jen's clients through some anonymized case vignettes and then to follow them through the various stages of therapy. Cognitive restructuring is the cornerstone of the intervention described, but the Breathing Retraining with linked imagery, wellness plans, and the support of family are all important. Work with trauma-related schemas is clearly described along with fascinating examples of techniques such as the Payoff Matrix. It was so encouraging to see specific chapters on treating PTSD within psychosis and within borderline personality disorder. The many challenges for clinicians are clearly described, and potential solutions demonstrated. A unique feature of this volume is that all the worksheets, handouts, and clinician tools are also translated into Spanish. This will improve treatment access to the Spanish-speaking client population in the United States and beyond.

This book will be read widely and should be available for every community psychiatry and mental health treatment clinician and to all inpatient staff, whether working in acute treatment units or in rehabilitation settings. Prepare to be inspired and to find new confidence in your clinical practice. There are nuggets of practical wisdom on virtually every page. I fully endorse this book and will be promoting it wherever I travel to give lectures or workshops.

That's enough from me, it's now time to start reading!

—Douglas Turkington, MD, FRCPsych
Professor of Psychosocial Psychiatry
Newcastle University
Newcastle-upon-Tyne, United Kingdom

PREFACE

Posttraumatic stress disorder (PTSD) is one of the most common disorders in persons with serious mental illness (SMI), leading to more severe psychiatric symptoms, greater impairment in psychosocial functioning, poorer physical health, and higher use of acute care services. Yet despite major advances in the treatment of PTSD in the general population and the devastating effects of trauma and PTSD on the well-being of individuals with SMI, for many years PTSD remained undiagnosed and unaddressed and therefore has continued to be a neglected treatment priority in the SMI population.

Only more recently has this begun to change, in part due to the development of our Cognitive Restructuring (CR) for PTSD program. Clinicians now have access to the tools for screening, detecting, and treating PTSD in their clients with SMI and therefore relieving them of the great burden of trauma on their lives. This volume is a practical guide to this evidence-based CR for PTSD treatment, which has been specifically designed to meet the unique needs of people with SMI.

The CR for PTSD program is a time-limited (12–16 weeks) intervention that targets PTSD through established cognitive behavioral therapy techniques shown to be effective for the treatment of PTSD in the general population. These techniques include psychoeducation; Breathing Retraining for coping with anxiety and physiological overarousal; and teaching cognitive restructuring as a step-by-step self-management skill to enable clients to identify and examine, challenge, and change trauma-related thoughts and beliefs that underlie their distressing PTSD symptoms. Designed to meet the particular needs and challenges of persons with SMI, the CR for PTSD program incorporates specific clinical techniques, including simplified skills and materials (and simplified methods for teaching them), collaboration with the client's primary treatment team, and opportunities to apply the Breathing Retraining and CR skills to other problematic psychiatric symptoms. The program is structured but flexible and can be used with clients across a broad range of SMI diagnoses and levels of functioning.

The CR for PTSD program can also play an important role in helping individuals make progress toward their recovery from SMI more generally. The intervention incorporates the defining characteristics of recovery-oriented services—including support for self-determination and choice and being person-centered, strengths-based, and trauma-informed. In multiple ways, the program facilitates different processes that contribute to recovery, including (based on the CHIME framework) Connection with others, Hope for a better future, Identity shifts to more positive and balanced self-concepts, new Meaning and sense of purpose in life, and Empowerment over one's life.

Rigorous, controlled research with persons with SMI diagnoses (e.g., schizophrenia, bipolar disorder, major depression, and borderline personality disorder) has shown that the CR for PTSD program is effective at reducing PTSD symptoms and diagnoses, depression, and other psychiatric symptoms and substantially improves overall functioning.

Part I of this volume is devoted to providing important background information to understand the interrelationship among trauma, PTSD, and SMI, which is critical to implementing the CR for PTSD program. Chapter 1 reviews the high prevalence and impact of trauma and PTSD on people with serious psychiatric conditions and lays out a comprehensive model for understanding how PTSD interacts with and worsens the course of SMI. Chapter 2 gives an overview of evidence-based treatments for PTSD, the rationale for the development of the CR for PTSD program, the intervention's theoretical underpinnings in cognitive models of PTSD and contributions to recovery from SMI, and a brief summary of research supporting this program. Chapter 3 covers the basics of trauma and PTSD assessment of persons with SMI, including a review of the defining symptoms and associated characteristics of PTSD, ways to distinguish PTSD symptoms from other SMI symptoms, and recommendations for easy-to-use and efficient methods for screening and identifying individuals with PTSD.

Part II of the book dives into the specifics of implementing the CR for PTSD program, beginning with Chapter 4 on the logistics of providing the intervention, which outlines where and when to implement the program and who can most benefit from it. The remaining chapters in this part of the book (Chapters 5–11) provide the nuts and bolts of how to deliver the CR for PTSD intervention. This begins with engagement and program orientation, development of a Wellness Plan, and the teaching and practice of Breathing Retraining in Chapter 5, followed by psychoeducation about trauma and PTSD and collaborative goal setting in Chapter 6. Chapters 7 through 9 get to the heart of the CR for PTSD program, in which cognitive restructuring is taught to clients as a self-management skill for dealing with all negative feelings and is eventually applied to helping them challenge and change inaccurate, distressing trauma-related and core beliefs responsible for their PTSD symptoms. Chapter 10 outlines specific helpful strategies that can be used to address common challenges that may come up in the program. Chapter 11, the final chapter in this part, provides information about fostering generalization of the CR for PTSD skills to clients' day-to-day lives as well as guidelines for termination. Within these chapters, there are abundant sample in-session dialogues with case vignettes that follow three unique clients (Leigh-Ann, Edmundo, and Donata) as they participate in the CR for PTSD program, and they bring to life and illustrate clinical techniques for teaching the program's specific skills.

Part III of the book includes two chapters focused on providing the CR for PTSD program to clients with special challenges, including those with psychosis (and associated negative symptoms and cognitive impairment; Chapter 12) and clients with borderline personality disorder traits or diagnosis (Chapter 13).

In Part IV of the book, we provide conclusions (Chapter 14) aimed at discussing the role of the CR for PTSD program in a recovery-oriented and comprehensive system of care for persons with SMI or in the armamentarium of treatment tools for independent clinicians who work with this population. We distinguish trauma-informed care from trauma-specific care (which targets PTSD directly), highlight the necessity of the latter as needed to truly address the critical unmet needs of those with SMI, and offer recommended steps to take toward increasing access to this intervention.

This volume provides critical and user-friendly resources and materials for delivering the CR for PTSD program and tracking clients' progress throughout it. Specifically, the book's Appendix includes the educational handouts and worksheets needed to guide clients in learning about PTSD, Breathing Retraining, and cognitive restructuring skills, as well as tools for helping clinicians evaluate clients' progress in therapy (such as tracking their trauma-related beliefs for change over the course of the program).

Furthermore, a special feature of the book is that in addition to providing the handouts and worksheets in the Appendix of the printed book; the online Appendix also contains the full range of educational handouts and worksheets for clients translated into Spanish. These additional materials provide clinicians with unique resources for treating Spanish-speaking individuals with SMI, who have high rates of trauma and PTSD but often do not have access to effective interventions, are often overlooked for participation in trauma-based services, and/or may not seek therapy due to a lack of availability of culturally appropriate treatment options in Spanish. The online Appendix (access to which is included via the hardcopy book) also contains a supplemental chapter (Chapter 15) that outlines a brief intervention for PTSD called BREATHE (for Brief Relaxation, Education, And Trauma HEaling) that can be implemented in settings (e.g., short-stay inpatient units) or situations (e.g., with unhoused individuals) where use of the full CR for PTSD program may not be appropriate. These resources can be accessed online (https://www.apa.org/pubs/books/treatment-posttraumatic-stress-disorder-serious-mental-illness): see the Resources tab.

In recent years, the growth of trauma-informed care in mental health treatment systems has resulted in a dramatic increase in awareness of trauma's pernicious impact on people with SMI. However, this increased awareness has not been accompanied by a concerted effort to address the most established (and most treatable) clinical syndrome associated with trauma—PTSD. This book provides clinicians with the necessary guidelines and resources to efficiently and effectively treat PTSD in the SMI population and to bridge the large gap between science and practice in serving these individuals. The time has come to alleviate the disproportionate burden of trauma and PTSD on the lives of persons with SMI.

ACKNOWLEDGMENTS

We greatly appreciate the many collaborators with whom we have worked over the years in developing and refining the Cognitive Restructuring (CR) for posttraumatic stress disorder (PTSD) program. We owe a debt of gratitude to our colleague Stanley D. Rosenberg, with whom we standardized and initially tested the CR for PTSD program for persons with serious mental illness (SMI). Portions of this book are drawn from an earlier book about this intervention (Mueser et al., 2009), which provided an explication of the CR program as applied to a broad range of special populations.

We have been influenced by and very much value the important work of Edna B. Foa. Dr. Foa's pioneering contributions to the treatment of PTSD, including both prolonged exposure and cognitive restructuring approaches, have had a major influence on the field and informed the development, structure, and pacing of the CR program, including the foundational components of psychoeducation and Breathing Retraining and the introduction of CR. If modern scientist–practitioners stand on the shoulders of the giants who preceded them, we stand firmly on her shoulders.

We also express our gratitude to our many colleagues who have worked with us in adapting the CR program for different clinical populations with PTSD and who have played critical roles in implementing the CR program in real-world settings, evaluating it, and championing it to increase access for those with SMI, including Kimberley Ahlgren, Angela Belleville, Steven Blum, Elisa Bolton, Michael Bradley, Patricia Carty, Kristen Davis, Delia Cimpean, Diane DiStaso, Rachel Fite, Lisa Fortuna, Virginia Fraser, Jessica Hamblen, Amy Hardy, Katie Hilton, Melissa Jadhav, Kay Jankowski, Aaron Katz, Chris Lerro, Weili Lu, Stephanie Marcello, Katie McDonald, Mark McGovern, Lauren Ng, Tom O'Hare,

Sarah Pratt, Lisa Razzano, David Roe, Harriet Rosenberg, Stephanie Sacks, Michelle Salyers, Margaret Sherrer, Steve Silverstein, Craig Steel, Barry Walsh, Andrea Wolloff, and Phil Yanos.

A big thank you to Julie Schwietert Collazo for working with us to provide professional Spanish translation of the CR program's handouts and worksheets included in this volume's online Appendix, which allows for much-needed increased treatment access for members of the Spanish-speaking community.

Finally, we are indebted to the many trauma survivors with whom we have worked over numerous years. We have deeply admired the strength and resiliency of these individuals and have learned immensely from the privilege of being let into their lives.

BACKGROUND AND OVERVIEW OF TRAUMA AND PTSD IN SERIOUS MENTAL ILLNESS

1

Trauma and PTSD in Serious Mental Illness

It is now widely recognized that emotionally traumatic events play an important role in the lives of people with serious mental illness (SMI). Early traumatic experiences such as sexual and physical abuse can increase an individual's chances of developing a major psychiatric disorder, such as schizophrenia, bipolar disorder, or severe major depression, which in turn can lead to further trauma after the onset of mental illness as a result of interpersonal victimization. Trauma exposure can also increase vulnerability to posttraumatic stress disorder (PTSD), which can contribute to more severe symptoms of SMI and greater impairments in functioning. Fortunately, there are effective treatments for reducing the burden of PTSD that were first developed and tested in the general population and more recently have been adapted and validated in persons with SMI, as described in this volume. This chapter is aimed at providing critical background information about trauma, PTSD, and the nature of their interactions with SMI to set the stage for the treatment of PTSD in the following chapters.

DEFINITION OF SERIOUS MENTAL ILLNESS

The term *serious mental illness* (SMI; also referred to as *severe mental illness*) is widely used when describing people who have a psychiatric disorder that results in significant and prolonged impairment in psychosocial functioning, including in areas such as role functioning (e.g., work, school, parenting), social functioning, and self-care and independent living skills. The psychiatric disorders most frequently associated with SMI are schizophrenia, schizoaffective disorder, bipolar disorder, and treatment-refractory major depression (Grubaugh

https://doi.org/10.1037/0000423-001
Treatment of Posttraumatic Stress Disorder in Serious Mental Illness: The Cognitive Restructuring Program, by K. T. Mueser and J. D. Gottlieb

et al., 2021; Parabiaghi et al., 2006). However, other psychiatric diagnoses may qualify as well, such as borderline personality disorder and schizotypal personality disorder, severe and chronic anxiety disorders, and PTSD. In this volume, we use the term *serious mental illness* mainly to refer to people with any of the four primary disorders listed earlier (schizophrenia, schizoaffective disorder, bipolar disorder, treatment-refractory major depression) or borderline personality disorder. Although substance use disorders are included as psychiatric disorders in classification systems such as the *Diagnostic and Statistical Manual of Mental Disorders* (5th ed.; *DSM-5*; American Psychiatric Association, 2013) and the *International Statistical Classification of Diseases and Related Health Problems* (11th ed.; *ICD-11*; World Health Organization, 2019) and often have a profound effect on functioning, substance use diagnoses alone are not generally included in definitions of SMI. However, it is common for people to have an SMI due to another mental illness and also to have a co-occurring substance use disorder.

There are some variations in the specific definitions of SMI (Martínez-Martínez et al., 2020). Nevertheless, the following broad definition provided by the Substance Abuse and Mental Health Services Administration (SAMHSA, 2017) captures the essence of the term: "having (within the past year) a diagnosable mental, behavior, or emotional disorder that causes serious functional impairment that substantially interferes with or limits one or more major life activities" (para. 3). In this volume, we adopt SAMHSA's broad definition of SMI and include anyone who has a psychiatric disorder that results in significant functional impairment.

PREVALENCE OF TRAUMA EXPOSURE IN SMI

The word *trauma* is part of everyday language and has many shades of meaning. For example, people may describe the impact of divorce, financial setbacks, or getting fired from a job as being *traumatic*. These types of stressors are discussed in the mental health literature as "adverse life events," and there is little question that the accumulation of such experiences can negatively impact health, mental health, and overall functioning (Avison & Gotlib, 1994; Lovallo, 2005). However, in this volume we use the term *trauma* to refer to a more limited and extreme class of events: the experience of an uncontrollable event perceived to threaten a person's sense of integrity or survival. This usage follows the definitions of trauma adopted by the *Diagnostic and Statistical Manual of Mental Disorders* (5th ed., text rev., *DSM-5-TR*; American Psychiatric Association, 2022) and the *ICD-11*, where a traumatic event is defined as any experience or witnessing of a direct threat of death, severe bodily harm, or psychological injury or knowledge that a traumatic event has occurred to a close family member or friend. People usually react to a traumatic event with intense distress, although such distress is not a required part of the definition.

Between 50% and 70% of all individuals living in the United States have experienced at least one traumatic event (Kessler et al., 1995, 2014;

Stein et al., 2000). Rates of trauma exposure for people with SMI far exceed those in the general population, and multiple traumas are common (Brady et al., 2003; de Vries et al., 2019; Grubaugh et al., 2011; Mueser, Salyers, et al., 2004). A review of 33 studies on interpersonal trauma reported that the mean prevalence of physical abuse in persons with SMI was 46%, and the mean prevalence of sexual abuse was 37%, compared with rates of 21% and 23%, respectively, in the general population (Mauritz et al., 2013).

The results of a large survey study using representative samples of people with SMI illustrate the high prevalence of interpersonal victimization in this population in both childhood and adulthood. This study included 779 persons with SMI receiving either inpatient or outpatient services in one of five treatment settings in the northeastern United States (Goodman et al., 2001). The study found that 49% of women and 29% of men had a history of childhood sexual abuse, with rates of physical abuse in childhood of 54% and 58%, respectively. In adulthood, 57% of women and 25% of men had been sexually assaulted, with corresponding rates of physical assault being 75% and 79%, respectively. Comparable findings were reported in a previous study (Mueser et al., 1998) using similar research methods in 275 persons with SMI from four treatment settings (two inpatient, two outpatient) in two states (Maryland and New Hampshire).

The high rates of interpersonal trauma in childhood for individuals with SMI are broadly consistent with abundant evidence that adverse childhood experiences increase the risk of developing a wide range of health and mental health conditions (Dube et al., 2010; Edwards et al., 2003; Felitti et al., 1998; Matheson et al., 2013). The findings are furthermore in line with research showing that interpersonal trauma in childhood, including sexual and physical abuse, has a major impact on the development of psychotic disorders such as schizophrenia and other SMI (Bendall et al., 2008; McGrath et al., 2017; Morgan et al., 2020; Varese et al., 2012). A broad range of hypotheses have been proposed to account for the influence of early trauma on the development of SMI (Kingdon & Turkington, 2004; Murphy et al., 2013; Read et al., 2001; Rosenfield et al., 2022), and it is likely that multiple pathways exist. For example, the developmental risk factor model of psychosis proposes that childhood adversity interacts with early neurodevelopmental abnormalities (due to factors such as genetic contributions, prenatal exposure to viral infections, poor nutrition, and obstetric hazards) and other factors in adolescence and early adulthood (e.g., urbanicity, migration, cannabis use) to increase risk to developing a psychosis-spectrum disorder (Murray et al., 2017).

In addition to the high prevalence of trauma preceding the onset of major psychiatric disorders, individuals are more likely to be exposed to traumatic events after developing a SMI as well (Dean et al., 2018; Maniglio, 2009; Monahan et al., 2017; Teplin et al., 2005). For example, a national cohort study from Sweden reported that individuals with a previously diagnosed psychiatric condition were 3.4 times more likely to be subjected to violence (defined as outpatient or inpatient treatment or death associated with an injury deliberately inflicted by another person) than their siblings with no diagnosed psychiatric condition (Sariaslan et al., 2020). Another study of 361 persons with SMI compared to 3,138 general population controls reported that 40% of clients versus 14% of controls had been the victim of a crime in the past year and that 19% of clients versus 3% of controls had been violently assaulted (Khalifeh et al., 2015). Rates of violent victimization are even higher among some subgroups of persons with SMI, such as those who are episodically homeless (Goodman et al., 1995; Roy et al., 2014).

Multiple factors may account for the high rate of trauma following the onset of SMI, including the following:

- Prior trauma exposure increases the risk of subsequent trauma exposure (both in the general population and in persons with SMI) resulting in a vicious cycle of revictimization.

- The symptoms of major mental illnesses and cognitive impairments can make individuals with SMI less able to recognize dangerous social situations, increasing their vulnerability to interpersonal trauma.

- The high prevalence of substance use disorders in people with SMI can result in victimization due to reduced ability to protect themselves when under the influence of alcohol and drugs and engagement in high-risk behaviors related to having an addiction.

- Most persons with SMI have limited economic means and live in low-income neighborhoods with higher crime rates.

PREVALENCE OF PTSD IN SMI

PTSD is a major psychological disorder that is diagnosed based on experiencing specific types of symptoms at least 1 month following exposure to a traumatic event (e.g., sexual or physical abuse/assault, witnessing violence to others, accidents, disasters, combat; American Psychiatric Association, 2013). Four clusters of symptoms are used to define PTSD, including (a) reexperiencing the trauma (e.g., intrusive memories of the event, flashbacks), (b) avoidance of trauma-related stimuli (e.g., people in situations that remind the person of the event), (c) physiological overarousal (e.g., exaggerated startle response, difficulty sleeping), and (d) altered thoughts or feelings (e.g., belief that other people cannot be trusted, pervasive feelings of anxiety). The lifetime prevalence of PTSD in the general population is estimated to be approximately 7% to 12% (Kessler et al., 1995, 2014; Kilpatrick et al., 2013), while approximately 3% to 4% of persons currently meet criteria for PTSD at any given moment (i.e., point prevalence; Kessler et al., 2005). PTSD most often develops during adolescence or early adulthood but can develop at any age. Women in the general population are more likely to develop PTSD than men (Goldstein et al., 2016).

By all accounts, the prevalence of PTSD in persons with SMI far exceeds that of the general population (Grubaugh et al., 2011; Mauritz et al., 2013;

Mueser, Rosenberg, et al., 2002; Seow et al., 2016), with most estimates ranging between 25% and 45%. For example, in one systematic review of 29 studies of PTSD in people with SMI (Zammit et al., 2018), the average prevalence of PTSD was found to be 33%. Another review of 33 studies (Mauritz et al., 2013) reported a population-weighted mean prevalence of PTSD in persons with SMI of 30%. One large epidemiological study with 34,653 participants reported that the rate of PTSD in people with borderline personality disorder was 30% (Pagura et al., 2010).

These high rates of PTSD among people with SMI have been reported in numerous studies throughout the world. For example, two relatively early studies conducted in the United States (Mueser et al., 1998; Mueser, Salyers, et al., 2004) with samples of 275 and 782 persons receiving treatment for SMI found rates of current PTSD 43% and 35%, respectively. The largest study to date in the United States of 3,445 veterans found that the prevalence of PTSD in veterans with schizophrenia was 22% and was 33% in veterans with bipolar disorder (Harvey et al., 2014). A study from Spain of 323 persons with SMI found that 38% met criteria for probable PTSD (Gottlieb et al., 2018). Similarly high rates of PTSD in this population have been reported in studies conducted in other countries, such as Australia (McFarlane et al., 2001), Brazil (Braga et al., 2005), Great Britain (Steel et al., 2011), Germany (Steinert et al., 2006), Hungary (Halász et al., 2013), Italy (Pollice et al., 2010), Morocco (El Jabiry et al., 2022), the Netherlands (Lommen & Restifo, 2009), Singapore (Sin et al., 2010), and South Africa (van Zyl et al., 2008).

Why Is PTSD so Common in Severe Mental Illness?

There are several reasons why the rates of PTSD are so much higher in people with SMI than in the general population. First, degree of trauma exposure is an important predictor of PTSD in the general population, with the number of traumatic events and the severity of trauma exposure increasing the likelihood of someone developing PTSD (Cougle et al., 2009; Gould et al., 2021; Liu et al., 2017). Similar associations between exposure to more types of traumatic events and specifically to childhood sexual abuse have been found to predict PTSD in persons with SMI (DeTore et al., 2021; Mueser et al., 1998; Mueser, Salyers, et al., 2004) and to be correlated with PTSD symptom severity (Lu et al., 2013). Thus, the higher rate of trauma in people with SMI (reviewed in the previous section) is consistent with their higher rate of PTSD.

Second, adverse childhood experiences and trauma in childhood and early adulthood increase the risk of someone developing a major mental illness such as a psychotic disorder (Read, 1997; Rosenfield et al., 2022). As early trauma exposure can also lead to PTSD, trauma may be acting as a "third variable" accounting for some of the increased comorbidity between PTSD and SMI. There may be other third variables that also serve to increase vulnerability to both disorders and explain further their high comorbidity. For example, lower levels of cognitive functioning increase the risk of developing both schizophrenia

(Kendler et al., 2016; MacCabe et al., 2013) and PTSD (Gilbertson et al., 2006; Kremen et al., 2007; Wigham & Emerson, 2015).

Third, prior psychopathology is an established risk factor that increases the chances of a person developing PTSD following exposure to a traumatic event (North et al., 1997; Pietrzak et al., 2014; Zlotnick et al., 2004). This means that when people have developed a SMI, they are more vulnerable to developing PTSD after a traumatic event than they would be if they did not have an SMI diagnosis. Consistent with this, although the prevalence of PTSD is increased in persons with first episode of psychosis (typically ranging between 5% and 20%; DeTore et al., 2021; Neria et al., 2002; Sin et al., 2010), PTSD rates are even higher among individuals with a previously established SMI (Mauritz et al., 2013; Seow et al., 2016), suggesting an increased susceptibility to developing PTSD after the onset of their illness.

Fourth, just as the onset of a SMI can increase the chances of developing PTSD, the onset of PTSD can also increase the risk of developing a SMI. Major depression is the most common comorbid disorder following the development of PTSD and is present in approximately 50% of cases (Flory & Yehuda, 2015). Furthermore, a prospective cohort study in Denmark showed that an inpatient or outpatient psychiatric diagnosis of acute stress disorder or PTSD significantly increased the person's chances of subsequently being diagnosed with either schizophrenia or bipolar disorder over the following 5 years (Okkels et al., 2017).

Last, there is strong evidence that PTSD is often associated with mild psychotic symptoms (e.g., hearing voices, overvalued ideas, paranoid beliefs) that cannot be explained by another psychiatric disorder such as schizophrenia or depression (Sautter et al., 2002; Seedat et al., 2003; Shevlin et al., 2011). Since psychotic symptoms are more frequently associated with SMI and are not mentioned as associated clinical features of PTSD in most diagnostic systems such as *DSM-5* (American Psychiatric Association, 2013), they may sometimes be misconstrued as due to another disorder, resulting in the misdiagnosis of some individuals with PTSD as having a psychotic disorder (Waldfogel & Mueser, 1988). The fact that PTSD is frequently underdiagnosed in people with SMI (see next section) makes this a distinct possibility.

Underdiagnosis of PTSD

Despite the high prevalence of PTSD in SMI, it is frequently not diagnosed in routine clinical services for this population (Brady et al., 2003; Brooker et al., 2016; Cusack et al., 2006; de Bont et al., 2015; Lu, Silverstein, et al., 2023; Mueser et al., 1998; Mueser, Salyers, et al., 2004). For example, in one large study of 776 clients with SMI receiving public mental health services who had probable PTSD based on screening with the PTSD Checklist (Weathers et al., 2013), only 13.7% had a diagnosis of PTSD documented in their medical records (Lu, Srijeyanthan, et al., 2022). Individuals with major depression were more likely to have a chart diagnosis of PTSD (18.8%) than those with bipolar disorder (6.3%) or schizophrenia (4.1%). In another study of a large mental health agency serving people with SMI in Madrid, Spain (Gottlieb et al., 2018), among 334 persons screened for trauma and PTSD, 124 (34%) were found to have probable PTSD with an average five lifetime traumatic events. Yet despite having received mental health services for an average of 16 years, none of them (0%) had a diagnosis of PTSD in their clinic chart.

The extent of the problem of overlooking PTSD in persons with SMI in routine clinical practice is demonstrated in a recent review of research on the topic (Zammit et al., 2018). Across 29 studies, only 2.3% of individuals with SMI had a diagnosis of PTSD in their medical records, compared with a PTSD prevalence rate of 33% based on systematic evaluation. Among those persons who were found to have PTSD following diagnostic assessment, only 11.5% had the diagnosis in their charts.

A variety of factors may explain the low rate of detection of PTSD in people with SMI. Historically, some in the professional mental health community have doubted the accuracy of self-reports of traumatic events such as sexual or physical abuse, hypothesizing that these reports were instead the result of psychotic distortions or delusions with abuse themes (Coverdale & Grunebaum, 1998). However, although there is now abundant evidence that reliable reports of trauma and PTSD symptoms can be obtained from those with SMI, even in persons with delusional ideation (reviewed in Chapter 3, this volume).

Clinicians have also been concerned that inquiring about traumatic experiences in vulnerable populations such as persons with SMI runs the risk of opening Pandora's box, or exacerbating symptoms and distress (Hardy & Mueser, 2017; Havens et al., 2012). However, it has now been well established that assessments of trauma and PTSD can be safely and effectively conducted with these individuals (also reviewed in Chapter 3, this volume).

Aside from the reluctance of clinicians to assess trauma and PTSD in persons with SMI, PTSD may be underdiagnosed because the characteristic symptoms can resemble or overlap with common symptoms of other psychiatric diagnoses. For example, difficulties with anger in PTSD are similar to the irritability and anger often seen during a manic episode of bipolar disorder or in borderline personality disorder (as discussed further in Chapter 3, this volume). Problems with sleep and other overarousal symptoms of PTSD may resemble the high activity level common during a manic episode. In persons with PTSD, social avoidance, interpersonal distrust, relationship problems, or exaggerated fears about safety may be mistaken for paranoia, negative symptoms of schizophrenia, or characteristics of borderline personality disorder. In PTSD, negative thoughts and beliefs about oneself and one's future and associated pervasive feelings of anxiety and depression may be construed solely as symptoms of major depression.

An additional reason for the underdiagnosis of PTSD is that flagrant symptoms of psychosis may overshadow the importance of PTSD symptoms, making them less likely to be recognized and assessed (Grubaugh et al., 2008). These findings are consistent with research showing that a diagnosis of PTSD is more likely to be missed in people with schizophrenia or bipolar disorder than in those with major depression (Lu, Srijeyanthan, et al., 2022). A final factor contributing to missed PTSD diagnoses in persons with SMI is related to the avoidance symptoms of PTSD. As people with PTSD tend to avoid trauma-related stimuli, they often avoid talking about their traumatic experiences unless directly queried. Thus, in the absence of direct inquiry by the clinician, trauma and PTSD are often not broached during clinical assessment.

CLINICAL CORRELATES AND FUNCTIONAL CONSEQUENCES OF TRAUMA AND PTSD

The high prevalence of trauma exposure and PTSD in people with SMI is related to a broad range of negative outcomes. For example, trauma exposure in this population has been found to be associated with an earlier onset of SMI (Dean et al., 2007), greater functional impairment and reduced response to treatment (Aas et al., 2016), more severe symptoms (Alameda et al., 2021), worse cognitive functioning (Wells et al., 2020), comorbid substance use disorder (Tomassi et al., 2017), and more frequent psychiatric hospitalizations (Lu et al., 2008; Rosenberg et al., 2007). Among the numerous clinical correlates of trauma, PTSD is, not surprisingly, one of the most common ones and is of particular importance for addressing the broad range of trauma sequelae in persons with SMI, as discussed in the following sections.

In those with PTSD compared to those without, general psychiatric symptom severity is greater (Abdelghaffar et al., 2018; Picken & Tarrier, 2011; Seow et al., 2016), with particular elevations in psychotic symptoms (Duke et al., 2010; Steel et al., 2011) and depression (DeTore et al., 2021; Mueser, Essock, et al., 2004; Resnick et al., 2003). Risk of suicide is substantially increased in people who have had psychotic experiences (DeVylder et al., 2015), a SMI (Nock et al., 2010), or PTSD (Gradus et al., 2010). Therefore, it is not surprising that individuals with SMI and PTSD are at high risk for suicidal ideation and behavior (Álvarez et al., 2012; Strauss et al., 2006). Also, as might be expected from more severe symptoms associated with PTSD in persons with SMI, these individuals have much higher levels of overall psychological distress (O'Hare et al., 2006; Steel et al., 2011) and poorer quality of life (Calhoun et al., 2006; Mueser, Essock, et al., 2004).

Common comorbid conditions independently associated with both SMI and PTSD tend to be even more frequent or more severe in clients who have both disorders, including cognitive impairment (Fan et al., 2008; Goodman et al., 2007; Halász et al., 2013; Pollice et al., 2010), substance use disorders (Brady et al., 2003; O'Hare & Sherrer, 2011a; Scheller-Gilkey et al., 2004), and medical problems (Calhoun et al., 2006; Mueser, Salyers, et al., 2004). As a result of the confluence of more severe symptoms and comorbid conditions, individuals with SMI and PTSD tend to have poorer psychosocial functioning than those with SMI only. PTSD is associated with worse interpersonal relationships (Mueser, Essock, et al., 2004), higher rates of unemployment (Mueser, Salyers, et al.,

2004; Ng et al., 2016; Russinova et al., 2018), and less benefit from evidence-based supported employment interventions (Mueser, Essock, et al., 2004). People with co-occurring SMI and PTSD are also more likely to be arrested (and have other legal problems) than those without PTSD (McCabe et al., 2012).

The broad range of challenges experienced by people with SMI and PTSD has important service implications. The impact of PTSD appears to further destabilize SMI and contribute to relapses, as discussed in more detail later in this chapter. The net consequence is that individuals with these comorbid disorders have more frequent psychiatric hospitalizations and are more likely to utilize emergency room services (Minsky et al., 2015; Mueser, Salyers, et al., 2004; Switzer et al., 1999). In addition, clients with PTSD are more likely to be placed in seclusion and restraints during inpatient psychiatric treatment (Steinert et al., 2006).

WHY FOCUS ON PTSD?

As reviewed in the previous sections, the evidence documents that people with SMI are more likely to have been exposed to trauma and more likely to have PTSD than in the general population and that the existence of these conditions, if left untreated, contributes to widespread and serious clinical, functional, medical, legal, and occupational consequences. These robust findings suggest that many individuals with SMI could benefit from interventions targeting trauma exposure and PTSD. An additional detailed rationale for focusing treatment efforts on PTSD in this population is provided in this section.

PTSD Is a Well-Established Psychiatric Disorder

PTSD is one of only two psychiatric diagnoses in modern psychiatric nosology that are defined in terms of psychological sequelae precipitated by a traumatic event. The second diagnosis is acute stress disorder (American Psychiatric Association, 2013). The symptoms of acute stress disorder are similar to those of PTSD, except that the diagnosis is given only within a month of the traumatic event, after which PTSD can be diagnosed. While the symptoms of acute stress disorder frequently remit spontaneously, PTSD symptoms tend to be more chronic and enduring (Kessler et al., 2022), suggesting that PTSD is a more suitable target for intervention between the two disorders.

Since the inclusion of PTSD in the *DSM-III* (American Psychiatric Association, 1980), thousands of scientific studies have been published on the psychopathology, epidemiology, neurobiology, and treatment of PTSD. Thus, much is known about the disorder, which can serve to guide efforts to treat it in people with SMI. In contrast, having been exposed to trauma is not a psychiatric disorder but rather a personal experience that can have a wide range of effects on individuals' lives depending on a multitude of factors, such as preexisting psychiatric conditions, social support, and coping style (Schmidt et al., 2017). There are no established treatments for trauma exposure because the impact of trauma is so variable on individuals. In fact, abundant evidence shows that the majority of people are resilient following exposure to a traumatic event and do not experience long-term negative psychological and psychosocial effects (Besser et al., 2014; Norris et al., 2009; Nurius et al., 2015; Pietrzak et al., 2014). Thus, much more is known about PTSD as a specific psychiatric disorder than about the effects of trauma, and this knowledge base about PTSD can serve to guide efforts to treat it in people with SMI.

High Prevalence of PTSD but Low Detection in Routine Clinical Practice

As reviewed in the previous sections, across numerous studies of people with SMI the prevalence of PTSD has been found to generally range between 25% and 45% (Seow et al., 2016; Zammit et al., 2018), far exceeding the 7% to 12% estimated prevalence in the general population (Kessler et al., 2014; Kilpatrick et al., 2013). Furthermore, PTSD is associated with greater symptom severity, more impaired psychosocial functioning, and worse quality of life in these individuals. At the same time, while PTSD is relatively common in people with SMI, it is frequently not identified in clinical practice and therefore is not treated.

The high prevalence of PTSD in persons with SMI, the substantial burden it imposes on the lives of people struggling with a SMI, and its frequent under-detection in individuals receiving care have clear treatment implications. The confluence of these factors suggests that efforts to systematically screen for PTSD in the SMI population and to treat it when present could have enormous effects on improving the quality of lives of the many people impacted by trauma and PTSD. The established feasibility of screening for PTSD in persons with SMI (described in Chapter 3, this volume) and research showing the positive effects of interventions for PTSD in this population (reviewed in Chapter 2, this volume) suggest that this is not a pipedream but a distinct possibility within our capability of achieving.

PTSD Is a Highly Treatable Disorder

Although untreated PTSD can have a profound impact on the quality and course of an individual's life, there is abundant evidence showing that it is a highly treatable condition. A variety of well-validated psychological interventions, primarily ones based on cognitive behavioral therapy, have been shown to be effective for the treatment of PTSD in the general population (Bisson et al., 2013; Ehring et al., 2014; Ronconi et al., 2015; Watts et al., 2013), and the list of effective treatments continues to grow. Effective interventions for PTSD tend to be relatively brief (typically requiring 9–15 sessions) but potent in terms of reducing PTSD symptom severity and associated depression and often resulting in remission of the PTSD diagnosis.

The fact that PTSD can be treated successfully in the general population with time-limited psychotherapeutic interventions provides realistic hope that similar interventions, adapted for the special needs of these individuals, may be effective in persons with SMI. Indeed, there is also growing evidence that PTSD can be effectively treated in persons with SMI using similar treatment approaches validated in the general population (Brand et al., 2018; Grubaugh et al., 2021; Van den Berg et al., 2015), including this Cognitive Restructuring for PTSD program.

PTSD Influences the Course of SMI

The final reason for focusing on PTSD is that treating the disorder may have far-reaching clinical effects beyond reducing PTSD symptoms. Specifically, treating PTSD may have a broader impact on improving the wide range of negative outcomes associated with SMI. This argument is based on the growing body of evidence showing that PTSD interacts with and worsens the course of SMI. This important interactive model is described next, the implications of which suggest that effective treatment for PTSD could improve the long-term outcome and recovery of people with SMI.

AN INTERACTIVE MODEL OF PTSD AND THE COURSE OF SMI

Based on the abundant research that PTSD in people with SMI is associated with more severe symptoms, more impaired functioning, and higher utilization of acute care services, Mueser, Rosenberg, et al. (2002) proposed a model that explains how PTSD interacts with and worsens the course of SMI. Since the initial model was published, further research has provided support for the model and for the hypothesized role of PTSD as a mediator of the negative effects of trauma on worse outcomes in this population (Cusack et al., 2013; Subica et al., 2011), and we have since updated the model so that it corresponds to the new version of the *DSM-5-TR*.

This model is an extension of stress-vulnerability models that have been proposed to account for variability in the onset and course of SMI (Mueser et al., 2013; Nuechterlein & Dawson, 1984; Zubin & Spring, 1977). Stress-vulnerability models propose that the onset and course of a major mental illness are the result of the dynamic interplay between a combination of biological, environmental, and personal (or psychological) variables. Psychobiological vulnerability to a mental illness, symptom severity, and impaired functioning are determined by a variety of biological factors (e.g., genetics, birth complications) and environmental influences (e.g., early trauma exposure, poverty). Once a mental illness has developed, this psychobiological vulnerability can be increased (hence worsening symptoms and precipitating relapses) by stress and substance abuse and can be decreased through medications, social support, and effective coping strategies for dealing with stress and persistent symptoms. Other illness management strategies—such as understanding the nature of the mental illness, collaborating with treatment providers, and developing a relapse prevention plan—can further buffer against the noxious effects of stress and improve the course of the disorder. As untreated PTSD in and of itself can be a debilitating

FIGURE 1.1. Interactive Model Between PTSD and Course of SMI

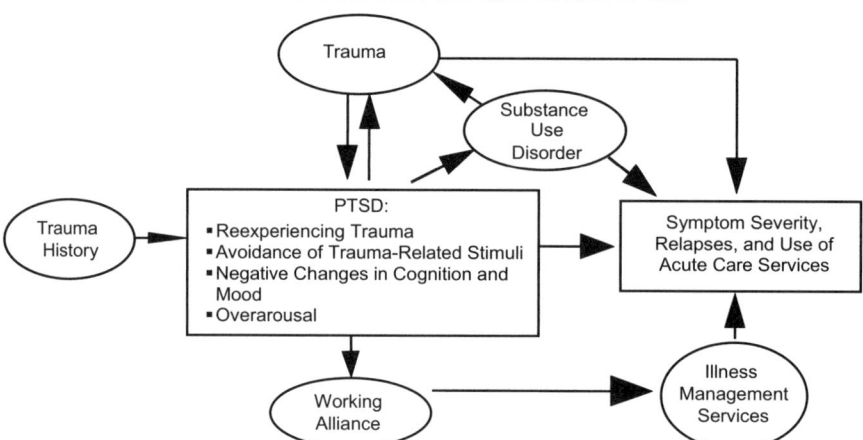

Note. PTSD = posttraumatic stress disorder; SMI = serious mental illness.

SMI, similar stress-vulnerability models have been proposed to understand factors that influence its course and outcome (Allen, 2005; McFarlane, 1996).

According to our interactive model, PTSD is a specific, treatable disorder that mediates the effects of trauma on negative outcomes associated with SMI. PTSD affects the course of SMI both directly through the impact of PTSD symptoms and indirectly through the effects of associated features of PTSD on stress-vulnerability factors that can influence the disorder. The model is illustrated in Figure 1.1.

Direct Effects of PTSD Symptoms on SMI

Each of the four different symptom clusters used to define PTSD (reexperiencing the trauma, avoidance of trauma-related stimuli, physiological overarousal, and altered thoughts and feelings) can directly influence the severity and course of the SMI. Reexperiencing symptoms such as intrusive memories, nightmares, and flashback are acutely distressing to people with PTSD, and based on the stress-vulnerability model they can be understood as chronic stressors that exacerbate individuals' symptoms and increase risk of relapse. In addition, in some individuals, the PTSD reexperiencing symptoms may be so intense that they overlap with psychotic symptoms of SMI such as hallucinations of trauma-related events and paranoid ideation (Ibáñez et al., 2014; Mueser & Butler, 1987).

The avoidance symptoms of PTSD often result in fewer social contacts with other people and reduced engagement in a broad range of other potentially rewarding activities, such as work, parenting, civic, or leisure and recreational activities. These symptoms can contribute to an avoidant coping style in individuals with SMI and PTSD, accompanied by higher levels of distress (McNeill & Galovski, 2015). This reduced participation in the social world has important implications for worsening the course of SMI. First, individuals with PTSD have less access to the beneficial effects of social support, depriving them of personally meaningful relationships, opportunities for reality testing, and the effects of supportive others on buffering the impact of stress. Second, lack of involvement in socially defined roles and other activities can result in reduced meaningful structure in people's lives, which act as a kind of stress precipitating psychotic and other symptoms (Rosen et al., 1981; Wong et al., 1987). For example, there is evidence that competitive employment reduces the chances of someone with SMI having a relapse and rehospitalization (Hoffmann et al., 2014; Kukla et al., 2012; Mueser, Becker, et al., 1997).

The overarousal symptoms of PTSD can have direct effects on worsening the symptoms of SMI. It is well established that chronic autonomic arousal is associated with more severe symptoms and worse functioning in people with SMI. Furthermore, the common PTSD symptom of sleep difficulties, either due to physiological overarousal or nightmares, may specifically interact with SMI. Insomnia and poor-quality sleep have been linked to more severe psychotic symptoms (Freeman et al., 2015) and worse social functioning (Blanchard et al., 2020) in people with SMI and can precipitate episodes of mania in those with bipolar disorder (Goodwin & Jamison, 2007).

Last, the altered thoughts and feelings symptoms of PTSD can have multiple effects on worsening symptoms and functioning in SMI. With respect to altered thoughts, cognitive biases such as distorted perceptions of threat, of oneself, and of one's future are common in PTSD (Ehlers et al., 2012; Naim et al., 2015). These PTSD-related biases may interact with or fuel other cognitive biases contributing to common symptoms in SMI such as delusions (Garety & Hemsley, 1994), hallucinations (Howes & Murray, 2014), and depression (Beevers et al., 2019). In terms of altered feelings, chronic negative feelings associated with PTSD such as depression and anxiety may further worsen these common negative affective states in persons with SMI, potentially increasing their vulnerability to suicide (Álvarez et al., 2012).

Indirect Effects of PTSD on SMI

The model also hypothesizes three different indirect pathways through which PTSD may contribute to a worse course of SMI, via its effects on increasing substance use problems, retraumatization, and interpersonal difficulties that interfere with developing a strong working alliance with treatment providers.

Substance Use Disorder

People with PTSD (both in the general and SMI populations) often use substances to self-medicate or escape distressing symptoms such as intrusive memories and problems sleeping (McCauley et al., 2012; Nishith et al., 2022). PTSD also contributes to the high rate of substance use disorders in persons with SMI (Cusack et al., 2013; Scheller-Gilkey et al., 2004), which have a direct effect on worsening the course of SMI (Noordsy et al., 2013). Furthermore, as previously discussed, the use of substances can lead to interpersonal victimization, both increasing PTSD symptoms and further worsening outcomes.

Retraumatization

It is well established that individuals with PTSD are at increased risk for retraumatization compared to those without PTSD (Nishith et al., 2000; Polusny & Follette, 1995), and similar associations have been reported in individuals with SMI and PTSD (Newman et al., 2010). The mechanisms underlying this seemingly paradoxical association are unclear, but it is plausible that the cognitive bias of overestimating threat impedes the ability of people with PTSD to correctly detect when they are in danger (Wilson et al., 1999); that is, if almost everything is perceived as a danger signal, there is no ability to discriminate the "signal" (danger) from the "noise" (no danger). In addition, an avoidant coping style, which is characteristic of PTSD, may result in some people ignoring or refusing to attend to potential danger signals and thereby falling prey to Santayana's (1905) observation that "those who cannot remember the past are condemned to repeat it" (p. 284).

Individuals with SMI are highly sensitive to the stressful effects of major events in their lives, both good and bad, which can precipitate symptom exacerbations and worsen functioning (Bebbington & Kuipers, 1992). Retraumatization of individuals who also have PTSD is an especially pernicious type of life event that can worsen outcomes, due both to the stressful nature of such experiences as well as to the effects on further worsening PTSD severity. Effective treatment of PTSD in people with SMI has been found to reduce the subsequent chances of interpersonal victimization (van den Berg et al., 2016).

Poor Therapeutic Working Alliance

The interpersonal nature of most traumatic events leading to PTSD results in problems establishing and maintaining close, trusting relationships with other people (Monson, 2005). This impact has the potential to influence not only friendships and intimate relationships but therapeutic relationships as well (Cloitre et al., 2004). The "working alliance" has been conceptualized as the therapeutic and collaborative relationship between a clinician and client (Horvath & Greenberg, 1989). There is abundant research showing that the working alliance is an important predictor of outcome across multiple psychotherapeutic approaches and populations (Martin et al., 2000). Mounting evidence also supports the association between a stronger working alliance and better outcomes in people with SMI (Browne et al., 2019). Research shows the importance of the working alliance across a broad range of interventions for these individuals (Brown, Cather, & Mueser, 2021), including the client's therapeutic alliance with psychiatric rehabilitation providers (Gehrs & Goering, 1994), with case managers (Solomon et al., 1995), with providers of supported employment (Corbière et al., 2017; Kukla & Bond, 2009), with cognitive remediation specialists (Cella & Wykes, 2019), with providers of integrated treatment for co-occurring substance use disorders (Barrowclough et al., 2010), with assertive community treatment team members (Calsyn et al., 2006), with clinicians providing family psychoeducation (Levy-Frank et al., 2011), and with providers of treatment for first-episode psychosis (Browne, Wright, et al., 2021).

Due to hallmark symptoms of distrust and avoidance, the presence of PTSD in people with SMI may interfere with their ability to form strong working relationships with treatment providers such as case managers, psychiatrists and other prescribers, clinicians providing psychoeducation and coping skills training, and rehabilitation specialists. As a poorer therapeutic relationship can result in minimal engagement and premature dropout from treatment, individuals with PTSD may receive fewer critical services for managing their mental illness effectively or may benefit less from those services. This problem may be particularly acute when PTSD is not detected by treatment providers and incorporated into collaborative treatment planning (Cusack et al., 2006; Mueser & Taub, 2008).

Treatment Implications of the Interactive Model

The interactive model points to how PTSD can worsen the symptoms, functioning, and use of acute care services in people with SMI, via both the direct effects of PTSD symptoms as well as other factors frequently associated with PTSD, including substance use problems, retraumatization, and difficulty with close relationships. The treatment implications of the model suggest that effective treatment for PTSD has the potential not only to reduce the considerable burden of PTSD symptoms but also to improve the long-term course of SMI. The fact that PTSD is a treatable disorder for the general population and, according to compelling research, can be effectively treated in people with SMI (Grubaugh et al., 2021) indicates that these implications are not theoretical but rather are grounded in hard evidence. Therefore, the Cognitive Restructuring for PTSD program outlined in this book is a practical, evidence-based, effective treatment program aimed at reducing or eliminating PTSD symptoms in people with a co-occurring SMI and at empowering individuals to regain control over their recovery and their lives.

CONCLUSION

The importance of trauma in the lives of people with SMI, both before and following the onset of their psychiatric disorder, cannot be overemphasized. The very high prevalence of PTSD in persons with SMI (between 25% and 45%), the numerous reasons that the disorder is so much more common than in the general population, and clinical correlates of PTSD (i.e., symptom severity, impaired psychosocial functioning, greater use of acute care treatment services) paint a clear and alarming picture of this problem. Yet despite the high prevalence of PTSD in persons with SMI, it is frequently not detected in routine clinical practice for reasons such as diagnostic overshadowing of other more prominent psychiatric symptoms, clinician fear of asking questions about traumatic events, and client avoidance of trauma-related stimuli. This substantial evidence makes a strong case for focusing treatment efforts on PTSD in people with SMI, as its treatment could reduce significant clinical burden in their lives.

Our interactive model of SMI and PTSD highlights the specific interactions between PTSD and the course of SMI, including both the direct effects of PTSD symptoms on SMI and indirect effects of PTSD on the illness (such as via substance use disorder, retraumatization, and problems forming a working alliance with treatment providers). The clinical implications of the model suggest that effective treatment of PTSD has the potential to both alleviate PTSD symptoms in this population and improve the long-term course of SMI, thereby helping clients move forward toward recovery.

2

Treatment of PTSD in People With Serious Mental Illness

The Cognitive Restructuring Program

The foundation for the Cognitive Restructuring (CR) for PTSD program lies in research on the treatment of PTSD in the general population and on cognitive theories of PTSD, informed by an understanding of the unique needs and challenges of persons with serious mental illness (SMI) and of the process of recovery from mental illness. Since its development, rigorous research has been conducted on the individual therapy-based CR for PTSD program, and two variants of the program have been created: a group-based format of the program and a brief (three-session) program (Brief Relaxation, Education, and Trauma Healing [BREATHE]; online Supplemental Chapter 15; manual contained in the online Appendix).

In this chapter, we review critical background information that led to the development of the CR for PTSD program and its incorporation of special considerations for working with people with SMI. We then provide an overview of the program, including its core components (psychoeducation, Breathing Retraining, cognitive restructuring). Next, we discuss the evolution of the mental health profession's conceptualization of recovery (which emphasizes the importance of people developing meaning and sense of purpose in their lives) and explicate the ways in which the CR program is a recovery-oriented service fostering specific recovery processes. We then review the empirical support for the CR program. The chapter concludes with a description of the group and BREATHE variants of the program, the supporting research on them, and considerations for implementing them in systems of care serving people with SMI.

https://doi.org/10.1037/0000423-002
Treatment of Posttraumatic Stress Disorder in Serious Mental Illness: The Cognitive Restructuring Program, by K. T. Mueser and J. D. Gottlieb

TREATMENT OF PTSD IN THE GENERAL POPULATION

Since the inclusion of PTSD in 1980 as a mental disorder in the third edition of the *Diagnostic and Statistical Manual of Mental Disorders*, the treatment of PTSD has been the focus of extensive research. Numerous psychotherapeutic interventions have been found to improve PTSD symptoms and, in many cases, to result in a sustained remission of the disorder (Cusack et al., 2016; Mavranezouli et al., 2020; McLean et al., 2022). Although pharmacological treatments such as antidepressant medications reduce the severity of PTSD symptoms (de Moraes Costa et al., 2020; Hoskins et al., 2021), in general psychological treatments have stronger effects.

While a variety of psychotherapies are helpful in improving PTSD, there is a broad consensus that trauma-focused cognitive behavioral interventions are the most effective approach, as reflected by the recommendations of multiple practice guidelines (American Psychological Association, 2017; International Society for Traumatic Stress Studies, 2018; National Institute for Health and Clinical Excellence, 2018; Phelps et al., 2022; Phoenix Australia Centre for Posttraumatic Mental Health, 2020). *Trauma-focused therapy* is a broad term used to describe psychotherapeutic treatments that include direct discussion of the traumatic event(s) experienced by the individual as a central component of the therapy. The most frequently studied and commonly available trauma-focused therapies include cognitive processing therapy (CPT), prolonged exposure (PE), and eye movement desensitization and reprocessing (EMDR) therapy. All of these approaches begin by providing some psychoeducation about the nature of trauma and PTSD symptoms, but they differ in other aspects. All of the approaches are usually provided in an individual psychotherapy format, with most courses of treatment lasting between seven and 16 sessions.

Cognitive Processing Therapy

CPT is a cognitive behavioral therapy approach aimed at helping individuals change trauma-related beliefs they have about themselves and others that contribute to anxiety, avoidance, and other symptoms of PTSD (Resick et al., 2024). During the first phase of CPT, participants write an impact statement to describe the effect that the traumatic event had on themselves and their view of the world. They are then taught the association between thoughts and feelings and learn how to identify stuck points, or exaggerated beliefs based on their traumatic experiences. In the second phase, participants learn how to evaluate evidence for and against these beliefs and have the option of writing a narrative of the traumatic event to provide further insight into their stuck points. In the third phase, clients learn how to change their trauma-related beliefs to more accurate ones and to explore and modify other stuck points that may have been overlooked. This last phase concludes with the person revising their initial trauma impact statement. Although CPT is the most frequently studied cognitive behavioral program for PTSD, other treatment programs for PTSD using the same principles of cognitive behavior therapy (or more specifically, cognitive restructuring) have also been shown to be effective (Marks et al., 1998; Tarrier & Sommerfield, 2004).

Prolonged Exposure Therapy

PE therapy involves helping people overcome their PTSD symptoms by counteracting their tendency to try to escape upsetting memories of traumatic experiences through imaginal exposure, during which the client focuses on describing the traumatic event in detail to the therapist, which usually results in a gradual reduction in associated anxiety. This is typically complemented by in vivo exposure, in which the person gradually learns how to approach and cope with feared but objectively safe real-life situations that are avoided because they remind the person of the traumatic event (e.g., for a client who was sexually assaulted, purchasing something from a male clerk at a store).

Emotional processing theory (Brown & Foa, 2022; Foa & Kozak, 1986) was developed to understand why PE therapy is effective for PTSD. This theory conceptualizes fear as a mental network comprised of representations of specific fear-related stimuli (including both external and internal stimuli) that serve to promote avoidance or escape from danger. This theory proposes that changes in the fear network, and hence PTSD symptoms, require two conditions: (a) the fear network must be activated and (b) the person must be exposed to information that is incompatible with the representations of fear in that network. The imaginal and in vivo exposure components of PE are both hypothesized to activate the fear network associated with the traumatic event, while the absence of any expected negative consequences related to either type of exposure (and the associated habituation of anxiety) provides the information that is incompatible with the fear network, resulting in a change in the network.

Eye Movement Desensitization and Reprocessing

EMDR therapy is an approach that combines some aspects of CPT and PE therapy with some novel components (Shapiro, 2017). The focus of the 60- to 90-minute therapy sessions is on creating a state of dual-focused attention aimed at facilitating the processing of the traumatic memory. For the procedure, the client recalls and focuses on a disturbing memory of the traumatic event and any associated thoughts or beliefs, while simultaneously engaging in eye movements by watching the therapist move their hand back and forth in front of them (most frequently) or another type of bilateral stimulation (e.g., listening to a tapping sound). The therapist periodically stops, and the client describes any associated emotional, cognitive, somatic, or imagery-related experiences and indicates their overall distress level and the degree of belief they have in their dysfunctional thought. The procedure is then repeated over subsequent sessions until the distress associated with the trauma-related memories has reduced or is gone.

A variety of different theories have been proposed to explain how EMDR therapy works (de Jongh et al., 2022). However, no one theory has strong support, and the mechanisms underlying its effects continue to be debated. As the imagery component of EMDR overlaps with the imaginal exposure part of PE therapy and as clients are encouraged to develop alternative ways of thinking about themselves and their traumatic experience, it is possible that some of the mechanisms underlying its effectiveness are shared with these other treatments for PTSD.

LIMITATIONS OF PTSD TREATMENT RESEARCH IN THE GENERAL POPULATION

Within the first 20 years (1980–2000) of research on the treatment of PTSD in the general population, strong evidence had emerged supporting several psychotherapeutic approaches, and the evidence base has continued to grow since then. However, this early research on the treatment of PTSD had significant limitations in terms of shedding light on effective interventions for people with PTSD who also have SMI.

First, most research studies of psychotherapeutic treatments for PTSD were conducted in either specialty clinics (e.g., treating PTSD following sexual assault), in Veterans Administration hospitals focusing on veterans with combat-related PTSD, or in general mental health outpatient settings (e.g., treating PTSD related to a variety of events, such as accidents, unexpected death of a loved one, etc.). Although people with SMI sometimes receive treatment in these types of settings, the majority do not. Most people with SMI receive their treatment from community mental health centers, where their care is managed by multidisciplinary treatment teams who provide a variety of services, such as pharmacological treatment, case management, psychiatric rehabilitation, and individual and group psychotherapy.

Second, most of the controlled research on psychotherapeutic treatments for PTSD has required study participants to meet an extensive set of inclusion and exclusion criteria that have in effect ruled out individuals with SMI and PTSD from participating in study trials. For example, common exclusion criteria for studies of psychotherapy for PTSD have been a diagnosis of schizophrenia, bipolar disorder, or active substance use disorder; cognitive impairment; psychotic symptoms; significant suicidal ideation; taking psychotropic medications; or having a recent change in pharmacological treatment—all common characteristics of the population of people with SMI. In addition, until recently, very little research on psychotherapy for PTSD has been conducted in settings where individuals with SMI most often receive treatment, such as community mental health centers.

As a result of these factors and despite the enormous advances in the psychotherapeutic treatment of PTSD over the first 20 years of research, the treatment of PTSD in persons with SMI remained largely unexplored. This predicament was summarized in an early review of the research literature by Spinazzola et al. (2005), who commented on the problem that most treatment research had been conducted on cases of "pure" PTSD with few or no comorbid conditions and other complexities, excluding more vulnerable and more representative samples of persons with PTSD. The authors wrote, "True advancement of the field will require a deliberate process of evaluation and adaptation of efficacious treatments with less restrictive, more clinically representative PTSD samples" (p. 427). The CR for PTSD program was developed to address this specific need.

DEVELOPMENT OF THE CR PROGRAM FOR PTSD IN SMI

The CR program was developed based on research on the treatment of PTSD in the general population, informed by consideration of the increased vulnerability of individuals with SMI. Some of the special needs of these individuals requiring attention include increased sensitivity to stress, frequent societal marginalization resulting in lower social support and more limited economic means, challenging symptom presentations (e.g., psychotic symptoms, labile mood, self-injurious behavior, suicidal ideation), cognitive impairment, and comorbid conditions (e.g., substance use disorders, physical illnesses). We sought to develop treatment guidelines for implementing this program that were robust enough to make a lasting impact on PTSD diagnosis and symptoms but that could also be flexibly carried out by trained clinicians in light of the broad range of challenges clients and their circumstances might present (Mueser, Rosenberg, et al., 2004).

Common Components of PTSD Treatment Programs

As we sought to capitalize on the extant research data on the treatment of PTSD in the general population when developing the CR for PTSD program and to not "reinvent the wheel," inclusion of several components of our program were relatively straightforward. By the late 1990s, when we began to develop the CR for PTSD program, the strongest evidence from controlled trials for the psychotherapeutic treatment of PTSD was for PE programs and cognitive-restructuring-based interventions (such as CPT). These two types of programs include three brief treatment components early in the intervention, all of which were incorporated into the CR program:

- providing an orientation at the beginning of the program to explain how it works, logistical details, and expectations (e.g., home assignments) to set positive expectations for the client's active participation the program;

- teaching a simple anxiety management skill (Breathing Retraining) to help the client cope with anxiety and other distressing PTSD symptoms that may get activated early in treatment; and

- providing psychoeducation about trauma and PTSD, including the prevalence of PTSD and common symptoms, to let clients know that they are not alone in their experience, they are not to blame for their symptoms, and there is hope for recovery from treatment.

Choice of Cognitive Restructuring Over Prolonged Exposure as a Primary Therapeutic Component

For over 20 years, there has been strong research evidence showing that both PE and CR-based therapies (like CPT and related therapies) are effective treatments for PTSD, with direct comparisons of the two types of interventions also indicating that neither approach is superior to the other (Bisson et al., 2013; Cusack et al., 2016). Furthermore, studies that have compared the impact of combining PE with a CR-based intervention (like CPT) versus providing either alone have found no additional benefit associated with the combined intervention (Foa et al., 2005; Marks et al., 1998; Resick et al., 2008). Thus, in order to develop the simplest, most evidence-based intervention for people with PTSD and SMI with the greatest potential for widespread dissemination, it made sense to have the primary therapeutic component of the program focused on providing either PE or a CR-based intervention alone. This decision also avoided the complexity of a combined intervention.

Effective interventions, such as CPT, that focus on cognitive restructuring are based on cognitive theories of PTSD that propose that the disorder arises from the difficulty people have integrating the traumatic event into their previous understanding of themselves and the world (i.e., their pretrauma schemas). These "shattered assumptions" result in an inability to encode the traumatic event in memory, leading to spontaneous, intrusive memories of it with alternating periods of intense distress and numbness (Horowitz, 1975, 1986; Janoff-Bulman, 1989, 1992). These early cognitive theories of PTSD have been elaborated on by Ehlers and Clark (2000; Ehlers et al., 2005, 2022) to emphasize the broad range of appraisals resulting from trauma that predict PTSD, including non-fear-based appraisals (e.g., "I'll never be able to live a normal life again," "I'm no good if I let this happen to me") and the dysfunctional meaning people attach to those experiences. Similar to other effective cognitive restructuring–based interventions, the aim with the CR for PTSD program was to help people learn to modify their schemas and integrate their traumatic experiences into their beliefs about themselves and the world.

We chose to focus the CR for PTSD program on cognitive restructuring rather than PE for several practical reasons (Mueser, Rosenberg, et al., 2004). First, considering that avoidance of trauma-related stimuli is one of the defining symptom clusters of PTSD, we expected that a cognitive restructuring approach to PTSD would be a more acceptable treatment for most clients than a PE approach. Indeed, there is evidence supporting this assumption. In a national survey of 301 people who screened positive for PTSD and were provided descriptions of four psychotherapeutic treatments and one pharmacological treatment for PTSD, the most common first-choice treatment was CPT (44%), whereas only 12% selected PE for their first choice (Jessica Hamblen, personal communication, 2023).

Second, in light of the anxiety people with PTSD typically experience when they anticipate exposure to situations that remind them of their traumatic experiences, we expected that engaging in and learning cognitive restructuring would be less stressful for clients with SMI and PTSD than participation in PE. For this same reason, we expected that delivery of CR (vs. PE) would be less stressful for therapists working with this client population as well. This is an important point considering the high levels of stress individuals with SMI often experience on a daily basis due to challenges such as persistent and severe symptoms, unemployment and poverty, stigma, poor housing, exposure to criminal victimization, and co-occurring substance use and medical conditions.

A third reason we chose to use cognitive restructuring in the CR for PTSD program rather than PE was based on research showing that PE is less effective in the treatment of PTSD when the dominant emotion experienced by the person is depression, guilt, or shame rather than anxiety (Foa et al., 1995; Pitman et al., 1991; Resick et al., 2002; Smucker et al., 2003). This is especially concerning given that guilt and shame are very common emotional reactions to sexual abuse and assault (Feiring et al., 2002; Kennedy & Prock, 2018; Street et al., 2005), two of the most common types of trauma experienced by people with SMI (Mueser et al., 1998). These findings are consistent with the fact that the primary mechanism underlying the effects of PE on PTSD is the habituation of anxiety during the extended imaginal exposure component of PE, whereas other emotions do not habituate with exposure. Cognitive restructuring, on the other hand, is more utilitarian in that it can address the broad range of emotions that occur in PTSD. This is also important considering that non-fear-based cognitive appraisals of traumatic events are often more predictive of the persistence of PTSD than fear-based (i.e., anxiety) ones (Ehlers & Clark, 2000; Ehlers et al., 2022).

Fourth, cognitive restructuring was chosen as the primary treatment component for the CR for PTSD program because of the likely higher level of in-the-field therapist experience with using this approach to treat individuals with SMI and therapists' presumed greater comfort with the approach. Broadly speaking, cognitive behavioral therapy 's core component of cognitive restructuring has a long history as a feasible and effective intervention for the treatment of the broad range of disorders typically found in people with SMI, as reflected by treatment manuals for major depression (Beck et al., 1979), bipolar disorder (Newman et al., 2002), schizophrenia (Beck et al., 2009; Byrne et al., 2006; Chadwick, 2006; Fowler et al., 1995; Granholm et al., 2016; Kingdon & Turkington, 2004; Morrison et al., 2004; Nelson, 1997), and borderline personality disorder (Linehan, 1993). Compared to the delivery of PE, collectively the field has much more experience using cognitive restructuring with people with SMI, including addressing challenges such as psychotic symptoms, mood lability, debilitating depression, low distress tolerance, and cognitive impairments. This lends support for the potential benefits of using a similar CR-based approach to treat PTSD. Furthermore, teaching clients the skill of cognitive restructuring can equip them with a personal self-management tool for dealing with other distressing symptoms and challenges for which it has already been shown to be useful, in contrast to PE, which does not involve teaching practical life skills.

Since the development and initial testing of the CR for PTSD program, several open clinical trials have been published showing that both PE and EMDR can be provided safely to persons with a psychotic disorder with positive outcomes observed (Frueh et al., 2009; Grubaugh et al., 2016; van den Berg & van der Gaag, 2012). In addition, a randomized controlled trial that was conducted in the Netherlands comparing the effects of PE, EMDR, and waitlist control in people with a psychotic disorder and PTSD found that interventions could be safely delivered (van den Berg et al., 2016) and were more effective at improving PTSD outcomes than the waitlist condition (van den Berg et al., 2015). A controlled comparative trial is currently underway in the Netherlands comparing the CR for PTSD program with a PE program and EMDR (Burger et al., 2022). These studies provide support for the feasibility and potential benefits of providing PE to some persons with SMI and PTSD. However, the research on PE has thus far been limited to individuals with a psychotic disorder such as schizophrenia and not the broader SMI population. Furthermore, the acceptability of PE as a treatment for PTSD in persons with SMI remains largely unknown at this point.

THEORETICAL FRAMEWORK FOR THE CR FOR PTSD PROGRAM

The CR for PTSD program is based on the cognitive/information processing model of PTSD (Ehlers & Clark, 2000; Ehlers et al., 2005, 2022). This model proposes that PTSD symptoms develop as a result of distorted, inaccurate, or self-defeating appraisals that people make about themselves, other people, and the world in general as they try to understand their traumatic experience(s) and get on with their lives. While these problematic appraisals provide important meaning to the person about the event, they are also distressing and lead to avoidance of trauma-related stimuli that can trigger those thoughts, which can cause important consequences in the realm of social and vocational functioning, relationships, health, and high-risk behaviors. Over time and with repeated avoidance of trauma-related situations that could provide disconfirming evidence about the accuracy of their thoughts, these appraisals become ingrained into firmly held beliefs (or schemas) that serve to further intensify the PTSD symptoms. As maladaptive appraisals are a common characteristic of major psychiatric disorders such as schizophrenia and bipolar disorder, individuals with SMI may be more vulnerable to such appraisals of traumatic events, increasing their risk for developing PTSD (Sherrer, 2011).

In Chapter 1 in this volume, we introduced an interactive model of SMI and PTSD that highlights the specific interactions between PTSD and the course of SMI (see Figure 1.1), including both the direct and indirect effects of PTSD symptoms on SMI. The CR for PTSD intervention was designed to both directly and indirectly address these impacted areas (such as substance use, poor working alliance, retraumatization, and so on) via identification and modification of distressing beliefs associated with them. See Figure 2.1 for an expanded interactive model

FIGURE 2.1. Interactive Model Between PTSD and Course of SMI With Associated Cognitions

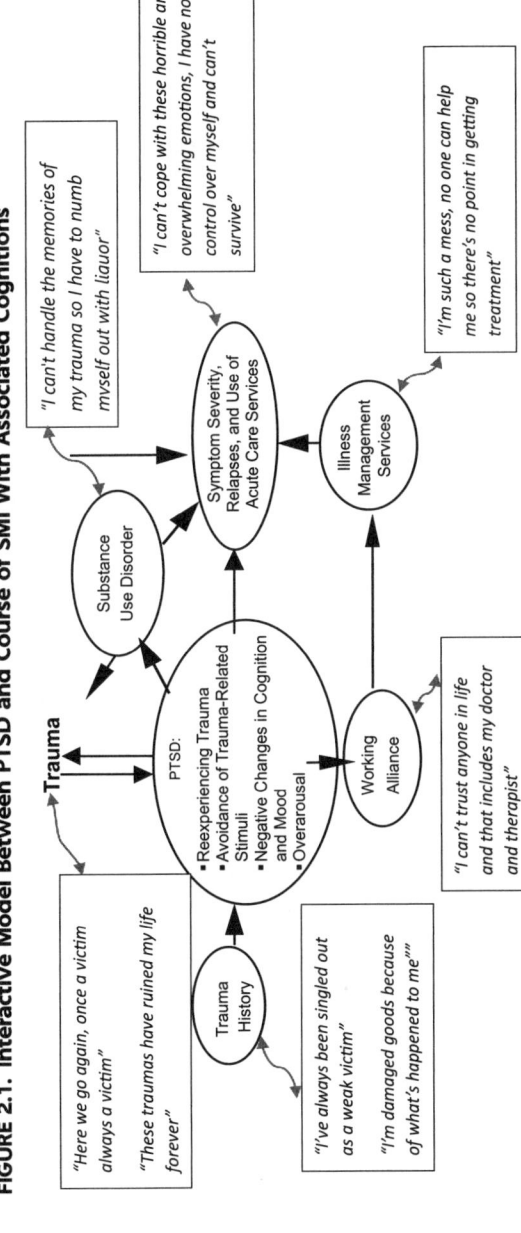

Note. PTSD = posttraumatic stress disorder; SMI = serious mental illness.

that includes sample trauma-based cognitions specific to the important areas that contribute to the maintenance of PTSD symptoms and associated problems in those with SMI.

The main goal of the CR for PTSD program is to provide information and teach skills aimed at modifying the core trauma-related beliefs that underlie PTSD symptoms. Each of the three treatment components of the program can assist in the challenge and adjustment of inaccurate and harmful trauma-related beliefs. Psychoeducation about PTSD provides valuable information to the client that PTSD is a well-established disorder that is both common and not the individual's fault. This information may offer a more benign interpretation for how people understand their PTSD symptoms and serve to correct dysfunctional beliefs such as "I must be going crazy because I keep having these flashbacks," "I'm weak. I should have gotten over it by now," and "I'm responsible for the traumatic event."

Teaching Breathing Retraining and encouraging clients to practice it every day, including when they are not feeling anxious, can reduce the chronic physiological overarousal that is characteristic of PTSD (e.g., racing heart, quickness of breath, muscular tension, perspiration) and along with it the pervasive sense of threat people often feel. As individuals feel calmer, less threatened, and safer in everyday social situations, they may become more exposed to information that is incompatible with or disconfirming of trauma-related beliefs about other people (e.g., "You can't trust anybody") or themselves (e.g., "I'm damaged goods. Nobody would be interested in me"), contributing to change in those beliefs.

Psychoeducation and Breathing Retraining both have the potential to change dysfunctional beliefs people have about their traumatic experiences without ever directly focusing on the beliefs themselves. Cognitive restructuring, on the other hand, directly targets dysfunctional thoughts and beliefs, including ones related to trauma, by teaching clients how to identify the thoughts underlying their distressing feelings, how to objectively examine their accuracy, and how to change them when they are inaccurate. In this program, cognitive restructuring is introduced and taught as a skill for dealing with negative feelings, which is then initially practiced on any upsetting feelings the person experiences. From there, attention is then turned to addressing and correcting trauma-related beliefs underlying the person's PTSD.

OVERVIEW OF THE CR FOR PTSD PROGRAM

The CR program is a 12- to 16-week individual cognitive behavioral therapy–based intervention for individuals with SMI and PTSD. The program sessions last about 60 minutes each and follow a semistructured format to facilitate learning, with home assignments collaboratively set at the end of each session for the client to practice skills taught in the session. PTSD and depressive symptoms are monitored routinely (every three sessions) using self-report measures, with scores discussed in sessions and incorporated into the therapy.

Initial sessions include an orientation, the development of a shared Wellness (safety) Plan, the teaching and practice of the aforementioned Breathing Retraining skill to manage anxiety and other PTSD symptoms, psychoeducation about the personal impact of PTSD, and collaborative goal setting.

From there, the program shifts into teaching cognitive restructuring, which is the primary therapeutic component of the intervention. To facilitate teaching this multidimensional skill, cognitive restructuring is broken down into two skills—the Common Styles of Thinking and the 5 Steps of CR—which are taught sequentially, with the second skill building on the first. This enables the client to gain some mastery over the first, simpler cognitive restructuring skill (Common Styles of Thinking) before moving onto the second, more complex and comprehensive skill (5 Steps of CR).

The Common Styles of Thinking skill begins with a discussion of the Thought–Feeling model (i.e., distressing feelings and associated behaviors people experience in different situations are related to their underlying thoughts in those situations, which may or may not be accurate). This sets the stage for examining the accuracy of thoughts when feeling upset or distressed. The therapist then explains that there are common ways that people jump to inaccurate conclusions leading to negative feelings, or Common Styles of Thinking, and a list of different Common Styles is reviewed together (e.g., catastrophizing, all-or-nothing thinking). Clients are taught that when they are experiencing a negative feeling, they can identify the underlying thought, check whether it is a Common Style of Thinking (inaccurate), and, if it is, change it to a more accurate (and less distressing) thought. Clients are generally able to grasp how the Common Styles skill works during the first session in which it is introduced, and they practice (and often find relief) identifying, evaluating, and changing distressing thoughts on their own as a home assignment.

When the client has gained some competence using the Common Styles of Thinking after one to three sessions, the 5 Steps of CR are introduced (using an accompanying worksheet). The steps include the following:

1. Describe the situation.

2. Identify the most distressing feeling in the situation.

3. Identify the most distressing thought associated with the feeling.

4. Evaluate the evidence for and against the thought (and consider whether it is a Common Style of Thinking and therefore inaccurate).

5. Take action: If the thought is not supported by the evidence, come up with a new and more accurate thought for the situation. If the thought is supported by the evidence, develop an Action Plan for dealing with the distressing situation.

The 5 Steps of CR skill builds on the Common Styles of Thinking skill but is more powerful and comprehensive in that it (a) provides the opportunity to uncover and explore the deeper core (and/or trauma-related) belief(s) underlying an initial distressing thought in order to help the client identify and then challenge these important thoughts in the subsequent steps of the skill (Step 3), (b) allows for detailed examination of evidence for and against the distressing belief (Step 4), and (c) includes an option for developing a behaviorally specific Action Plan based on problem solving when the client concludes that the evidence does in fact support their upsetting thought (Step 5). This makes the 5 Steps of CR a more broadly utilitarian skill for dealing with all negative feelings.

Throughout these midtreatment CR sessions, the therapist guides the client through the 5 Steps of CR, using various distressing situations from the client's life. After a few sessions of in- and between-session 5 Steps practice, the content used to work on distressing situations and beliefs shifts to more of a trauma-related focus. In these sessions through the end of the intervention, using the 5 Steps of CR, the client and therapist are focused on exploring, evaluating, challenging, and modifying upsetting and often inaccurate core and trauma-based beliefs. Toward the end of the CR for PTSD program, the therapist works with the client to identify someone who can support them in continuing to use the 5 Steps of CR when needed (e.g., primary therapist, case manager, family member, or friend). A joint session with that identified person, the PTSD therapist, and the client is scheduled to review the CR for PTSD program skills and plan for ongoing support and further skill generalization (see the CR for PTSD Session-by-Session Agenda for Clinicians handout in the Appendix for further details about the outline of treatment components and the intervention timeline).

THE CR FOR PTSD PROGRAM'S CONTRIBUTION TO RECOVERY FROM SMI

Over the past 3 decades, there has been a sea change in how recovery from SMI is conceptualized and understood, which has been accompanied by dramatic change in the stance taken and interventions used by the mental health profession. In past years, recovery was strictly defined in medical terms to refer to the complete and permanent remission of the characteristic symptoms of mental illness and elimination of associated impairments and functioning. Clinicians and researchers alike believed that recovery from SMI was either exceedingly rare or impossible and often told this spirit-breaking news to patients and their families (Deegan, 1990). Individuals with SMI were believed by professionals to be incapable of articulating their own needs and desires or of engaging in rational decision making and were thus regarded as passive recipients of treatment at best, often requiring coercive measures to ensure their compliance with treatment, as determined by "experts." Due to their presumed unreliability, client reports of traumatic experiences were usually ignored, labeled as delusions, or ascribed to personality disorders or other characterological defects. Clients who declined treatment or reacted to professionals with common PTSD symptoms, such as anxiety, avoidance, or anger, were dealt with harshly by liberal use of seclusion and restraints, including both physical and chemical restraints (Jennings, 1995). Tragically for many of these individuals, the mental health system that was supposed to help them heal instead failed them by retraumatizing them further.

In more recent years, traditional medical definitions of recovery have been challenged and largely replaced with more nuanced conceptualizations that emphasize recovery as a personal process of regaining or recovering a sense of meaning, purpose, and identity in one's life, despite having a mental illness (Anthony, 1993; Slade, 2009; Substance Abuse and Mental Health Services Administration, 2012). For example, one widely used definition of recovery is provided by Deegan (1988), a clinical psychologist, trauma survivor, and person who lived experience of SMI:

> Recovery is a process, a way of life, an attitude, and a way of approaching the day's challenges. It's not a perfectly linear process. At times our progress is erratic and we falter, slide back, regroup, and start again. The need is to establish a new and valued sense of integrity and purpose within and beyond the limits of the disability; the inspiration is to live, work, and love in a community in which one makes a significant contribution. (p. 15)

As understanding of recovery in the mental health field evolved to recognize that the nature and experience of recovery differs across individuals, so have attitudes about the capability and importance of the active involvement of people with SMI in their own treatment. It is now widely accepted that not only are individuals with SMI able to collaborate with providers in determining and planning their own treatment but playing such an active role in their treatment is critical to achieving the best outcomes possible (Mueser, Corrigan, et al., 2002). Furthermore, it is now recognized that people with SMI have the same basic human rights of all people to make decisions about their own lives, including decisions about their treatment and ways to best pursue their personal recovery. Recovery-oriented services are mental health programs that embrace the vision of recovery described above, respect the personal agency of each client, and help them progress toward developing more meaningful, purposeful, and rewarding lives.

The CR Program as a Recovery-Oriented Service

Although a variety of core characteristics of recovery-oriented practices for SMI have been identified by different investigators (Davidson et al., 2009; Farkas, 2007; Le Boutillier et al., 2011; Zuehlke et al., 2016), there is a broad consensus about the importance of four defining elements: trauma-informed, self-determination and choice, person-centered, and strengths-based. We describe next how the CR program is a recovery-oriented service that incorporates each of these characteristics.

Trauma-Informed

The importance of trauma in the lives of people with SMI is now widely recognized, including the fact that trauma was ignored by the mental health system for many years (and still is by some providers) and that many individuals have been retraumatized by the system itself (e.g., involuntary hospitalization, use of seclusion and restraints; Ashcraft & Anthony, 2008). Recovery-oriented services are trauma-informed in that they demonstrate an awareness of the impact of trauma on individuals and show special sensitivity to inadvertently retraumatizing them (Huckshorn & Lebel, 2013). The CR program goes beyond the trauma-informed nature of most recovery-oriented programs in that it provides treatment for the most common and scientifically validated consequence of trauma: PTSD. In fact, the focus of the CR program on PTSD is unique among recovery-oriented interventions in that it is trauma-specific and employs evidence-based methods shown to be effective at reducing PTSD symptoms and associated distress.

Self-Determination and Choice

Farkas (2007) described support for self-determination and choice as the cornerstone of all recovery-oriented services. The symptoms of mental illness and associated life challenges can have a devastating effect on individuals' self-confidence and self-efficacy for shaping and controlling their lives, and its effects are exacerbated by the stigma (and self-stigma) of mental illness and negative experiences with mental health providers. Bolstering clients' self-determination and autonomy is critical to countering these effects and helping them regain control over their lives, including their treatment. The CR program supports the individual's self-determination in several ways. Personal goals for desired life changes are set by the client early in the program and are actively pursued and monitored with the therapist over the course of the program, providing concrete evidence that change is possible and building self-efficacy. Psychoeducation about PTSD is provided to clients to equip them with information they need to make informed decisions about their treatment with their other providers. All CR program sessions begin with the therapist and client setting the agenda for their meeting together and end with the collaborative development of a home assignment for the client based on that session, reflecting an equitable sharing of control over the therapy between therapist and client.

Person-Centered

Just because someone has a mental illness it does not mean the person is the illness. Recovery-oriented services recognize and celebrate the individuality and growth of each person and are geared to their unique values, preferences, and goals (Roe & Chopra, 2003). In the CR program, the therapist takes an interest in the client as a person, not a diagnosis, and focuses on understanding and helping them improve their lives. Personal goals are set by each client, and although the program covers specific information and skills, all of the teaching is individually tailored to the person and informed by their unique circumstances and preferences.

Strengths-Based

Just as a person-centered approach sees the whole person and not just a diagnostic label, strengths-based services do not narrowly focus on deficits and impairments but instead take a broader view of recognizing and building on each client's positive qualities, skills, and resources, while also developing new areas of strength (Slade et al., 2015). First, during the psychoeducational sessions, coping strategies that the client uses to manage troubling symptoms or other problems (e.g., social situations, work) are explored and encouraged when effective. Second, the two primary skills that clients are taught in the program (Breathing Retraining and cognitive restructuring) not only are effective at reducing PTSD symptoms but also are intended for dealing with a wide range of different life situations long after the program has ended and thus become new strengths available to the client.

How Does the CR Program Foster Recovery?

The CR program includes the critical elements that characterize recovery-oriented programs. This leads to the question of what are the mechanisms through which the CR program helps individuals make progress in their own personal recovery?

Extensive research has been conducted aimed at understanding the experience of recovery in individuals with a mental health condition. Although each person's experience is unique, common processes involved in recovery have been identified. Perhaps the most widely accepted research on this topic identified five different processes associated with the experience of recovery, summarized with the acronym CHIME: connectedness, hope and optimism, identity, meaning in life, and empowerment (Leamy et al., 2011). We briefly describe next how the CR program influences each of these five processes, thereby fostering recovery.

Connectedness, or feeling and having closer relationships with others while experiencing less alienation and loneliness, is prominent in the process of recovery. Improving social relationships is a common goal of clients in the CR program, which can contribute to connectedness in multiple ways. The person-centered, structured, and collaborative nature of the CR program (including the therapist's interest in the client's life and goals, the transparent and systematic teaching of skills, and the shared decision making about the tasks of therapy) often results in the client experiencing a strong personal connection with this clinician. As difficulty trusting other people is a common problem with trauma survivors, this experience can let clients know that trusting relationships with other people are possible and encourage them to try to let others in their lives. Psychoeducation about trauma and PTSD can normalize the symptoms and challenges clients have, letting them know they are not alone or "crazy" and helping them to feel less cut off from others. Cognitive restructuring can help clients challenge and change inaccurate trauma-related beliefs that can interfere with close and rewarding relationships, such as beliefs that they are defective or weak or that others will take advantage of them.

Hope and optimism for the future are vital to recovery as they are needed for individuals to take risks and make changes in their lives that may feel scary but ultimately have the potential to improve their lives. In the CR program, the therapist is always on the lookout for opportunities to instill hope in the client for a better future, whether it is about coping with PTSD symptoms, overcoming debilitating depression, improving their relationships, or returning to work. When teaching cognitive restructuring, pessimistic (often trauma-related) beliefs about the future can be challenged and changed to more accurate beliefs that allow the possibility of a better future.

Identity changes in terms of how individuals view themselves are a major process in recovery, with negative self-identities dominated by mental illness and a sense of inferiority or failure giving way to more complex, balanced, and positive self-identities (Lysaker & Lysaker, 2008; Roe & Davidson, 2005; Yanos et al., 2011). The CR program fosters healthy changes in identity in multiple ways. Learning about the nature and prevalence of PTSD in the psychoeducational sessions often results in changes in negative appraisals that clients have about themselves based on their reactions to the trauma, such as being weak and ineffectual due to having not recovered from the effects of the traumatic event. Further changes in identity often occur during cognitive restructuring, such as when core beliefs about oneself that have their origins in traumatic events are systematically examined and changed (e.g., "I'm easy prey because I was abused as a child and married to a physically abusive man," "I'm a bad person because I didn't stop my sexual abuse when I could have").

Meaning and sense of purpose in life are often lost or disrupted when someone develops SMI and has difficulty pursing their previous goals or is prevented from continuing to engage in meaningful activities. Developing new meaning in life is integral to the recovery process. Traumatic events can further have radical effects on purpose in life, sometimes dominating and robbing the person of all other meaning. Closely examining (via cognitive restructuring) the meaning people attach to their traumatic experiences—which is frequently based on faulty logic not supported by the available evidence—often results in positive changes in the meaning people derive from their lives. For example, the primary meaning in the life of a woman with a history of sexual abuse and assault may be the avoidance of further victimization, based on the belief that no one can be trusted. This belief may be altered via cognitive restructuring by challenging the client's overestimation of risk of revictimization, allowing space for more rewarding and diverse types of meaning in life to develop.

Empowerment involves the growing sense of control individuals feel over their own mental illness and their lives, which is crucial to marshalling efforts to pursuing their personal vision of recovery (Russinova et al., 2011). The CR program supports the growth in empowerment in multiple ways: Perhaps the most important way is by teaching clients specific skills (Breathing Retraining and cognitive restructuring) that give them greater control over the disruptive effects of distressing emotions, including those directly related to PTSD and other negative feelings as well.

RESEARCH ON THE CR FOR PTSD PROGRAM

Research on the CR for PTSD program has included both open (noncontrolled) clinical trials aimed at evaluating the feasibility and preliminary outcomes of the program and randomized controlled trials (RCTs) comparing the effects of the program with different control groups.

Open Clinical Trials of the CR for PTSD Program

Two open clinical trials of the CR for PTSD program have been conducted in treatment settings serving people with SMI, one in rural New Hampshire (NH) and Vermont (VT; Hamblen et al., 2004; Mueser, Rosenberg, et al., 2004; Rosenberg et al., 2004) and the other in urban New Jersey (NJ; Lu et al., 2009). The primary purposes of these studies were to evaluate the safety and feasibility of providing the CR program and to explore whether participation was associated with changes in PTSD and other symptoms. We defined completion of six or more sessions as sufficient exposure to the program to be clinically meaningful based on the fact that clients would have received three sessions of cognitive restructuring (in addition to the initial three orientation/Breathing Retraining/psychoeducation/goal-setting sessions), which was presumed to be the most critical component of the program. Dropout from the program was defined as completing fewer than six sessions.

These two studies employed similar methods to screen and confirm PTSD among the clients with SMI and to determine eligibility for participation in the CR for PTSD program. Inclusion/exclusion criteria for both studies were (a) psychiatric diagnosis of schizophrenia spectrum disorder, psychosis NOS (not otherwise specified), bipolar disorder, or major depression; (b) in treatment for SMI, as defined by the respective states where the studies took place (NH, NJ, VT); (c) current diagnosis of PTSD based on a structured clinical interview; (d) not presenting a grave threat to self or others; (e) no psychiatric hospitalization or suicide attempt within past 2 to 3 months; and (f) interested in participating in treatment and willing to give informed consent.

Both studies also used similar methods to train and supervise clinicians in providing the CR for PTSD program (e.g., weekly group supervision), to monitor therapist fidelity to the intervention, and to evaluate the effects of the program on PTSD and other symptom outcomes assessed at baseline, posttreatment, and 3-month follow-up (the NJ study also conducted a 6-month follow-up). The two studies differed primarily in the setting and population served and in the clinicians providing the program. The NH–VT open trial was conducted in relatively rural New England with a White, non-Latinx sample of participants, with the program provided mainly by PhD-level research-trained clinicians. In contrast, the NJ study was conducted in a relatively urban area with a more racially and ethnically heterogeneous sample of participants, with frontline master's-level clinicians providing the intervention.

Table 2.1 summarizes the sample characteristics of the participants in the two studies, the dropout rates from the program, and the PTSD outcomes at

TABLE 2.1. Characteristics and Outcomes From Two Open Clinical Trials of the CR for PTSD Program in Persons With SMI

Study	Location	No. of participants	Clinicians	Dropout	Result
Rosenberg et al. (2004)	Rural New Hampshire and Vermont	22 54% women 100% White 45% schizophrenia, schizoaffective, or psychosis not otherwise specified 55% bipolar or major depression	4 PhD 1 MA	14%	PTSD severity fell 18 points on CAPS at posttreatment and 23 points at 3-month follow-up. 50% had PTSD at 3-month follow-up.
Lu et al. (2009)	Urban New Jersey	19 58% women 42% non-Latinx White 38% Black 11% Latinx 16% schizophrenia or schizoaffective 86% bipolar or major depression	6 MA-level frontline clinicians	24%	PTSD severity fell 10.3 points on PDS at posttreatment, 15.9 points at 3-month follow-up, and 18.4 points at 6-month follow-up. 69% had PTSD at posttreatment, 33% had PTSD at 3-month follow-up, and 58% had PTSD at 6-month follow-up.

Note. CR = cognitive restructuring; PTSD = posttraumatic stress disorder; SMI = serious mental illness; CAPS = Clinician-Administered PTSD Scale for *Diagnostic and Statistical Manual of Mental Disorders, Fourth Edition* (Blake et al., 1995); PDS = PTSD Diagnostic Scale (Foa et al., 1993).

posttreatment and the follow-ups. The results of both open clinical trials provided strong support for the safety and feasibility of the CR for PTSD program, with significant adverse events not observed and the overall rate of retention in treatment high (86% in NH–VT, 76% in NJ). Furthermore, participants in the program showed significant improvements in their PTSD symptoms at posttreatment and at the follow-ups in both the severity of their PTSD symptoms and PTSD diagnosis. For example, 31% to 67% of participants no longer met diagnostic criteria for PTSD at either the posttreatment or follow-up assessment. Additionally, participants who received the CR program improved during the 16-week intervention period as well as at follow-ups in other psychiatric symptoms, especially depression (not shown in table).

These findings indicated that the CR for PTSD program was safe, well tolerated, acceptable, and beneficial to clients with SMI and PTSD, including those from diverse racial and ethnic backgrounds. Furthermore, the apparently beneficial effects of the CR program on PTSD and other symptoms found when it was delivered mainly by PhD-level clinicians in the NH–VT study were confirmed when it was delivered by frontline master's-level clinicians in NJ.

RCTs of the CR for PTSD Program

Three RCTs of the CR for PTSD program have been completed. The first two studies were conducted in locations similar to the two open clinical trials in NH–VT and NJ described previously and used methods similar to the methods used in those trials. All of the studies took place at mental health centers that served people with SMI but did not provide trauma-focused treatments. In addition, as mentioned earlier, an in-progress RCT in the Netherlands is evaluating the impact of the CR program (in comparison with PE and EMDR) in people with PTSD and psychotic disorders (Burger et al., 2022). Highlights of the findings from the three completed RCTs are provided next.

NH–VT RCT

This study was conducted at five sites in NH and VT and compared the CR for PTSD program with treatment as usual (TAU), with the CR for PTSD program delivered mainly by PhD-level clinicians (Mueser et al., 2008).

Participants and Assessments

The same inclusion/exclusion criteria were used as in the NH–VT and NJ open trials except that individuals with substance dependence were not included (clients with substance abuse were included). A total of 108 participants were enrolled, of whom 77% were women, 84% were non-Latinx White, and 84% had a major mood disorder (16% had a psychotic disorder). In addition, 25% of the clients also had borderline personality disorder. Most (75%) clients had severe PTSD, as defined by a Clinician-Administered PTSD Scale (CAPS) total score of 65 or over.

Assessments were conducted by raters who were blind to participants' treatment assignment at baseline, posttreatment, and 3- and 6-month follow-ups on PTSD symptoms and diagnosis using the CAPS. Trauma-related beliefs were assessed with the Posttraumatic Cognitions Inventory (Foa et al., 1999), and understanding of symptoms was assessed with the PTSD Knowledge Test (Pratt et al., 2005). A variety of other interview-rated and self-report measures were used to assess changes in symptoms. In addition, to explore whether participants with lower levels of cognitive functioning benefitted differently from the CR for PTSD program than those with normal cognitive functioning, a neurocognitive battery was administered at baseline to that group.

Findings

Of the clients randomized to the CR for PTSD program, only 19% dropped out before participating in six or more sessions, and thus 81% received adequate exposure to the program. The results indicated that although participants in both groups improved from baseline to the subsequent assessments on all the PTSD outcomes (symptoms, diagnosis, knowledge, trauma-related beliefs), clients who received the CR program improved significantly more. Clients in the program also improved significantly more in other psychiatric symptoms than the TAU group, especially in depression. Moreover, the effects of the program were especially strong on clients with severe PTSD. The impact of the program was unaffected by level of cognitive impairment among the participants (Mueser et al., 2018). Participants with borderline personality disorder benefitted as much from the program as those without the disorder (Kredlow et al., 2017).

Two other analyses shed further light on how the CR for PTSD program works. First, an analysis examined whether improvements in trauma-related beliefs mediated the greater improvements in PTSD symptoms between the CR and TAU conditions. Results indicated that PTSD symptom improvements were fully mediated by changes in trauma-related cognitions in the CR group, consistent with the cognitive model on which the program is based. Second, an analysis was conducted to evaluate whether CR participants who completed more home assignments had better outcomes than those who completed fewer assignments. This hypothesis was confirmed, as those who completed more assignments had better PTSD symptom (and other) outcomes than those who completed fewer, underscoring the importance of facilitating client follow-through on home assignments to get the greatest clinical benefit from the CR program.

NJ RCT

This RCT was conducted at five sites in NJ with a more racially and ethnically heterogeneous sample of participants than the NH–VT RCT and used frontline master's-level clinicians rather than PhD-level clinicians to deliver the interventions. Because of the strong effects of the CR for PTSD program in the NH–VT RCT, the NJ RCT compared the CR program with a brief (three-session) program that included the psychoeducational and Breathing Retraining components of the CR program but not the cognitive restructuring component. An educational video was also developed to facilitate the psychoeducation in the brief program. Thus, this study was designed to provide information about the specific benefits of the cognitive restructuring component of the CR program (Mueser, Gottlieb, et al., 2015).

Participants and Assessments

Similar inclusion/exclusion criteria to the NH–VT RCT were used. A total of 201 participants enrolled in the study, of whom 69% were female, 56% African American, 18% Latinx, 33% had a psychotic disorder, and 67% had a major mood disorder; 27% also had borderline personality disorder. All (100%) clients had severe PTSD as defined by the CAPS.

Assessments were conducted over a 1-year period using a similar battery of assessments as the NH–VT RCT, with overall functioning and quality of life also measured.

Clinician Training

A training program was developed for the frontline master's-level clinicians who delivered the interventions. Clinicians first participated in a 2-day training in the intervention that combined didactics with role-playing. They then engaged a client with SMI and PTSD as a practice case, audio recorded sessions for review, and participated in weekly group supervision meetings. Intervention-trained supervisors reviewed and rated each session soon after it was completed with our CR for PTSD Fidelity Scale and provided the clinician with written quantitative fidelity ratings and qualitative feedback prior to the next client session. Clinicians were deemed "certified" in delivery of the CR for PTSD program if they scored an average of at least 3.5 (on a 5-point total score: 1 = *poor*, 2 = *borderline*, 3 = *satisfactory*, 4 = *good*, 5 = *excellent*) on our Fidelity Scale on this practice case. If clinicians scored below an average of 3.5, they took on a second practice case. Clinician certification was required before treating study cases.

A total of 22 clinicians were trained in the program, of whom 20 (91%) met certification criteria with their first practice case (Lu et al., 2012). The remaining two clinicians met certification criteria with their second practice case. In addition to the high rate of certification following the first practice case, clients who received the CR for PTSD program from these clinicians during training showed steady reductions in PTSD symptoms (on the PTSD Checklist—PCL; Blanchard et al., 2013; Weathers et al. 2013) and depression (on the Beck Depression Inventory–II; Beck et al., 1998, 1996) over the course of treatment.

Findings

Seventy-three percent of participants attended six or more sessions and were thus exposed to the CR for PTSD program. Statistical analyses indicated that clients in both programs (the full CR for PTSD program and the brief program) improved on all of the outcomes from baseline to the posttreatment and 6- and 12-month follow-ups. However, those in the full CR program improved more than those in the brief program on all the PTSD outcomes and overall functioning.

Participants in both treatment conditions improved similarly on other psychiatric symptoms and quality of life. As in the NH–VT RCT, those with borderline personality disorder benefitted as much from the CR program as those without the disorder (Kredlow et al., 2017).

Closer examination of changes in PTSD symptoms between the two treatment programs suggests that despite the overall better outcomes for the CR for PTSD program, the brief treatment did confer some clinical benefit. These differences are illustrated in Figure 2.2. The apparent clinical benefit associated with the brief program in this study led to the refinement of the brief intervention and standardization of it as the BREATHE program, as described in the online Supplemental Chapter 15 to this book.

FIGURE 2.2. Changes in PTSD Outcomes Over Time for Participants With SMI in Two RCTs of the CR for PTSD Program Compared With TAU (NH–VT Study) or Brief PTSD Program (NJ Study)

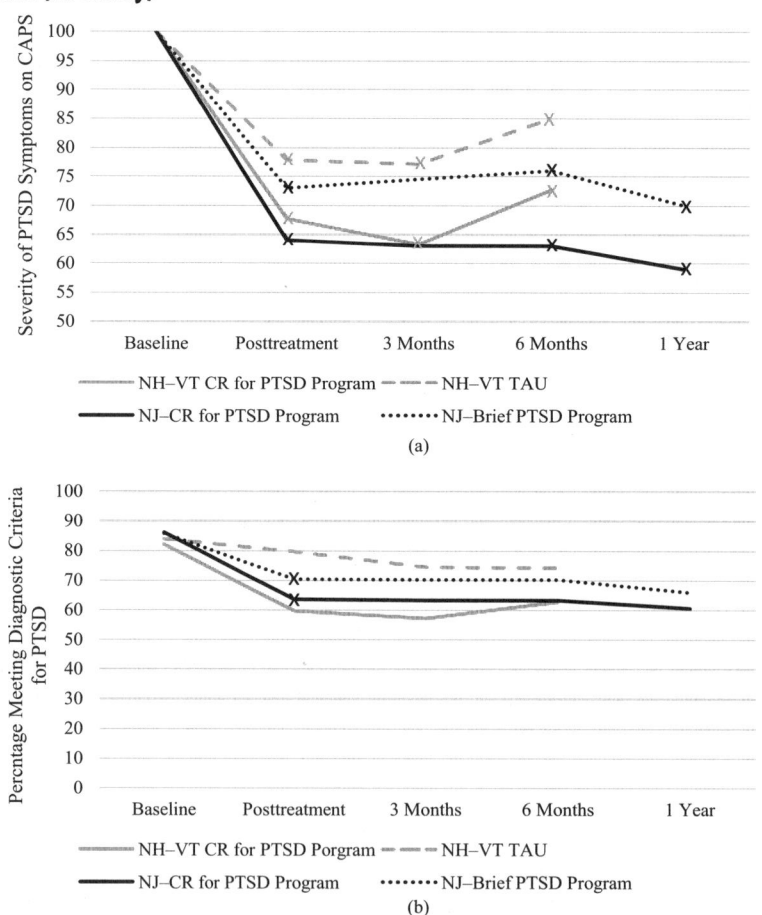

Note. (a) PTSD symptom severity on the Clinician-Administered PTSD Scale (CAPS total). (b) PTSD diagnosis based on the CAPS. Data based on Mueser, Gottlieb, et al. (2015) and Mueser et al. (2008). PTSD = posttraumatic stress disorder; SMI = serious mental illness; RCT = randomized controlled trial; CR =cognitive restructuring; TAU = treatment as usual; NH = New Hampshire; VT = Vermont; NJ = New Jersey.

U.K. RCT

This study was conducted at two National Health Service trusts serving people with SMI located in the South of England (Steel et al., 2017). The CR for PTSD program was compared with TAU in 61 participants with schizophrenia or schizoaffective disorder, with PTSD symptoms and diagnosis assessed with the CAPS at baseline and 6- and 12-month follow-ups. Trained clinicians implemented the CR program, and fidelity to the model (although conducted and evaluated somewhat differently than within our RCT study fidelity system described earlier) was monitored throughout the trial.

Although many of the methods in the study were similar to those used in the NH–VT and NJ RCTs, they differed in three ways. First, the sample in the U.K. RCT was restricted to participants with schizophrenia spectrum disorders and PTSD, whereas the two U.S. RCTs also included participants with major mood disorders, borderline personality disorder, and PTSD. Second, most of the participants in the NH–VT RCT (75%) and all the participants in the NJ RCT (100%) had severe PTSD on the CAPS, whereas relatively few participants in the U.K. RCT had severe PTSD. Third, the two U.S. RCTs included only participants with PTSD secondary to the typical traumatic events experienced in the general population (e.g., physical or sexual abuse/assault), whereas the U.K. RCT also included participants with PTSD secondary to psychotic symptoms (i.e., PTSD diagnosis related to the traumatic experiences, such as hearing voices telling the person to kill himself or being forcibly secluded and restrained due to psychotic behavior).

Somewhat surprisingly, no differences between the CR for PTSD and TAU groups were seen in PTSD or any of the other outcomes at either of the follow-ups, with both groups showing significant reductions in PTSD and other symptoms. While it is unclear why significant differences were not found in the U.K. RCT compared with the two RCTs conducted in the United States, one possible explanation is the significantly lower levels of baseline PTSD severity in the U.K. RCT (CAPS total = 52.3) compared with the NH–VT and NJ RCTs (CAPS total = 75.3 and 85.9, respectively). In the NH–VT RCT, the effects of the CR program were found to be stronger for the majority of participants with severe PTSD compared with the subgroup with moderate levels of PTSD. Although it has been suggested that the CR program may be less potent in clients with schizophrenia and PTSD (Sin & Spain, 2016), analyses of the NH–VT and NJ RCTs exploring differences between primary SMI diagnosis and improvement in the CR program found no interactions, suggesting that participants with both psychotic and nonpsychotic disorders benefit comparably from the program.

GROUP THERAPY VERSION OF THE CR FOR PTSD PROGRAM

Following the initial work on developing the individual-based CR for PTSD program, a group version, the CR for PTSD group, was developed, pilot tested, and subsequently implemented at a number of agencies. This program was first developed in collaboration with clinicians at the Mental Health Center of Greater Manchester, NH. The CR for PTSD group was designed to treat groups of six to eight persons with SMI and PTSD and to be led by two clinicians.

The same basic structure and organization of the individual-based CR for PTSD program was used for the CR for PTSD group, including provision of the orientation, Wellness Plan, Breathing Retraining, and psychoeducation components of the program over the first three sessions, followed by the two cognitive restructuring components (Common Styles of Thinking, the 5 Steps of CR) taught over the next 13 sessions. Two additional components were added to address coping skills and recovery planning. Specifically, three more sessions were devoted to teaching strategies for coping with common persistent PTSD symptoms, such as intrusive memories of the event and difficulty sleeping. Two sessions were also added to the end of the program aimed at helping participants develop a personal recovery plan for the future. Thus, the CR for PTSD group was designed to be provided over 21 weekly or twice weekly sessions.

Two open clinical trials of the CR for PTSD group in persons with SMI and PTSD have been conducted that provide preliminary support for the program— one study with 80 participants at a community mental health center (Mueser et al., 2007) and another study with 14 participants at a VA Medical Center (Sacks et al., 2017). Across both studies, retention of participants in the group was good, indicating high satisfaction with the program. Furthermore, in both studies participants showed significant improvements in PTSD symptom severity and depression from baseline to posttreatment, gains that were maintained at the 3-month follow-up in the study with follow-up assessments (Mueser et al., 2007).

BRIEF RELAXATION, EDUCATION, AND TRAUMA HEALING (BREATHE) PROGRAM

As previously described, the BREATHE program, a brief three-session program based on the Breathing Retraining and psychoeducation components of the CR for PTSD program, was found to be a surprisingly effective treatment for PTSD in persons with SMI when it was compared with the full CR program in the large NJ RCT study (Mueser, Gottlieb, et al., 2015). In addition to the NJ RCT, two open clinical trials exploring the effectiveness of the BREATHE program have been conducted with people with SMI and PTSD, including 18 clients living in St. Louis, Missouri (Nishith et al., 2015) and 211 clients living in Chicago, Illinois (Mueser et al., in press). Uptake of the BREATHE program was excellent in both studies. In addition, assessments conducted at baseline, posttreatment, and 3 months later indicated significant improvements in PTSD symptom severity and depression. These studies provided further support for the clinical utility of the brief, BREATHE program for treating PTSD in people with SMI and suggest that it may be a valuable treatment option in certain settings, either as a stand-alone intervention for PTSD where it may not be feasible to deliver the CR for PTSD intervention or as a first step toward implementing the full CR program.

These considerations are discussed in more detail in online Supplemental Chapter 15 about the BREATHE program.

CONCLUSION

There has been substantial research on effective treatments for PTSD in the general population; however, the problem of overly restrictive eligibility criteria for clinical trials unfortunately culminated in the exclusion of most people with SMI from these past investigations of psychosocial treatments for PTSD. The CR for PTSD program was developed to address the need for an effective, evidence-based treatment for PTSD that could be provided flexibly and with a minimum of stress to the vulnerable population of clients with SMI. The CR program is based on cognitive restructuring rather than prolonged exposure, given presumed higher acceptability to clients (and potentially clinicians) and the lower stress associated with these intervention components, among other considerations.

The CR for PTSD program is an individual-based cognitive behavioral intervention provided over 12 to 16 weekly sessions and focusing on three therapeutic components: psychoeducation, Breathing Retraining, and a unique version of cognitive restructuring, used to assist clients in identifying and modifying general distress as well as inaccurate and upsetting core and trauma-related beliefs.

The CR program is informed by the mental health field's newer understanding of recovery from SMI as a personal growth process, incorporates the core characteristics of recovery-oriented services (being trauma-informed, person-centered, strengths-based, and supporting self-determination and choice), and facilitates the individual's recovery by fostering the CHIME acronym's five specific processes of recovery: improving Connectedness, instilling Hope for a better future, promoting positive and healthy shifts in personal Identity, creating new Meaning and sense of purpose, and Empowering people to regain control over their own lives.

Research on the CR program, including two open clinical trials and three RCTs, supports it as an effective, evidence-based intervention. Two variants of the CR program are also briefly discussed in this chapter, including the group version of the program (the CR for PTSD group) and a brief (three-session) program based on the Breathing Retraining and psychoeducational components of the CR program (the BREATHE program).

3

Understanding and Assessing Trauma and PTSD

We begin this chapter with a brief description of the diagnostic criteria for posttraumatic stress disorder (PTSD) and its common clinical correlates, followed by a review of the safety and accuracy of trauma and PTSD assessments in persons with serious mental illness (SMI). We next provide tips for distinguishing between the symptoms of PTSD and SMI and briefly consider the misdiagnosis of other disorders when PTSD has not been previously assessed. We then give clinical guidelines for the assessment of PTSD and other related areas and recommendations for responding to client distress during the assessment process. Next, we outline the role of monitoring selected outcomes over the course of the Cognitive Restructuring (CR) for PTSD program, including PTSD symptoms, depression, trauma-related cognitions, and personal goals. Last, we address how psychotic symptoms and adverse mental health treatment experiences can be understood as traumatic events and consider possible treatment options.

ONSET AND DEFINING FEATURES OF PTSD

The diagnosis of PTSD entails the assessment of the experience of a psychologically traumatic event or events and the evaluation of specific symptoms that define the disorder.

Definition of *Traumatic Event*

The definition of *traumatic event* has varied over different editions of the *Diagnostic and Statistical Manual of Mental Disorders* (*DSM*) series, and in the *Diagnostic and Statistical Manual of Mental Disorders* (5th ed.; *DSM-5*; American Psychiatric

https://doi.org/10.1037/0000423-003

Treatment of Posttraumatic Stress Disorder in Serious Mental Illness: The Cognitive Restructuring Program, by K. T. Mueser and J. D. Gottlieb

Association, 2013), it requires exposure to an event involving death or the threat of death, serious injury, or sexual violence. Exposure can include directly experiencing or witnessing the event. Learning about the event occurring to a close family member or friend is also included in the definition of traumatic if it was violent or accidental but not if it occurred due to natural causes. People who have direct extreme exposure to the immediate consequences of a traumatic event, such as first responders to an accident or disaster, are also considered to be exposed to a traumatic event. Seeing images of the traumatic event (e.g., in the media, in pictures) or hearing personal accounts of people who directly witnessed or experienced the event is not considered traumatic per the *DSM*.

Symptoms and Onset of PTSD

The *DSM-5* diagnosis of PTSD requires that the defining symptoms are present at least 1 month after the traumatic event occurred. PTSD symptoms often develop rapidly following an event and then persist or worsen over the following month. Sometimes PTSD symptoms emerge following a period of time after the event (delayed-onset PTSD).

As mentioned in Chapter 1, the diagnosis of PTSD requires the presence of four clusters of symptoms that must cause clinically significant distress or impairment in social, occupational, or other important areas of functioning. The specific diagnostic criteria for PTSD are summarized in Exhibit 3.1, and the symptoms are described in more detail in this section.

EXHIBIT 3.1

DSM-5 **Criteria for Posttraumatic Stress Disorder in Adults**

A. Exposure to one or more events involving serious injury, sexual violence, threatened death, or death in one of the following ways:

1. Experiencing the event directly.

2. Witnessing the event in person happen to someone else.

3. Learning that the event occurred to a close person (if threatened or actual death, event was violent or accidental).

4. Exposure to the adverse details of a traumatic event (e.g., a dead body after an accident), excluding exposure via media (e.g., TV, photos).

B. Two or more of the following intrusion (or reexperiencing) symptoms related to the traumatic event:

1. Recurrent, involuntary distressing memories of the event.

2. Upsetting dreams related to event either in terms of content or feeling.

3. Flashbacks in which the person temporarily feels or acts as though the event is happening again.

4. Psychological distress when exposed to internal or external reminders of the event.

5. Significant physiological reactions when exposed to internal or external reminders of the event.

(*continues*)

EXHIBIT 3.1

DSM-5 **Criteria for Posttraumatic Stress Disorder in Adults** (*Continued*)

C. One or more of the following avoidance symptoms related to the traumatic event:

   1. Avoidance of (or attempts to avoid) distressing thoughts, feelings, or memories related to the event.

   2. Avoidance of (or attempts to avoid) situations that remind the person of the event, such as places, people, conversational topics, activities, or feelings.

D. Two or more of the following negative changes in thoughts and feelings related to the traumatic event:

   1. Inability to remember important aspects of the event (not due to factors such as substance use or head injury).

   2. Exaggerated negative beliefs about oneself, others, or the world.

   3. Inaccurate beliefs about the cause or consequences of the event resulting in self-blame or blaming others.

   4. Consistent negative emotions such as anxiety, shame, or anger.

   5. Reduced interest or participation in important activities such as self-care, parenting, or leisure activities.

   6. Feeling detached, estranged, or not connected to other people.

   7. Difficulty feeling positive emotions such as love or happiness.

E. Two or more of the following overarousal symptoms related to the event:

   1. Irritable behavior and anger outbursts with little or no provocation.

   2. Self-destructive or reckless behavior.

   3. Hypervigilance.

   4. Exaggerated startle response.

   5. Difficulties with concentration.

   6. Problems sleeping such as difficulty falling asleep or staying asleep.

F. The symptoms in Items B to E have lasted more than a month.

G. The symptoms cause or worsen impairment in important areas of functioning (e.g., work, social relationships) or cause clinically significant distress.

H. The problem cannot be explained by the physiological effects of alcohol, drugs, or a medical condition.

Note. Data from American Psychiatric Association (2013).

The first group of symptoms are intrusion symptoms, which occur when the individual reexperiences the traumatic event. The most common of these symptoms are recurrent and unexpected distressing memories of the event, such as an image of what happened suddenly popping into the person's mind. Another common intrusion symptom is the experience of intense distress when exposed to trauma-related cues, such as a sexual abuse survivor seeing a story on the news about a sexual abuse case and becoming very upset or emotionally dysregulated. Sometimes people have distressing dreams or nightmares that in terms of content or theme are related to the traumatic event. Less often people experience actual flashbacks, in which the person momentarily feels or acts as though the traumatic event were happening again.

The second cluster of symptoms is avoidance of trauma-related stimuli. People often avoid situations involving external cues that remind them of the traumatic event, such as the neighborhood where a bad accident occurred or physical intimacy with a new partner when previously sexually assaulted earlier in life. People may also try to avoid or quickly escape from upsetting thoughts, memories, or feelings related to the traumatic event, such as not talking about a loved one who recently died unexpectedly.

The third group of symptoms include negative alterations in cognition and mood that emerge as related to the traumatic event. Negative beliefs or unrealistic expectations about themselves (e.g., "I am bad," "It was completely my fault that I was raped," "I have no future") or other people (e.g., "No one can be trusted") are common. There may be chronic negative feelings (e.g., fear, shame) and difficulty experiencing positive feelings, leading to reduced interest and participation in activities and feeling detached from others. People may also be unable to recall important aspects of the traumatic event.

The fourth cluster of symptoms reflect problems with overarousal associated with the experience of the traumatic event. One of the most common and distressing of these symptoms is difficulty sleeping (despite desire and need for sleep). Having an exaggerated startle response, hypervigilance, and difficulties concentrating are also common overarousal symptoms, as are irritability and outbursts of temper.

Common Clinical Correlates of PTSD

PTSD is associated with a broad range of other symptoms, problems, and comorbid psychiatric disorders. The most common clinical correlate of PTSD is depression (Shah et al., 2012), with about 50% of people with PTSD having major depression (Flory & Yehuda, 2015). In line with this, among people with SMI, rates of PTSD tend to be highest in persons with major depression, followed by bipolar disorder, and then schizophrenia and schizoaffective disorder (Mueser et al., 1998; Mueser, Salyers, et al., 2004). Relatedly, PTSD is associated with higher suicidal ideation and attempts, with comorbid depression accounting for the greatest increase in vulnerability (Álvarez et al., 2012; Panagioti et al., 2012).

As mentioned earlier, people with PTSD are also more prone to substance use disorders (McCauley et al., 2012). At least some of this comorbidity can be explained by attempts to self-medicate PTSD symptoms such as intrusive memories and difficulty sleeping (Nishith et al., 2001), which usually provide only temporary relief at best. Furthermore, as discussed in Chapter 1 (see An Interactive Model of PTSD and the Course of SMI section), substance use can have untoward effects on increasing retraumatization due to the reduced ability of people to protect themselves when under the influence of substances and their tendency to spend time with people who are more likely to victimize them.

Mild psychotic symptoms (when they cannot be attributed to another psychiatric disorder such as schizophrenia or major depression) are another common symptom in people with PTSD (Braakman et al., 2009; Seedat et al., 2003). Hallucinations (e.g., hearing voices) and delusions (e.g., paranoia) are the most common psychotic symptoms in PTSD (Butler et al., 1996) and are associated with more severe PTSD symptoms (Mueser & Butler, 1987). Psychotic symptoms may be linked to the nature of the traumatic event, such as hearing the voice of the perpetrator of one's childhood physical abuse, but may also be unrelated to the event (Braakman et al., 2009). Research indicates that PTSD with psychotic features is not related to a family history of psychosis, suggesting the symptoms do not reflect an underlying psychotic disorder (Sautter et al., 2002). Among individuals with SMI, trauma history and PTSD have frequently been reported to be associated with more severe psychotic symptoms (Chapter 1, this volume).

Complex PTSD

Early and repeated interpersonal trauma (e.g., childhood physical or sexual abuse) has an especially pernicious effect on long-term psychological functioning. Complex PTSD has been proposed as a diagnostic category to reflect the broader range of impact of early trauma beyond PTSD symptoms, including disturbances in consciousness, self-perception, and social relationships (Herman, 1992). Whether complex PTSD should be a separate diagnosis from PTSD (or subdiagnosis) has been a topic of extensive debate. Proponents of the diagnosis argue that it reflects the broad range of consequences associated with early and repeated traumatization beyond the symptoms of PTSD, such as effects on interpersonal relationships and self-esteem, that may require different or modified interventions than for PTSD (Courtois & Ford, 2009; Karatzias et al., 2019, 2023). Other experts note that research on complex PTSD suggests it is a severe variant of PTSD but not a distinct diagnostic entity (Landy et al., 2015; Resick et al., 2012; Wolf et al., 2015) and point to the lack of evidence showing that different interventions are needed to effectively treat it (De Jongh et al., 2016).

The debate about whether complex PTSD should be a separate diagnosis from PTSD is further reflected in the differences between how PTSD is defined in *DSM-5* and the *International Statistical Classification of Diseases and Related Health Problems* (11th ed.; *ICD-11*; World Health Organization, 2019; see also Cloitre, 2020). In *ICD-11*, PTSD is defined in terms of the three symptom clusters of reexperiencing, avoidance, and overarousal symptoms (described previously), with complex PTSD defined as requiring those same symptoms plus disturbances in emotion regulation (e.g., heightened emotional reactivity, dissociative symptoms, emotional numbing), negative beliefs about oneself related to the event, and difficulties with social relationships or feeling close to others (World Health Organization, 2019). In *DSM-5*, the diagnosis of PTSD was modified to require negative alterations in thought and mood in addition to the three core PTSD symptom clusters used to define PTSD in *DSM-IV* and *ICD-11*, but complex PTSD was not included as a separate diagnosis. Thus, many of the unique symptoms used to define complex PTSD in *ICD-11* are incorporated into the *DSM-5* definition of PTSD.

In our experience treating PTSD in persons with SMI with the CR for PTSD program (prior to the publication of *DSM-5*), we have found that problems with emotion regulation, negative beliefs about oneself, and difficulties with social relationships are nearly always present, suggesting that most of these clients would meet *ICD-11* criteria for complex PTSD. These symptoms may be so common because they reflect major challenges experienced by most people with SMI, including those without PTSD. When teaching clients about PTSD in this CR for PTSD program, we use the *DSM-5* definition because it is simpler and easier for clients to grasp, and it avoids the connotation that some types of PTSD (i.e., complex PTSD) are more complicated and difficult to treat than others.

ACCURACY AND SAFETY OF TRAUMA AND PTSD ASSESSMENT IN SMI

Recall that mental health treatment providers have historically been reluctant to inquire into the traumatic experiences and PTSD symptoms in people with SMI for two reasons. First, clinicians have believed that psychotic distortions or delusions with themes involving sexual or physical abuse in this population could result in unreliable self-reports of trauma and PTSD (Coverdale & Grunebaum, 1998). Second, there have been concerns that inquiring about past trauma could be stressful and upsetting to individuals, potentially destabilizing their mental illness and resulting in symptom relapses (Hardy & Mueser, 2017). Fortunately, as discussed next, there is ample evidence that both accurate and safe assessments of trauma and PTSD can be conducted with clients with SMI (Brown et al., 2014).

Given the private nature of many interpersonal traumas such as sexual abuse, external verification of reports of victimization is often difficult or impossible to ascertain. However, the reliability of reports over time can be more easily determined. Numerous studies show that self-report measures of trauma exposure in clients with SMI have high levels of test–retest reliability (Carr et al., 2018; Jiang et al., 2018; Kim et al., 2013; Meyer et al., 1996; Mueser et al., 2001; Wolford et al., 2008) and convergent validity (Cristofaro et al., 2013). The validity of self-report measures of trauma in persons with SMI is further supported by research showing they are predictive of the results of structured clinical interviews of PTSD (de Bont et al., 2015; Jiang et al., 2018; Kim et al., 2013).

Self-report measures of PTSD such as the PTSD Checklist (PCL; Weathers et al., 2013) and the PTSD Symptom Scale–Self-Report (Foa et al., 1993) have also been shown to have high test–retest reliability and strong validity in predicting gold-standard diagnoses based on interviews with the Clinician-Administered PTSD Scale (Weathers et al., 2018) in persons with SMI (Grubaugh et al., 2007; Mueser et al., 2001; Roberts et al., 2021; Sin et al., 2012). Further support for the validity of PTSD assessment in this population is provided by evidence that the dimensionality of PTSD symptoms in people with SMI is similar to that in the general population (Lu, Yanos, et al., 2022; Penney et al., 2023; Schäfer et al., 2011).

Finally, just as how the reliability and factor structure of PTSD assessments are similar between the SMI and general populations, so are measures of trauma-related cognitions. Specifically, evaluation of common trauma-related thoughts and beliefs with the Posttraumatic Cognitions Inventory (PTCI; Foa et al., 1999) has shown it has similar psychometric properties and dimensionality in individuals with psychotic and related disorders as in the general population (Lu, Mueser, et al., 2023). Taken together, the evidence indicates that reliable and valid assessments of both trauma exposure and PTSD can be conducted in persons with SMI and that these assessments are low-risk and generally well received by clients with SMI.

DISTINGUISHING SMI SYMPTOMS FROM PTSD

PTSD symptoms may appear to overlap with three common symptoms of SMI: psychotic symptoms, negative symptoms, and manic or hypomanic symptoms. Specific exploration may reveal that a particular symptom is more likely the result of an SMI, PTSD, or both (OConghaile & DeLisi, 2015).

Psychotic Symptoms

The relationship between psychotic symptoms of psychiatric disorders such as schizophrenia or major mood disorders and PTSD is complex, and a definitive resolution as to which disorder is causing a symptom is not always possible. Psychotic symptoms such as hallucinations and delusions are defining features of schizophrenia spectrum disorders but are also common during manic or depressive episodes of major mood disorders. At the same time, mild psychotic symptoms can be a clinical feature of PTSD (Ibáñez et al., 2014), and there is evidence for a subgroup of persons with PTSD and psychotic symptoms (Braakman et al., 2009; Shevlin et al., 2011). Nevertheless, the following guidelines may be useful.

The PTSD symptoms of intrusive memories or flashbacks can sometimes be confused with visual hallucinations, and additional probing is needed to clarify the nature of the symptom. Flashbacks are usually very brief periods of time in which the person temporarily relives the traumatic event and is no longer oriented to the present time and place. Flashbacks are relatively rare in PTSD but are sometimes confused with the more common symptom of intrusive memories of the traumatic event, in which a memory unexpectedly pops into the person's mind but there is no loss of orientation. An intrusive memory can be distinguished from a visual hallucination through questioning to determine whether it is (a) a distinct memory of a traumatic event and (b) experienced as a mental picture in the person's mind rather than perceived as part of the external world. Flashbacks can be distinguished from hallucinations by determining whether the experience (a) is part of a specific traumatic event and (b) involves a temporary loss of orientation to time and place. Hallucinations do not involve a loss of orientation.

Psychotic symptoms related to a loss or traumatic event can also occur in grief reactions (Baethge, 2002; Ratcliffe, 2021) and PTSD. For example, an individual with PTSD may experience auditory hallucinations following the sudden unexpected loss of a loved one. Someone with PTSD due to being a victim of gang violence during adolescence may develop persecutory delusions about current gang threats in their new neighborhood. Exploration of the specific nature of the symptom can shed light as to whether it is most likely due to one or the other or both disorders.

Psychotic Distortions of Traumatic Events

Psychotic distortions related to traumatic events reported by the client can also occur, raising questions about whether any of the events actually took place. For example, the client may provide a plausible description of a traumatic event experienced, but after further discussion, psychotic distortion may render the overall account implausible. For example, one client ("Donata," who is introduced with her case vignette details in Chapter 4, this volume) described multiple instances of physical abuse as a child from her parents, who had drug addiction problems. She then went on to describe being kidnapped by drug dealers and forced to fly a helicopter at gunpoint as a teenager.

When a client, such as Donata, has a delusional elaboration of what appears to be a plausible traumatic experience and also reports many other PTSD symptoms, we recommend proceeding with providing the CR for PTSD program and focusing primarily on the plausible part of the client's trauma account during the early sessions. On the other hand, when a client's entire account of traumatic events is patently delusional (e.g., being abducted by aliens) or highly implausible (e.g., being a victim of Satanic ritual abuse), the clinician should not treat the event as the index trauma for assessing PTSD. Rather, the clinician should explore whether the client experienced other (more plausible) traumatic events that have resulted in PTSD symptoms.

Negative Symptoms

The negative symptoms of schizophrenia—including apathy, avolition (difficulty initiating goal-directed behavior), anhedonia (loss of pleasure), and blunted affect (diminished emotional expressiveness)—may appear to overlap with the PTSD symptom clusters of avoidance of trauma-related stimuli and alterations in cognition and mood. Conducting a more detailed inquiry can usually determine which type of symptom it is. This is an important distinction to make as most research indicates that comorbid PTSD in schizophrenia is not related to more severe negative symptoms (DeTore et al., 2021; Seow et al., 2016), and some reports suggest it is associated with less severe negative symptoms (Strauss et al., 2011).

PTSD avoidance symptoms and the negative symptoms of apathy and avolition are similar in that they both involve a failure to initiate and sustain behaviors necessary for optimal functioning in areas such as relationships with others, role functioning (e.g., work, school, parenting), or self-care. The role of anxiety is most useful in distinguishing avoidance symptoms from apathy and avolition. Avoidance in PTSD is driven by the anxiety associated with specific situations, places, and people that remind the person of their traumatic experiences.

In contrast, lack of motivation or the degree of effort perceived to be required by the person, and not anxiety, underlie apathy and avolition.

Blunted affect can sometimes be mistaken for the reduced positive feelings or numbness symptoms of PTSD. However, blunted affect is defined in terms of behaviors (diminished emotional expressiveness in facial expression and voice tone), whereas reduced positive emotions and numbness are defined in terms of emotions. Research shows that blunted affect is not correlated with reduced emotional experience in persons with SMI (Kring & Elis, 2013), and thus it does not indicate numbness or reduced positive feelings in PTSD. Direct inquiry about the individual's feelings in different situations can distinguish between blunted affect and these PTSD symptoms. See Chapter 12 in this volume for suggestions about how to work with clients with psychotic and other schizophrenia-spectrum symptoms in the CR for PTSD program.

Manic or Hypomanic Symptoms

Several of the overarousal symptoms of PTSD can be mistaken for or overlap with symptoms of a manic (or the slightly milder variant of hypomanic) episode, including difficulty sleeping and anger outbursts. Physiological hyperarousal in PTSD frequently interferes with the person's ability to get to sleep and stay asleep, despite a desire to do so. Problems with sleep can contribute to a constant state of fatigue and are a major source of distress to many people with PTSD. Decreased need for sleep, on the other hand, is a common symptom of mania that differs from the PTSD symptom of difficulty sleeping in that the individual feels fully rested after only a few hours of sleep (e.g., 2–3 hours) and has no desire to sleep more. Careful questioning of the client's attempts to sleep, desire to sleep, and degree of feeling rested after sleeping can distinguish between these two symptoms.

Anger outbursts are another symptom of PTSD that overlaps with the symptom of irritability in mania. The key to determining whether irritability or anger is due to mania or PTSD lies in evaluating whether other symptoms of mania are also present. Other common symptoms of a manic episode include periods of abnormally positive (even euphoric) mood, increased goal-directed behavior, pressured speech, inflated self-confidence, grandiosity, and decreased need for sleep. If a client with irritability or anger outbursts has several other manic symptoms, the simplest explanation for the symptom is that it is part of a manic episode. On the other hand, if most of the other symptoms of a manic episode are absent and the person has many PTSD symptoms, then the irritability or anger outbursts can be attributed to PTSD.

MISDIAGNOSIS OF SMI

As noted in Chapter 1 in this volume, while it is often common for people to have co-occurring SMI diagnoses, the apparent or real overlap between PTSD symptoms and the symptoms of other SMIs can sometimes result in the misdiagnosis of the SMI, such as in the case of bipolar disorder and borderline personality disorder (BPD), as discussed in this section. This is particularly common when trauma history and PTSD have not been properly assessed before. Relatedly, clients themselves sometimes question the accuracy of their primary SMI diagnosis (e.g., schizophrenia) after learning that they have PTSD. See Chapter 12 in this volume for a discussion of how to address these concerns when providing the CR for PTSD program.

Bipolar Disorder

As described in the previous section, some of the overarousal symptoms of PTSD can resemble or overlap with symptoms of mania, such as sleep disturbance and anger outbursts. These PTSD symptoms alone are unlikely to result in a misdiagnosis of bipolar disorder, but they can in circumstances when a broader range of manic symptoms are triggered by antidepressant medications, as described next.

Antidepressants can precipitate manic symptoms, both in individuals who have bipolar disorder and in those with depression only (Baldessarini et al., 2013; Barbuti et al., 2017). When this occurs in someone who did not have a previous diagnosis of bipolar disorder, the antidepressant is usually discontinued, and if needed, a mood stabilizing medication may be temporarily prescribed (Goldberg & Ernst, 2016). If the manic episode ends after the antidepressant is stopped, a diagnosis of bipolar disorder is not given. However, if manic symptoms persist despite ceasing the antidepressant, a diagnosis of bipolar disorder can be given (American Psychiatric Association, 2013), which is when a misdiagnosis of bipolar disorder may occur. Clients with undiagnosed PTSD who have had manic symptoms precipitated by an antidepressant may display characteristic PTSD symptoms (e.g., difficulty sleeping, anger outbursts) after stopping the antidepressant, which can be mistaken for symptoms of mania (e.g., decreased need for sleep, irritability), resulting in an incorrect diagnosis of bipolar disorder. Although it is unclear how often this occurs, we have personally identified and treated several such cases in our own clinical experience.

To evaluate whether unrecognized PTSD symptoms may have contributed to a misdiagnosis of bipolar disorder in individuals who have had a manic episode triggered by antidepressant medication, the clinician needs to first explore whether the client has had other manic episodes when not taking antidepressants. If no other manic episodes can be identified, then the diagnosis of bipolar disorder may be incorrect, and persistent symptoms such as sleep difficulties and irritability may be more parsimoniously explained by the PTSD diagnosis.

Borderline Personality Disorder

When systematic surveys of trauma and PTSD are conducted in populations of persons with SMI, it is common to find that many individuals with undiagnosed PTSD have a chart diagnosis of BPD (Mueser et al., 1998). Several of the symptoms and problems associated with PTSD may contribute to a misdiagnosis of BPD when PTSD is undetected. Severe reexperiencing symptoms of PTSD (e.g., intrusive memories, flashbacks, and severe distress when exposed to cues that remind the person of the event), combined with PTSD avoidance and hyperarousal symptoms, may resemble the affective instability, anger difficulties, and suicidal and impulsive behavior characteristic of BPD. PTSD-related alterations in cognition and mood may resemble the identity disturbance and chronic feelings of emptiness found in BPD. Similarly, difficulties with close interpersonal relationships due to the symptoms of PTSD and trust issues related to trauma may be attributed to the diagnosis of PTSD when PTSD is not assessed. This overlap is demonstrated in the case study of "Leigh-Ann" (one of this book's three client vignettes), as her medical record contains notes suggesting BPD traits (see Chapter 4, this volume).

Given the apparent overlap in symptoms between PTSD and BPD and the underdiagnosis of PTSD in routine treatment, clinicians should maintain a healthy skepticism regarding long-standing chart diagnoses of BPD in individuals who have recently been assessed and diagnosed with PTSD.

ASSESSMENT OF TRAUMA AND PTSD

A thorough assessment serves as the cornerstone of all cognitive behavioral therapy approaches. Comprehensive assessment is aimed both at determining whether an individual has PTSD and at evaluating common characteristics associated with the disorder and its impact on the person's life and well-being. It also plays an important role in monitoring symptom severity throughout treatment and in guiding specific session content and focus. For the CR for PTSD program, this includes conducting a lifetime history of trauma exposure, assessing PTSD symptoms related to the most upsetting traumatic event(s), examining trauma-related thoughts and beliefs, and evaluating other symptoms frequently correlated with PTSD (e.g., depression). In addition to these domains of assessment, the clinician should have a basic understanding of the client's other psychiatric symptoms, substance use problems, current psychosocial functioning, psychiatric history, and current treatments.

As conducting a trauma history is necessary to determine whether someone has PTSD, these two assessment components are usually done in tandem. The most efficient approach to establishing whether an individual with SMI is likely to have PTSD is to administer a brief screening assessment of traumatic events and then associated PTSD symptoms. As explained next, we recommend routine screening for trauma and PTSD for all clients with SMI, either when they are beginning services (e.g., at a community mental health center, with a new therapist) or when they are in treatment if they have not previously been screened.

Screening for PTSD

As reviewed in Chapter 1 in this volume, although the prevalence of PTSD in persons with SMI is consistently higher than in the general population (Abdelghaffar et al., 2018), PTSD is frequently not identified in typical treatment settings (Zammit et al., 2018) for a variety of reasons. For example, due to the nature of PTSD, clients tend to avoid spontaneously talking about their traumatic experiences and PTSD symptoms. In addition, as described in the previous section, the symptoms of PTSD can easily be mistaken for another psychiatric disorder. Given the variability in clinical presentation, there is no typical person with PTSD, and thus therapists cannot rely on their clinical acumen to identify cases of PTSD. Rather, routine screening for PTSD is recommended for all persons with SMI.

Screening for trauma and PTSD can be conducted with a brief clinical interview requiring about 15 to 20 minutes. The interview begins with a structured checklist of traumatic events the person may have experienced and is followed by a second structured assessment of current PTSD symptoms related to the event indicated by the client as their most distressing traumatic experience. Immediately before administering the screen, it is useful to prepare the client by briefly explaining the nature and purpose of the questions that will be asked. For example, a clinician can say the following:

> I would like to spend a few minutes talking with you about some difficult or stressful experiences that you might have had in your life and their effects on you. This is important information for me to have to provide you with the most effective treatment possible.

When inquiring about trauma, the clinician should avoid asking overly broad questions, such as "Have you ever experienced trauma?" Clients often answer "no" to such broad questions but are willing to acknowledge having experienced specific traumatic events. Clinicians should also refrain from using emotionally loaded language that is open to interpretation when asking about trauma, such as "physical or sexual abuse," "molestation," or "rape." For example, the question "Were you physically abused as a child?" requires the client to draw inferences about the boundaries of abuse versus discipline, which may be experienced as stigmatizing one's family or call forth denial in other ways. Similarly, for some people the word *rape* means the use of violence to force another person to have sexual intercourse against their will, whereas for others it refers to any sexual activity that is foisted upon someone against their will or when their capacity to consent is diminished.

In addition to using behaviorally specific language when asking about traumatic experiences, the clinician should adopt a neutral, matter-of-fact tone when talking about trauma and PTSD symptoms to convey that it is common to talk about such things with clients and that nothing the client says will shock or upset the clinician. Maintaining a relatively emotionally neutral stance when discussing trauma and avoiding strong responses or extensive displays of empathy or sympathy gives clients the freedom to talk openly about their experiences without worrying about how the clinician will react. This is not to say that clinicians should appear cold or uncaring; rather, they should clearly show that they are listening attentively and demonstrate concern through a muted expression of sincere empathy and validation.

Recommended Screening Instruments

A variety of measures have been developed to assess exposure to traumatic events in the general population, and many have also been used with people with SMI. Some of these measures are quite brief, evaluating lifetime experience of as few as 10 traumatic events, such as the Brief Trauma Questionnaire (Schnurr et al., 1999) and the Traumatic Life Events Questionnaire (Kubany et al., 2000), while others are more extensive and may include upwards of 40 items, such as the Stressful Events Survey (Goodman et al., 1998, 1999). A comprehensive list of instruments for assessing trauma exposure can be found at a website maintained by the National Center for PTSD at https://www.ptsd.va.gov/professional/assessment/index.asp.

We recommend using a brief self-report instrument to determine trauma exposure. To address this need, we developed a questionnaire (the Difficult Life Events Inventory) that contains 18 items representative of common traumatic events as defined by *DSM-5* criteria and that uses behaviorally specific language while avoiding loaded terms such as sexual abuse. The Difficult Life Events Inventory provides a user-friendly example of a brief questionnaire that can be used to obtain a trauma history when screening for PTSD and is displayed in Exhibit 3.2.

EXHIBIT 3.2

Difficult Life Events Inventory

Instructions: For each of the different events listed below, please indicate whether you have experienced the event before ("Yes") or have not experienced the event before ("No").

1. Have you ever been involved in a bad accident in which you were injured or someone else was hurt or killed (like a car accident, fire, or near drowning)?	Yes	No
2. Have you ever been involved in combat or directly exposed to warfare?	Yes	No
3. Have you ever had a family member or close friend die unexpectedly due to something like an accident, suicide, murder, drug overdose, or catastrophe (such as earthquake)?	Yes	No
4. Have you ever been robbed by someone with a weapon or witnessed such a robbery?	Yes	No
5. Have you ever been hit or assaulted by a stranger or someone you didn't know well?	Yes	No
6. Have you ever seen a stranger or someone you didn't know well assault or kill someone else?	Yes	No
7. Has anyone ever threatened to physically hurt or kill you?	Yes	No
8. When you were growing up, were you ever punished physically in a way that caused bruises, bleeding, or some other injury?	Yes	No
9. When you were growing up, did you ever see other family members fighting with each other in a way that caused bruises, bleeding, or some other injury?	Yes	No

---

(continues)

EXHIBIT 3.2

Difficult Life Events Inventory   (*Continued*)

10. Have you ever been hit, punched, slapped, or physically hurt in some other way by your spouse, partner, boyfriend, girlfriend, or other intimate person?	Yes	No
11. Before you were 16 years old, did anyone who was five or more years older than you touch you in a sexual way or make you touch them in a sexual way?	Yes	No
12. Before you were 16 years old, did anyone who was less than 5 years older than you touch you in a sexual way or make you touch them in a sexual way (or engage in any sexual act) against your will?	Yes	No
13. After you became 16 years old, has anyone ever touched you in a sexual way or made you touch them in a sexual way (or engage in any sexual act) against your will?	Yes	No
14. Has anyone ever followed you, kept track of you, or stalked you in a way that made you afraid about your safety?	Yes	No
15. Have you ever been in a natural disaster (like an earthquake, hurricane, tornado, forest, fire, or flood) where you feared for your life or saw others injured or killed?	Yes	No
16. Have you ever been present during a terrorist attack (like a bombing), mass shooting, or some other type of mass violence in which you feared for your life or saw others injured or killed?	Yes	No
17. Have you ever experienced or seen any other events that were life-threatening, caused injury to yourself or others, or were otherwise extremely frightening or disturbing (like being kidnapped or suddenly seeing a dead body)?	Yes	No
18. In your line of work, have you ever seen or repeatedly heard about disturbing details of distressing events experienced by others (like repeatedly hearing or seeing details about crime or war victims or dealing with seriously injured people or human remains)?	Yes	No

Of the different events listed above that you reported experiencing, which event is currently the most distressing one to you now in your day-to-day life?

Event: _____.

Following administration of the trauma screening questions, if the client has endorsed more than one event (which is common, given the previously discussed prevalence and high rates of trauma exposure in this population), the client should be asked which of the different traumatic events that were endorsed is the most distressing one currently in the person's day-to-day life. If the client is unsure about which event is most distressing, the clinician can probe by asking which event the client most often has sudden, unwanted memories or thoughts about. Intrusive memories of a traumatic event are one of the most common symptoms of PTSD and are usually a strong indicator of which event is currently most upsetting to the client.

Note that the trauma screening questions we recommend yield information about whether a client has experienced varying types of traumatic events (e.g., an accident, sexual abuse as a child) but not the number of events within a single category. This is for practical reasons, as attempting to identify all the traumatic events experienced by a client with SMI would take much more time and would likely be very taxing to the client. For some types of trauma, multiple different events are more likely to be the norm than the exception (e.g., physical or sexual abuse as a child), although this can also occur in adulthood (e.g., domestic violence). In these cases, it is common for PTSD symptoms to be related to multiple different events within a category of trauma. When this occurs, the clinician can evaluate the client's PTSD symptoms related to any of the events experienced within the trauma category and need not focus on one event.

After identifying the most distressing traumatic event (or type of event), the clinician administers a brief questionnaire to evaluate the client's PTSD symptoms in relation to that specific traumatic event (this will serve as the index trauma). Several different self-report instruments have been developed and validated for screening individuals for PTSD. The most widely used and researched screen is the PTSD Checklist (PCL) for *DSM-5* (Weathers et al., 2013), which can be obtained for free online (https://www.ptsd.va.gov/professional/assessment/adult-sr/ptsd-checklist.asp#obtain). The PCL has good psychometric properties in persons with SMI, including internal and test–retest reliability and convergent validity with structured diagnostic interviews for PTSD (Mueser et al., 2001).

The PCL contains 20 questions that map onto the four *DSM-5* PTSD symptom clusters related to the most distressing traumatic event. For each question, the client indicates how much the symptom has bothered them over the last 3 months (other versions of the PCL cover the past week, as discussed later in this chapter). The response options are rated on a 5-point scale ranging from 0 = *not at all* to 4 = *extremely*. For example, Question 1 asks the person if they have "Repeated, disturbing memories, thoughts, or images of the stressful experience?"

The most common way to score the PCL is to sum the scores of the 20 symptom items, resulting in a total ranging from 0 (*no symptoms*) to 80 (*all symptoms present at an extreme level*). Research shows that a total score of 33 or over indicates that the person probably has PTSD (Bovin et al., 2016).

Diagnosis of PTSD

Validated screening measures such as the PCL are strongly predictive of a diagnosis of PTSD in people with SMI (Grubaugh et al., 2007; Mueser et al., 2001; Roberts et al., 2021), as determined by standardized clinical interviews such as the Clinician-Administered PTSD Scale for *DSM-5* (Weathers et al., 2018), the Posttraumatic Stress Diagnostic Scale for *DSM-5* (Foa et al., 2016), or the Structured Clinical Interview for *DSM-5* (First et al., 2015). Thus, clients who screen positive for PTSD on the PCL can be considered to have probable PTSD and can likely benefit from the CR for PTSD program. Nevertheless, it is recommended that clinicians take some additional steps to confirm that the client's symptoms are consistent with a diagnosis of PTSD.

This can be accomplished by the clinician having a brief discussion with the client about their responses to the trauma questionnaire and PCL. The clinician should begin by briefly reviewing the results of the trauma screen (e.g., the Difficult Life Events Inventory), with a particular focus on the event indicated by the client as most distressing (the index trauma). The clinician should inquire about the event enough to get a general understanding about its nature, including what happened and when. For example:

THERAPIST: You indicated that before you were 16, someone older than you forced you to have sexual contact with them. Can you tell me just a little more about what happened? How old were you when this first happened? And who was the person involved?

If the client has difficulty describing the index trauma or it is hard for the clinician to understand it, the clinician can alternatively ask the client to briefly describe some of the upsetting memories they experience related to the event. The objective here is to not to have the client go into so much detail about the event that it is highly distressing but to get enough information for the clinician to grasp what happened to the client and to understand their posttraumatic reactions to the event. It is important for the clinician to have a basic understanding of the event reported by the client in order to work with them effectively in the CR for PTSD program and help them make better sense of their traumatic experience. If the clinician cannot establish the basic details of the traumatic event (e.g., who, what, where, when, etc.) or identify one clear memory of the event the client has, a diagnosis of PTSD cannot be confirmed, and the CR program is not recommended.

After briefly reviewing the most distressing (index) traumatic experience reported, the clinician should review the client's ratings for the PTSD symptoms on the PCL, occasionally pausing to ask for recent examples of particularly severe symptoms. This review provides assurance that the individual has specific PTSD symptoms and also confirms which symptoms are most distressing to the client. This information is useful as the intervention progresses, specifically when providing psychoeducation about PTSD and later when using cognitive restructuring to target these symptoms.

When the clinician has confirmed the client's PTSD diagnosis through a discussion of their index trauma and PTSD symptoms (and hence their basic eligibility for the CR for PTSD program), the clinician can either describe the program to the client as a treatment option and proceed with treatment (if interested) or refer the client to another clinician for potential treatment. See Chapter 4 for a discussion and recommendations for how to refer individuals with probable or confirmed PTSD to a clinician who can provide the CR program.

MONITORING AND MANAGING CLIENT DISTRESS DURING PTSD ASSESSMENT

Although most clients tolerate the assessment of trauma and PTSD well and many are relieved to be finally talking about these issues, some experience modest increases in distress during this process. Indications of such distress may include tearfulness, reports of anxiety or fear, cognitive disorganization, reported or observable increases in physiological arousal, or increased severity of psychotic symptoms. When this occurs, the clinician should empathize with the client's distress, normalize, and offer some comforting and encouraging words. Two examples are provided as follows:

THERAPIST: I completely understand how difficult this is for you to talk about. You've had these feelings inside you for a long time, and now you're finally talking about them. I think you're taking an important step toward dealing with these hard experiences.

THERAPIST: It is hard to talk about these things. Other people have had difficult life experiences like you and have had the same symptoms as you. You are not alone. I also want you to know that there are effective treatments for these problems and that other people with similar experiences have been able to go on to live rewarding and meaningful lives, despite all they have been through.

Occasionally, the distress experienced by a client during the assessment of trauma and PTSD is so strong that a short break is needed to help the person calm down. It can be helpful for the therapist to lead the client in a relaxation exercise, such as Breathing Retraining, before resuming (see Chapter 5, this volume, for Breathing Retraining details). This is preferable to having the therapist prematurely end the assessment with the intention of completing it at a later time, which can inadvertently increase the client's fear of talking about traumatic events and make subsequent assessment and treatment even more challenging.

RECOMMENDED ASSESSMENT OF DOMAINS RELATED TO PTSD

It can be useful, when time and resources permit, for clinicians to assess two other domains related to PTSD before beginning treatment: trauma-related thoughts and depression. This information can inform treatment planning and delivery of the CR for PTSD program, and assessment responses can serve as excellent clinical material to use for practice of the specific intervention skills. For these two domains, standardized self-report measures exist that have been validated in the SMI population. The most efficient general approach to administering these questionnaires is to briefly explain their purpose to the client and to have the client complete them on their own (either print versions or online versions). For clients who have lower reading ability or difficulties with attention, the clinician can read the questions out loud. For example:

THERAPIST: I'd like to ask you to complete a few more brief questionnaires. The first one is about common thoughts and beliefs people have after they have experienced a traumatic event. The second measure is about depression. Your responses to these questionnaires will help me with planning and working with you in the CR for PTSD program. How does that sound to you?

Trauma-Related Thoughts and Beliefs

Trauma-related cognitions can be evaluated with the PTCI (Foa et al., 1999). The PTCI includes 36 items that assess common negative thoughts and beliefs about oneself ("I have no future"), self-blame ("Somebody else would not have gotten into this situation"), and the world ("Other people cannot be trusted"). A confirmatory factor analysis of the PTCI in 432 persons with SMI and PTSD found four factors of trauma-related cognitions (Lu, Mueser, et al., 2023). The first three factors corresponded to the same factors the PTCI was designed to assess (negative cognitions about self, the world, and self-blame); the fourth factor reflected the ability of the person to cope with negative feelings (e.g., "I can't deal with even the slightest upset"). The PTCI is sensitive to change following the CR for PTSD program (Mueser et al., 2008; Mueser, Gottlieb, et al., 2015). A brief, nine-item version of the PTCI was recently developed that was found to have the same three-factor structure as the original 36-item version (Wells et al., 2019).

Depression and Suicidality

The most common symptom associated with PTSD is depression. In addition to PTSD symptoms, the CR for PTSD program has been shown to reduce depressive symptoms as well in people with SMI (Mueser et al., 2008; Mueser, Gottlieb, et al., 2015). Assessing the client's level of depression prior to initiating treatment and monitoring it along with PTSD symptom severity during the therapy (as discussed later in this chapter) are important for gauging the client's level of distress, assuring the client's safety, and maintaining optimal pacing of the sessions. We recommend using the Beck Depression Inventory–II (BDI-II; Beck et al., 1996) as a brief (21-item) self-report measure of depression experienced over the past week. The BDI-II has been used with a wide range of different clinical populations, including in the CR program for persons with SMI.

Suicidal ideation is a common correlate of depression and PTSD that warrants addition assessment if detected at the initial evaluation. The presence of suicidal ideation can be identified with the BDI-II (Item 9: Suicidal Thoughts or Wishes). A response to this question indicating moderate endorsement (Item 2: I would like to kill myself) or strong endorsement (Item 3: I would kill myself if I had the chance) should be followed by a careful evaluation of the person's suicidal intent (e.g., believing life is not worth living, having plans for suicide, etc.).

It should be noted that the presence of thoughts about death or suicidal thoughts alone in a client should not postpone treatment with the CR for PTSD program, nor should self-injurious behavior without suicidal intent, provided that safety plans are put in place for monitoring the symptoms and responding to any increases. In our two large controlled studies of the CR for PTSD program, we excluded individuals who had recently (within the past 3 months) made a suicide attempt or had a psychiatric hospitalization but included all other eligible clients regardless of suicidal ideation (Mueser et al., 2008; Mueser, Gottlieb, et al., 2015). Among persons with PTSD and BPD in these studies, suicidal ideation was relatively common, with 57% endorsing some degree of suicidality on Item 8 of the BDI-II at the baseline assessment (Kredlow et al., 2017). There were no suicides among the study participants. More generally, trauma-focused therapy such as the CR for PTSD program is more likely to reduce suicidality and associated distress in clients with PTSD and other psychiatric conditions than increase risk of suicide (De Jongh et al., 2016).

GOAL SETTING AND TRACKING IN THE CR FOR PTSD PROGRAM

The high distress associated with PTSD is often the most important motivation for clients to participate in the CR for PTSD program. However, some reduction in acute distress is common during the first three therapy sessions due to normalizing the nature of PTSD through psychoeducation and teaching the Breathing Retraining skill. Thus, it is important to help clients establish longer term, more meaningful goals to sustain their engagement in the program and to increase motivation to do the hard work of learning cognitive restructuring and tackling their trauma-related thoughts and beliefs.

In our experience, the process of setting goals is most effectively accomplished toward the end of the third session of the CR for PTSD program. By this point, the client has a better understanding of PTSD and the ways it has affected them, and they can more clearly articulate how they would like their life to be different as a result of participating in the program (i.e., treatment goals). The most motivating goals are functional in nature, such as being able to work, return to school, be a better parent, and improve relationships with loved ones (or develop new and more rewarding relationships). Potential goals for treatment can be developed collaboratively with the client and recorded on the Goal Tracking Sheet, which can be updated as needed over the course of the program. (Reminder: All worksheets and educational handouts mentioned in this volume are provided in the Appendix.)

TRACKING CHANGES IN PTSD AND OTHER OUTCOMES DURING TREATMENT

Routinely tracking changes in PTSD and other outcomes over the course of therapy serves two broad purposes. First, as the severity of PTSD and depression usually decreases steadily following initiation of the CR for PTSD program (Lu et al., 2012), conducting routine assessments and reviewing them together can be reinforcing to both the client and therapist by showing that their efforts are paying off. Second, monitoring outcomes can provide valuable information about the effectiveness of the intervention and identify specific areas in need of targeted intervention in therapy. For example, midway through the program, routine monitoring could reveal that the client continues to experience frequent, distressing memories of the traumatic event that disrupt their daily activities. The therapist could use this information during the therapy session as a starting point for further understanding the nature of these intrusive memories and the reasons they are so upsetting to the client. This could be followed by initiation of cognitive restructuring to examine, challenge, and change trauma-related beliefs that underlie the client's specific PTSD symptom.

PTSD and Depression

We recommend routinely monitoring PTSD symptoms (with the past-week version of the PCL, using the same index trauma as for the initial assessment) and depression severity (with the BDI-II) over the course of the CR for PTSD program. Administering these self-report measures after every three sessions provides useful information about symptoms that can be incorporated into the program without the symptoms becoming the dominant focus of therapy (i.e., in Sessions 1, 4, 7, 10, 13, and 16 or last). The clinician can record and graph the results of each assessment on the PTSD Assessment Tracking Sheet and Depression Assessment Tracking Sheet.

Tracking PTSD and depression is most useful when it occurs at the beginning of the session, immediately following setting the agenda. After the client has completed the measures, the therapist should immediately review them, score them (sum up scores and add to graph), and initiate a brief discussion about them. When reviewing the responses on the questionnaires, the therapist should acknowledge specific symptoms that the client reports are especially distressing, allowing the client to elaborate if needed. The clinician should discuss with the client the overall change in symptom severity from the prior assessment, then resume with the regular structure of the specific session by reviewing the home assignment, and return later in the session, if desired, to work on specific distressing symptoms, typically via the CR skill.

Most clients who participate in the CR for PTSD program experience significant reductions in their PTSD symptoms and depression over the first three sessions (Lu et al., 2012). However, some do not, and a few clients report increases in symptoms. It is important for the clinician to reinforce the client for any improvements in symptoms, while also reframing any lack of change or worsening in symptoms as part of the overall change process to encourage continued effort and attendance in the program. Such encouragement is especially vital at the beginning of the program as the therapeutic alliance is developing. Guidelines for discussing changes in PTSD and depression symptoms after the first three sessions are provided in Chapter 6 in this volume.

Trauma-Related Cognitions

Therapists will find it useful to begin keeping track of trauma-related cognitions during the initial assessment (with the PTCI, as previously described) and adding additional trauma-related beliefs as they are identified in subsequent sessions using the Therapist Tracking Sheet for Client's Trauma-Related Cognitions (Appendix). It is common for such beliefs to become evident during the early psychoeducation sessions of the CR for PTSD program (e.g., in Session 3, the client reports thinking that she will never be able to have a romantic relationship again because she is "damaged goods"). Identifying and keeping track of specific trauma-related thoughts over the course of the CR program can ensure that important beliefs underlying PTSD symptoms are targeted and changed through cognitive restructuring.

Therapists may also find it helpful to track changes in trauma-related cognitions by administering the PTCI several times over the course of therapy. Persistently endorsed trauma-related beliefs (e.g., "I am a weak person," "You never know who will harm you") can then be directly addressed through cognitive restructuring. As the primary method for addressing trauma-related thoughts in the CR program is cognitive restructuring, after the initial administration of the PTCI before treatment it need not be administered again until at least several sessions into the teaching of cognitive restructuring (e.g., Session 7 or 8) and then as needed thereafter.

PSYCHOTIC SYMPTOMS AND TREATMENT EXPERIENCES

The experience of psychotic symptoms such as hallucinations (e.g., telling you that you are no good or instructing you to kill yourself) or delusions (e.g., believing other people are plotting against you or controlling your mind), have long been described by individuals as terrifying (Dunkley et al., 2015; Kaplan, 1964; Lu, Mueser, et al., 2017). Similarly, coercive treatment experiences during a psychotic episode such as involuntary hospitalization, being placed in seclusion and or restraints, and being forced to take medication have also been described by individuals as frightening and traumatizing (Jennings, 1994; Millet, 1991). Over 30 years ago, it was observed that the traumatic nature of these experiences could lead to a syndrome similar to PTSD (McGorry et al., 1991; Shaner & Eth, 1989).

Research has confirmed that psychotic symptoms and coercive treatment experiences can result in PTSD symptoms similar to those following more typical traumatic events studied in the general population (Rodrigues & Anderson, 2017). Furthermore, PTSD symptoms can occur not only following treatment for a first episode of psychosis (Mueser & Rosenberg, 2003; Tarrier et al., 2007) but also after multiple psychotic episodes (Lu et al., 2011). In addition, research shows that individuals with PTSD symptoms related to psychosis or treatment tend to have higher levels of distress, including depression, and worse psychosocial functioning than those who do not have PTSD symptoms related to such experiences (Lu et al., 2011; Mueser et al., 2010; Picken & Tarrier, 2011). Psychotic symptoms appear to be the most common cause of psychosis-related PTSD symptoms, followed by coercive treatment experiences.

Although it is evident that PTSD symptoms can occur due to psychotic experiences and coerced treatment, it is less clear whether these events constitute valid traumatic events for diagnosing PTSD according to *DSM-5*. The *DSM-5* criteria for a traumatic event imply that the event was external to the individual, raising the question of whether internal events such as psychotic symptoms would meet the criteria. In addition, also implicit in the *DSM-5* definition is that the individual's appraisal of and emotional reaction to the event are consistent with the nature of the threat posed, also suggesting such events might not meet criteria for a traumatic event.

We do not address the treatment of PTSD secondary to a psychotic episode in this book for several practical reasons. First, in contrast to PTSD as previously discussed in this chapter, much less is known about the nature and course of PTSD symptoms related to a psychotic episode. Second, less attention has been paid to the treatment of PTSD symptoms related to experiencing a psychotic episode. One approach to treating PTSD symptoms following a first onset of psychosis is included in the psychotherapy component (individual resiliency training [IRT]) of the NAVIGATE program (Meyer-Kalos et al., 2015), a comprehensive multicomponent intervention for first episode of psychosis (Mueser, Penn, et al., 2015). IRT is a broad-based psychotherapeutic intervention composed of different modules addressing topics related to psychoeducation, illness self-management, and skills for recovery. The "Processing the Psychotic Episode" module is aimed at reducing posttraumatic reactions to the psychotic episode. The module includes a combination of helping the individual write a personal narrative related to their experience and teaching cognitive restructuring to address persistent negative beliefs about the self and one's future. Although the NAVIGATE program was found to improve clinical and psychosocial outcomes over 2 years significantly more than usual care in a large cluster randomized controlled trial including 34 sites and 404 persons with first episode of psychosis (Kane et al., 2016), the specific effects of this treatment component of IRT were not evaluated. The specific clinical guidelines for the "Processing the Psychotic Episode" module are in the IRT treatment manual (https://navigateconsultants.org).

Based on our experience with the NAVIGATE program study, we believe that the treatment guidelines provided in this volume are effective in treating PTSD symptoms related to the experience of a psychotic episode. For clinicians who want to evaluate PTSD symptoms related to a psychotic episode, Exhibit 3.3 provides recommended questions for exploring traumatic responses to psychotic experiences and coercive treatments.

EXHIBIT 3.3

Suggested Probe Questions for Exploring Psychotic Symptoms and Treatment Experiences as Traumatic Events

Symptoms

Have the symptoms of your psychiatric illness ever caused you to feel extremely anxious or terrified? Please briefly describe what happened.

When your symptoms were severe, did you ever (for any yes, the clinician explores the degree of distress associated with the symptom and upsetting memories of symptom currently experienced)

- believe that people or groups of people wanted to hurt you?

- believe that people were out to get you or were plotting against you?

- believe that forces or people outside yourself could make you harm yourself?

(continues)

EXHIBIT 3.3

Suggested Probe Questions for Exploring Psychotic Symptoms and Treatment Experiences as Traumatic Events   (*Continued*)

- hear voices that threatened to hurt you, which made you afraid?
- hear voices that told you other things that were upsetting?
- see, feel, or smell things that scared you?
- do anything violent, strange, or embarrassing?
- hurt yourself or try hurting yourself?
- fear that you would lose your mind or lose touch with reality?

Treatment Experiences

Have you ever been given a treatment that frightened you, that you were afraid would hurt you, or that actually did hurt you? Please briefly describe what happened.

Have you ever (for any yes, the clinician explores the degree of distress associated with experience and upsetting memories of it currently experienced)

- been forcibly taken to the hospital or to jail?
- been threatened by a treatment provider in order to make you do something you didn't want to do as a part of your treatment?
- experienced a serious problem or side effect from taking a psychiatric medication?
- been placed in a seclusion room in a hospital?
- been placed in physical restraints (e.g., tied down in a bed)?
- been forced to take medication?

CONCLUSION

Routine screening of trauma history and PTSD is recommended for all clients with a SMI. Assessments of trauma and PTSD in persons with SMI (such as the PCL-5) are both reliable and valid, can be conducted safely with no increased risk to the client in about 15 minutes, and are highly predictive of clinical diagnosis of PTSD. Some challenges may arise when assessing trauma and PTSD for which clinical recommendations are made, including distinguishing between the symptoms of the major mental illness and PTSD symptoms, managing client distress during assessment, and experiencing PTSD symptoms due to frightening symptoms or upsetting treatment experiences during a psychotic episode. While screening and assessment provide critical information about eligibility for the CR for PTSD program, ongoing monitoring of selected outcomes (PTSD, depression, and trauma-related thoughts) over the course of the program can inform treatment delivery and provide reassurance that progress is being made.

THE COGNITIVE RESTRUCTURING FOR PTSD PROGRAM

4

Logistics of Implementing the CR for PTSD Program

The Cognitive Restructuring (CR) for PTSD program is a time-limited individual cognitive behavioral intervention for persons with serious mental illness (SMI) and PTSD symptoms, typically provided across a 3- to 6-month period. A total of 12 to 16 sessions are usually provided, with most sessions conducted on a weekly basis. Sessions are organized in a structured, predictable fashion to facilitate learning, while a collaborative approach to teaching is used to ensure the client's full engagement in treatment. All teaching in the program is individualized, with a wide range of strategies available to the therapist to accommodate different symptoms and associated challenges in clients, such as psychotic symptoms, severe depression, parasuicidal behaviors, and cognitive impairment.

As described in Chapter 2 in this volume, the CR for PTSD program includes three therapeutic components designed to reduce PTSD symptoms: (a) providing psychoeducation about trauma and the nature of PTSD in order to normalize common reactions to trauma and PTSD symptoms and to reduce feelings of self-blame and weakness; (b) introducing Breathing Retraining as a skill for managing anxiety and for reducing the hyperarousal symptoms of PTSD; and (c) teaching CR as a self-management skill for examining, challenging, and changing trauma-related thoughts and beliefs that underlie PTSD symptoms. As CR targets the cognitive biases that characterize PTSD and contribute to its long-term perpetuation over time, the preponderance of the 16 sessions are devoted to teaching this skill to clients. While the focus of the initial trauma-related CR work and ongoing symptom tracking is on the specific event from the trauma/PTSD screening (the index trauma), over time other traumatic events can be readily addressed using the CR skill as well, within the course of the 12 to 16 sessions. A session-by-session overview of the CR for PTSD program is provided in Table 4.1.

https://doi.org/10.1037/0000423-004

Treatment of Posttraumatic Stress Disorder in Serious Mental Illness: The Cognitive Restructuring Program, by K. T. Mueser and J. D. Gottlieb

TABLE 4.1. Session-by-Session Overview of the CR for PTSD Program

Session no.	Topic	Purpose
1	Orientation Wellness Plan Breathing Retraining	• To inform the client what the CR for PTSD program is and what to expect • To make a plan to help the client maintain their mental health during the program • To teach a skill for reducing anxiety and hyperarousal symptoms
2	Education about trauma and PTSD: Part I	• To teach the effects of trauma on people's lives • To teach the symptoms of PTSD • To help the client understand how PTSD has impacted their life
3	Education about trauma and PTSD: Part II Goal setting	• To teach other common ways that trauma and PTSD affect people • To help the client understand how PTSD has impacted their life • To help the client set personal goals related to participating in the program
4	The Thought–Feeling model Common Styles of Thinking	• To teach how our experiences impact our beliefs about the world • To teach how our thoughts can lead to feeling distressed • To teach that our thoughts are not always accurate and that this is common • To teach and practice a simple first-level cognitive restructuring skill for recognizing and changing common but inaccurate ways of thinking that often lead to distressing feelings
5–6	The 5 Steps of CR	• To teach and practice a powerful cognitive restructuring skill for dealing with upsetting thoughts and feelings that happen on a day-to-day basis
6–14	Continuing with the 5 Steps of CR Addressing trauma-related and core beliefs	• To help the client get comfortable with the 5 Steps of CR skill so that they can use it in many situations in their daily life • To help the client use the 5 Steps of CR to address upsetting trauma-related and core beliefs • To help the client problem-solve and deal with their PTSD symptoms and other stressful situations
15	Reviewing treatment gains and a postprogram support plan: Inviting the primary clinician (or other supportive person)	• To help the client share with their primary clinician (or other support) what they have learned in the program • To help the client demonstrate the 5 Steps of CR skill to their primary clinician

(continues)

TABLE 4.1. Session-by-Session Overview of the CR for PTSD Program (*Continued*)

Session no.	Topic	Purpose
16	Reviewing goals Next steps Termination	• To help the client develop a plan with their primary clinician (or other support) for how to keep using these skills going forward • To review with the client what they learned in the program and what was helpful • To review the client's progress toward goals made in Session 3 • To confirm the client's plan for continuing to use the skills going forward to improve even more

Note. CR = cognitive restructuring; PTSD = posttraumatic stress disorder.

In this chapter, we address logistical aspects of implementing the CR for PTSD program. At the end of the chapter, we introduce three case vignettes of clients with SMI and PTSD who were enrolled and treated in the CR program. We provide background information about these three clients, the nature of their trauma history and PTSD symptoms, and their goals for participation in the program. Throughout the remainder of this volume, we provide client–therapist dialogues that articulate the delivery of specific intervention skills and provide details about the course of therapy for these individuals to illustrate how the different treatment elements of the program are individualized to each person.

FREQUENCY AND DURATION OF TREATMENT SESSIONS

Between 12 and 16 individual sessions are recommended for clients participating in the CR for PTSD program. Like all time-limited cognitive behavioral therapy programs, clients are informed about the planned duration of the program from the outset of treatment, and planning for termination is integrated throughout the program. Some clients show rapid improvement in their PTSD symptoms within the first eight to 10 sessions, and the client and therapist may agree that an early termination of the program in Session 12 is warranted. However, it is much more common that clients need and benefit from the full 16 sessions of the program.

Sessions of 50 to 60 minutes are generally scheduled on a weekly basis, preferably at the same time on the same day of the week to develop a routine for the person's participation in the program. If preferred or needed, slightly shorter sessions may be conducted (e.g., 40 minutes) or slightly longer sessions (e.g., 70–75 minutes). Missed sessions can occur due to reasons such as illness or vacation, although it is recommended that sessions that fall on a holiday should not be cancelled but rather rescheduled for another time the same week. If a client misses an appointment without giving prior notification, the therapist should follow up as soon as possible, seek to identify the problem, and work with the client to reschedule the session and problem solve any obstacles to their following through on it. Given that a hallmark symptom of PTSD is avoidance, it can be helpful for the therapist to have open and empathic communication with the client about how to circumvent avoidant behavior as it pertains to session attendance.

An alternative to conducting 16 weekly sessions is to taper the last several sessions more gradually. For example, the first 13 sessions can be done on a weekly basis, with the last three sessions conducted every other week. Some clients prefer this because it allows a sense of a slower, less abrupt termination, and they can experience what it is like going for a longer period of time on their own between therapy sessions (as well as having more time to practice the skills between sessions). Other clients prefer going through the whole program in consecutive weeks so that they can reach the end sooner. The therapist can mention this option early in the program and then revisit it later with the client to determine their preference.

Some clients may want to continue participating in the CR for PTSD program beyond 16 sessions, either because they believe they could improve more with additional sessions, or they feel dependent upon the therapist for support in using the skills they have learned in the program. With these clients, we typically recommend sticking to the 16-session limit on the program for two reasons. First, many clients continue to improve their ability to use the CR skill after the program ends, in part due to reduced dependency on the therapist for helping them use the skills, and they experience further improvements in their PTSD symptoms. Second, toward the end of the program, the therapist works collaboratively with the client to identify at least one supportive person in the client's life who can help them use the skills they have learned in the program (e.g., their primary clinician, case manager, family member, friend; see Chapter 11, this volume, for further details). Thus, even after the intervention ends, clients can continue to be supported in using their skills.

There are some circumstances where an extra session or two is warranted, which can be determined on a case-by-case basis. Some examples of when extra session(s) might be appropriate include the following: when a client has a medical issue that disrupts the consistent flow of treatment, when the termination date falls near a trauma-related anniversary, and/or when the client has been working diligently overall but CR skill uptake took a bit longer to click and so an additional session or two is indicated to provide more practice focused on trauma-based thoughts. The plan for any additional sessions should always be worked out and agreed upon ahead of time, with a commitment from the client to a specific agenda for the additional sessions, focused on using the CR skill to address trauma-related beliefs.

WHO CAN BENEFIT FROM THE CR FOR PTSD PROGRAM?

Most individuals who have SMI, who have either a formal diagnosis of PTSD, or who have screened positive for a probable diagnosis of PTSD (based on a PTSD Checklist–5 [PCL-5] score of 33 or higher; see Chapter 3, this volume) that has been reviewed by a clinician can benefit from the CR for PTSD program. However, there are several considerations that need to be weighed regarding if and when to engage clients in the program, as discussed in this section. Recommended eligibility criteria for treating clients in the CR program are summarized in Exhibit 4.1.

Client Motivation for Treatment

First and foremost, the client has to want to participate in the program. This means the client understands what the nature of the program is and what it entails and is willing to try it. Because of the suffering associated with PTSD symptoms and the fact that the CR for PTSD program does not require recounting the traumatic events or other elements of exposure therapy, it is usually not difficult to motivate clients to participate in the program. However, there are circumstances in which despite the distress associated with PTSD symptoms, the client has difficulty committing to participating in the program. For example, if individuals are experiencing an unusually high level of stress in their life—such as being homeless and living on the streets, being in the middle of a legal case, having an ill family member who must be cared for, or having significant medical problems themselves—they may not be able to focus their

---

EXHIBIT 4.1

Recommended Inclusion Criteria for Treating Clients in the CR for PTSD Program

- Has been diagnosed with PTSD or probable PTSD with screening measure (e.g., PCL-5 total score ≥ 33), followed up with a review by a clinician.
- Is interested in participating in treatment for PTSD.
- To the extent possible, has had stable psychiatric symptoms for at least a month.
- Has had no psychiatric hospitalization or suicide attempt within the past 2 months.
- Is not experiencing an acutely stressful, temporary life situation (e.g., recent death of loved one, recent housing displacement).
- Does not have a severe substance use disorder that would interfere with an agreement of sober attendance at CR for PTSD sessions and sober skills practice (also known as home assignments).
- Has sufficiently intact cognitive functioning to participate in sessions and understand information and skills (with some reasonable modification; see Chapter 12, this volume).
- Is not currently participating in treatment program for trauma or PTSD.

Note. CR = cognitive restructuring; PTSD = posttraumatic stress disorder; PCL-5 = PTSD Checklist–5.

attention on participating in the program, and treatment may need to be postponed to another time when their life seems more manageable.

Although clients need to be interested in treatment, this is not to say they have to be highly motivated to participate in the program. Ambivalence about treatment is quite normal for people with PTSD. Clients may be fearful that participation in the CR for PTSD program will be stressful and difficult as it will dredge up memories of highly painful experiences they would rather try to forget. Alternatively, clients may be skeptical that the treatment will be effective and worth the effort. A common symptom of PTSD is not believing that one has much of a future, and lack of hope is a common symptom of depression, so it is natural that some people with PTSD are dubious about the potential for treatment to improve their lives.

When working with such ambivalent clients, the therapist need not convince them to commit to participating in the entire CR for PTSD program. If the person is interested in treatment but is unsure about committing to the whole program, the therapist can explore with the client whether they are willing to participate in a few sessions and then reevaluate with the therapist whether they want to continue with the program or stop there. For example, the therapist could negotiate with the client to participate in the first three sessions of the intervention, which covers psychoeducation about PTSD and the Breathing Retraining skill, and to then meet to evaluate whether to continue with the program. In most cases, once rapport is established and clients find the initial sessions and skills useful, they tend to be willing to continue onward.

Symptom Stability

To the extent possible, it is preferable if the primary symptoms of the client's SMI are relatively stable for at least a month or two before engaging them in the CR for PTSD program. If the client has experienced a recent symptom exacerbation or relapse (e.g., emergence or significant worsening of psychotic symptoms, marked increase in depression with accompanying impairment in self-care), it can be helpful to wait a few weeks until the symptoms have reduced before beginning the CR program. Some clients may have persistently unstable symptoms, and waiting until their symptoms stabilize may not be feasible. For these individuals, we recommend proceeding with the program, as their PTSD may be contributing to their poor symptom stability and effective treatment may reduce the severity of their overall symptoms.

Although it is preferable that clients' symptoms be as stable as possible before beginning the CR for PTSD program, this does not mean that clients with persistent and even severe symptoms cannot participate (and benefit), including those with frank psychotic symptoms such as hallucinations and delusions, severe depressive symptoms, or persistent non-life-threatening self-injurious behaviors. In fact, it is quite likely that untreated PTSD symptoms are contributing to these other symptoms, and treatment in the CR program may lead to reductions in these symptoms as well as PTSD symptoms.

As discussed in the previous chapter, suicidal ideation is relatively common in people with SMI and PTSD, and effective treatment of PTSD has the potential to reduce these symptoms. When suicidal ideation is detected in a client, it is important for the therapist to take the necessary steps to conduct additional assessment to evaluate the seriousness of the symptom and to initiate safety plans accordingly if significant threat is present (see Chapter 3, this volume). If the suicide risk assessment indicates the need for a special safety plan, it is best to postpone initiation of the CR for PTSD program until after the client's suicidality has subsided, is stable, and no longer poses a major risk.

Related to the issue of symptom stability, if the client has had a recent inpatient psychiatric hospitalization, we recommend waiting for at least 2 months after the person has been discharged to begin the CR for PTSD program. Similarly, if the client has had a recent suicide attempt (also known as action beyond ideation), a 2-month waiting period is also recommended before beginning the program.

Problematic Substance Use

Substance use problems are common in people with SMI as well as people with PTSD, so it is not surprising that they are also common in people with both disorders. In our experience, most people with substance use disorders can be engaged and successfully treated in the CR for PTSD program. It is important for the clinician to assess and be aware of the client's use history and current behaviors as soon as possible in this intervention.

When a pattern of problematic substance use is identified, this needs to be discussed with the client, built into the Wellness Plan developed in the first session, and monitored over the course of the program. The therapist also needs to initiate a discussion with the client about the importance of regularly attending the CR for PTSD sessions as well as practicing the intervention skills when they are not under the influence of alcohol or drugs. Substance use in people with PTSD is often an attempt to cope with distressing PTSD symptoms. If individuals are going to be successful in learning the skills taught in the program, they need to be willing to try to practice those skills when they experience their PTSD symptoms instead of immediately resorting to using substances. If clients are not willing to try this, it is preferable to postpone their involvement in the CR program.

Although problematic substance use is usually not an obstacle to successful treatment of PTSD in the CR program, severe substance dependence, especially physical dependence, can be. The lives of individuals with physical dependence on alcohol, opiates, or stimulants, such as cocaine or amphetamines, often revolve around maintaining their substance use habits, and it is difficult for anything else, including PTSD treatment, to take priority over the addiction. In our experience, although individuals with substance dependence can often be engaged in the CR program, it is difficult to retain them in treatment.

When considering the treatment needs of people with SMI, PTSD, and severe drug or alcohol use disorder, clinicians should look for natural opportunities in the course of their substance use disorder to engage them in treatment for PTSD.

For example, such individuals may require inpatient treatment to be safely withdrawn from the substances they are dependent upon. As active use often dampens PTSD symptoms, abstinence from substances is frequently associated with a worsening of PTSD symptoms, which can increase the person's risk for a relapse of their use. These periods of detoxification from alcohol or drugs and temporary abstinence can present an important opportunity to engage the person in PTSD treatment (McGovern et al., 2010), which may have the added benefit of reducing their risk of relapse back into substance use. In addition, the cognitive restructuring skills in the program can be readily applied to clients' beliefs and behaviors related to their substance use, which can serve as a potential method of insight and reduction of use.

Cognitive Functioning

Impaired cognitive functioning is common in people with SMI. In addition, lower intellectual functioning is associated with an increased risk of developing PTSD following a traumatic event (McNally & Shin, 1995). Thus, some degree of impaired cognitive functioning is common in people with SMI and PTSD.

Lower cognitive functioning is not an exclusion criterion for participation in the CR for PTSD program. As long as individuals are able to actively participate in sessions with the therapist and have basic comprehension abilities, they can benefit from the program. Prior research on this program has found that individuals with cognitive impairment clinically benefit from the program as much as those with more intact cognitive abilities (Mueser et al., 2018).

When significant cognitive impairment is present in a client with PTSD and SMI, the therapist should be mindful of strategies for accommodating these challenges into the CR for PTSD program. For example, psychoeducational information may need to be simplified and the amount of information reduced, and there may need to be less reliance on the handouts and worksheets. Individuals with significant cognitive impairment may benefit from closer coordination of the CR program with other treatment providers or family members, who may be able to facilitate the person's practice of home assignments or prompt their use of skills in naturally occurring situations. More detailed adaptations for working with clients with cognitive impairment can be found in Chapter 12 in this volume.

Ongoing Exposure to Trauma

Some individuals with PTSD may be motivated to participate in the CR for PTSD program but may be exposed to ongoing trauma in their lives that can threaten their safety, complicate treatment, and reduce the benefit they get from it. Examples of situations in which people may be exposed to ongoing trauma include being homeless, having a severe substance use disorder that increases high-risk behavior (e.g., exchanging sex for drugs) or potential for victimization, or having a partner or family member perpetrating ongoing physical or sexual abuse. In addition to potential risks to safety, exposure to ongoing trauma can distract people from focusing on their PTSD symptoms, make it more difficult to attend the CR program sessions regularly, and reduce their ability to practice the skills taught in the program. In addition, when the ongoing trauma is the same or similar to the index trauma associated with the person's PTSD (e.g., domestic abuse by the same or different partner as the index trauma), continued exposure can make it more difficult to use cognitive restructuring to challenge and change core beliefs about the trauma underlying the PTSD symptoms (e.g., "I'm to blame for what happened") because the ongoing experience of trauma may appear to support those beliefs.

When a client with PTSD who is exposed to ongoing trauma wants to participate in this intervention, the primary question the clinician needs to address is, "Are there viable steps that can be taken (or are currently underway) to reduce or eliminate the client's current exposure to trauma?" If there is a practical chance that the client's exposure to trauma can be minimized soon and efforts to reduce the risk are already underway or can be initiated by the CR for PTSD therapist or other member of the treatment team, then the best option would be to postpone beginning the intervention until the person is in a safer situation. For example, homelessness is episodic for many individuals with SMI, and waiting until the individual has stable housing may be preferable, provided the waiting period is not too long. An individual with a severe substance use disorder may agree to participate in an inpatient addiction treatment program, resulting in sobriety following discharge and an opportunity to begin the CR program then. A person in a domestic violence situation may have decided to leave or already be in the process of leaving, and so postponing initiating treatment may be relatively straightforward.

If there do not appear to be currently viable options for reducing the client's ongoing exposure to trauma, we recommend clinicians nevertheless try to provide the CR for PTSD program. As reviewed in Chapter 1 in this volume, PTSD can lead to a cycle of revictimization (Mueser, Rosenberg, et al., 2002), and thus treatment of PTSD has the potential to break that cycle of violence. Indeed, it has been shown that successful treatment of PTSD in people with SMI results in a reduction of their subsequent exposure to traumatic events compared with those who did not receive treatment (van den Berg et al., 2016). There are multiple strategies that clinicians can use to maximize their effectiveness when working with clients who are exposed to ongoing trauma and when helping them cope with and overcome their PTSD. Exhibit 4.2 summarizes some of these strategies.

SCREENING, IDENTIFICATION, AND REFERRAL OF CLIENTS WITH PTSD

As discussed in Chapter 3 in this volume, PTSD is common in people with SMI but is frequently underdiagnosed and hence undertreated. In addition, there is no typical client with PTSD that therapists can reliably detect. Furthermore,

EXHIBIT 4.2

Strategies for Working With Clients Exposed to Ongoing Trauma

- Incorporate ongoing trauma exposure into the Wellness Plan and monitor as needed.
- Offer more frequent sessions (e.g., twice per week) during periods of relative calm to teach the CR for PTSD program skills more quickly when the client is less distracted and more able to focus on learning.
- Engage with existing treatment team members to create safety plans and strategies for increased support of the client.
- As needed, help connect the client to new services and treaters to offer assistance (shelters, case management services, etc.).
- Look for opportunities to use the 5 Steps of CR to work on distressing feelings related to ongoing traumas and then to develop Action Plans aimed at addressing those situations.
- Consider offering the three-session BREATHE program (brief modification of CR for PTSD program; see Supplemental Chapter 15, this volume) and then reevaluate PTSD 1 month after completion to determine need for further treatment with the full CR for PTSD intervention.

Note. CR = cognitive restructuring; PTSD = posttraumatic stress disorder; BREATHE = Brief Relaxation, Education and Trauma Healing.

some of the symptoms of PTSD can masquerade as symptoms of SMI (i.e., psychotic symptoms, severe mood lability, etc.), making it even more difficult to recognize without direct questioning. Therefore, routine screening for trauma and PTSD of all individuals with SMI is recommended to identify the broad range of clients who could benefit from the CR for PTSD program.

Routine Screening of Trauma and PTSD

Brief and efficient methods for screening clients for PTSD are described in Chapter 3 in this volume. It is recommended that routine screening of trauma and PTSD be incorporated into standard intake procedures of mental health agencies serving persons with SMI and that procedures be established for referring individuals with probable PTSD to treatment. For agencies implementing routine screening of trauma and PTSD, it is also recommended that clinicians be encouraged to systematically screen all individuals they are currently serving who were on their caseloads before routine screening at intake is initiated. A similar approach is recommended for therapists in private practice serving people with SMI.

When routine screening in a mental health agency leads to the identification of a case of probable PTSD, the client needs to be referred to a clinician who can provide the CR for PTSD program (unless the screening was conducted by a clinician who received training in this program). To facilitate this referral, the intake clinician or primary therapist conducting the screening should inform the client that they have PTSD and explain that they would like to refer the client to a clinician who has expertise in the treatment of PTSD. The intake or primary clinician should be prepared to provide the client with some information about PTSD (such as that PTSD is a relatively common disorder that happens after someone has been exposed to traumatic events), describe some of the common symptoms of PTSD (e.g., intrusive memories), and assure them that there are effective treatments for PTSD, including one offered at the agency (the CR program). As clients may be unsure of whether they want to receive treatment for their PTSD, the screening clinician should emphasize that the purpose of a referral to the PTSD clinician is for clients to learn more about PTSD and the CR program so they can make an informed decision about whether they want to participate.

TREATMENT SETTING

The CR for PTSD program can be provided in any treatment setting that serves people with SMI for at least intermediate periods of time (e.g., 4–6 months). Therefore, it would not be feasible to implement the program in a shorter term treatment setting, such as an acute care inpatient hospital, where clients are hospitalized for periods of time ranging from only several days to several weeks. Community mental health centers, day treatment programs, some partial hospitalization programs, and private practice are examples of treatment settings where the CR program has often been implemented.

Longer term institutional settings may also be appropriate places to provide the CR for PTSD program. For example, psychiatric hospitals providing inter-mediate or long-term care and prisons with inmates receiving treatment for SMI are all viable settings where the program can be delivered. Similarly, any long-term residential setting serving this population would be an appropriate setting for providing the program.

Remote Delivery of the CR for PTSD Program

In this volume, we primarily focus on providing the CR for PTSD program in in-person sessions. However, following the COVID-19 pandemic and the shift of many psychosocial treatment services to virtual delivery, we have gained significant experience in providing the program remotely, usually through Zoom or other videoconferencing technology. In line with other general evi-dence showing that remote delivery of cognitive behavioral interventions can be just as effective as in-person sessions, we have found that the CR program can be similarly potent. See Table 4.2 for tips for remote delivery of this intervention.

INTEGRATION WITH OTHER INTERVENTIONS

Most people with SMI who are receiving treatment participate in care from multiple providers. For example, it is common for clients at community mental health centers to receive services from at minimum a psychiatrist (or other

TABLE 4.2. Considerations and Tips for Remote Delivery of the CR for PTSD Program

During the session	Use of handouts and worksheets	Other considerations
Before meeting with the client, establish a videoconferencing plan (including private time and space) and conduct a dry run.	As needed, send handouts for upcoming session either by email, internal medical record system, or regular post.	Some clients may need special training in the use of videoconferencing platforms before they begin the CR for PTSD program. Use of headphones may facilitate privacy and reduce distraction during sessions.
Encourage the client to stay on video throughout and use gentle troubleshooting to address challenges in this area.	Use the screen-sharing function as much as possible during session to show the handouts in order to increase engagement and collaboration.	Use the whiteboard function available on most remote platforms to write or draw on a shared page so that notes and other information can be collaboratively developed during sessions.
Stay flexible! If the technology is not working that day or if the client has difficulty using internet technology, be ready to switch to the phone to complete the session.	When using electronic handouts, convert them into a fillable PDF form when possible so that worksheets can be directly typed into and printers are not needed.	If using a phone, work through handouts and worksheets together. If the transmission of handouts and worksheets is not feasible, encourage clients to set up similar makeshift materials on their phone or on their computers, if possible, or to write notes on a piece of paper (e.g., tracking of Breathing Retraining practice, the 5 Steps of CR skill listed, etc.).

Note. CR = cognitive restructuring; PTSD = posttraumatic stress disorder.

medication prescriber) and a case manager and often several other professionals, such as a primary therapist, a nurse, and/or a rehabilitation practitioner (e.g., supported employment specialist). It is essential that the client's involvement and progress in the CR for PTSD program be integrated with other parts of the individual's treatment for several reasons.

First, all members of the treatment team need to be aware that the person is receiving treatment for their PTSD and be supportive of their participation in the CR for PTSD program. Not all clinicians are enlightened as to the necessity of treating PTSD in people with SMI, and some may harbor concerns that involvement in the intervention will be stressful and potentially cause a symptom exacerbation, relapse, or other problems. Helping treatment team members understand the client's need for treatment and the way the CR program works can ensure their support of the client's decision to address their trauma history and PTSD. Providing feedback to treatment team members about the client's progress during the intervention can allay concerns about untoward effects of therapy as they learn about the client's improvement in PTSD and related symptoms.

Second, integration of treatment in the CR for PTSD program with other services the client is receiving can help prepare other team members for responding to possible questions that may arise during the intervention. For example, clients may ask their psychiatrist why they had not been previously diagnosed with PTSD or what symptoms a particular medication is prescribed to treat. As PTSD symptoms diminish during the CR program, clients may express interest in vocational services to their case manager as their motivation to work increases.

Third, ongoing contact with other treatment providers can be useful in enlisting their help in supporting the client in learning the information and skills taught in the CR for PTSD program. For example, a case manager or residential counselor could facilitate or prompt the use of Breathing Retraining during an interaction in which the client is highly anxious or upset about something. Similarly, many clients benefit from having another treatment provider who can help them use the cognitive restructuring skill to deal with negative feelings that arise between CR program sessions and remind them about their home assignment to practice skills.

It is recommended that the therapist providing the CR for PTSD program have contact with other treatment providers at least once every 2 weeks over the course of the program. This contact can be accomplished through brief visits to regular treatment team meetings, short phone calls, or other in-person (or remote) meetings with relevant treatment team members. Charting clients' progress in the intervention in the medical record alone is not sufficient to meaningfully integrate this treatment with other services provided, as such notes may not be routinely reviewed by other team members and notes alone do not permit discussion of pertinent issues. Clinicians in private practice should similarly attempt to have brief contact with other providers at least every 2 weeks to ensure the CR program is well coordinated with other mental health services the client is receiving.

It is preferable that clients not be currently receiving another psychotherapeutic treatment for their PTSD, such as prolonged exposure therapy (Foa et al., 2019), cognitive processing therapy (Resick et al., 2017), eye movement and desensitization and reprocessing therapy (Shapiro, 2017), seeking safety (Najavits, 2002), or psychodynamic or psychoanalytic trauma interventions. Participation in these treatments could influence which trauma-related issues clients choose to bring up in the CR for PTSD program, giving the therapist an incomplete understanding of the effects of trauma on their lives and core beliefs underlying their PTSD symptoms. Involvement in more general individual or group supportive therapy while participating in the CR program, however, is acceptable.

THERAPIST QUALIFICATIONS

Therapists providing the CR for PTSD program should have a good understanding of and experience working with the SMI diagnoses of the clients they are treating, most often schizophrenia, schizoaffective disorder, bipolar disorder, major depression, and borderline personality disorder. This includes familiarity with the basic symptoms of each disorder, their course, and their treatments, including pharmacological treatment. Therapists should also have a good working knowledge of PTSD, including characteristic symptoms, associated problems, and effective treatments.

The CR for PTSD program is based on a cognitive behavioral treatment approach, and therefore some background in cognitive behavioral therapy is important for therapists learning the program. As the clinical methods for providing the CR program are clearly laid out in this volume, clinicians with prior experience delivering cognitive behavioral interventions may learn how to implement the program without extensive training. Clinicians without (or with less) prior cognitive behavioral therapy experience are encouraged to seek training, consultation, and/or supervision from qualified individuals (including the authors) when learning and implementing the CR program. We have demonstrated that master's-level frontline clinicians with minimal prior cognitive behavioral experience can be trained to high levels of fidelity in the CR program after just one completed practice case over a 3- to 6-month period, following participation in an initial training workshop, weekly supervision/consultation over the course of the first client case, and written feedback on audio recorded sessions delivered by someone with CR for PTSD program expertise (Lu et al., 2012).

CLINICAL CASE VIGNETTES

To illustrate how the different elements of the CR for PTSD program are provided in therapy and are individualized to each unique person, we introduce three vignettes of clients who were referred to and engaged in this program (personal details have been altered to protect privacy). In subsequent chapters, we provide client–therapist dialogues illustrating specific CR program techniques and follow up on the progress of these three clients over the course of their participation in this intervention.

Leigh-Ann

Leigh-Ann is a 24-year-old, White, cisgender female who is single with no children. She moved around quite a bit as a child with her family and also as a young adult on her own.

As a young adolescent when she was living in another state, she was a victim of childhood sexual abuse perpetrated by her friend's father on approximately 6 to 10 occasions over about 2 years. More recently, at age 22, she was raped in the laundry room of her apartment complex by a male neighbor.

Since then, she has again relocated to a different state and is living on her own in a studio apartment. She is unemployed but looking for work in the restaurant industry, where she has some past experience. She has a primary diagnosis of bipolar I disorder. Her clinic chart also notes borderline personality traits, including emotion dysregulation; intense, unstable interpersonal relationships; and some self-harm behaviors, including cutting.

Leigh-Ann has recently initiated mental health services at a local community mental health clinic, where she was referred to the CR for PTSD program. Given her sexual trauma history, her index traumas are linked, described by her on her PCL-5 as "being molested as a teen then raped as an adult," with a baseline total score of 47.

She reports a history of vocational and interpersonal difficulties related to her bipolar and PTSD symptoms (and potentially related to the aforementioned borderline personality disorder traits), including lack of close, positive friendships and family relationships; distrust of others, especially men; frequent triggering by anxiety and flashbacks causing emotional dysregulation; and functional interference related to depression symptoms. Leigh-Ann's CR for PTSD program goals are to better manage her PTSD to be able to hold a job for longer and enjoy it more and to try to find more social contacts she can trust to decrease her loneliness.

Edmundo

Edmundo is a 41-year-old, Latinx cisgender male who lives with his female partner and their three children (ages 4–12). He has a vocational background in construction but is currently unemployed as a result of an ongoing shoulder injury from a severe car accident last year that necessitated a 2-week hospitalization. His primary diagnosis is major depressive disorder. He has a history of methamphetamine abuse as an adolescent but has not used in 10 years. However, he reports intermittent binge drinking during times of stress.

Edmundo grew up in an impoverished urban neighborhood with high levels of gang violence, into which he was recruited as a young adolescent. As a result, he has reported having witnessed violent assaults and murders. In addition, his younger brother died by suicide 3 years ago, following guilt related to his own gang-related activities.

Edmundo had initially connected with the mental health center for help with his Social Security Disability Insurance application, as he requested assistance and treatment for his physical injuries from the car accident as well as his psychiatric symptoms. When referred to the CR for PTSD program, he first indicated his most distressing traumatic event was the car accident but later disclosed that he was most upset by his history of gang life and its association with his brother's unexpected suicide. His first PCL score was 43.

Edmundo's goals for the CR for PTSD program include wanting to understand and manage his PTSD symptoms so he can find meaningful work again. He also wants to better deal with what he describes as a challenging and sometimes volatile relationship with his partner, which he attributes somewhat to his unresolved feelings about his brother's death. He says his partner complains that she cannot get close to him and that he "shuts down."

Donata

Donata is a 64-year-old cisgender gay female of mixed ethnic heritage who has never been married and has one estranged adult son. She currently lives in a supportive housing community specifically for seniors with psychiatric conditions. Her primary diagnosis is schizophrenia, and she has a fairly extensive alcohol use disorder history spanning approximately 25 years; however, she has been sober for the last 12 years.

Donata experienced an impoverished childhood that included physical abuse and neglect by her parents, who likely had severe but untreated psychiatric conditions and were involved in heavy drug use and potentially some informal drug dealing as well. As a result, Donata's childhood and adolescence included periods of inappropriate activity and abuse perpetrated by her parents' social circle and possible sexual abuse from her older brother as well. In addition, she was bullied at school by her classmates.

She has a history of distressing command hallucinations of voices telling her what to do and severely criticizing her, as well as paranoid thoughts about people wanting to hurt her. As Donata's paranoia is related to the features of her traumatic events, there seems to be some delusional elaboration of these events as well. As a result of her longtime untreated PTSD and psychotic symptoms, she has had several inpatient hospitalizations over the years and is an ongoing client of mental health services.

Her initial PCL-5 at baseline was 60 with an index trauma of "my parents and their friends beating me up and making me run drugs for them by flying helicopters when I was growing up." Donata currently experiences distracting and highly critical hallucinations and as a result tends to avoid public places and interactions with others. She has identified her primary goals for the CR for PTSD program as follows: (a) coping better with stress and traumatic memories that her voices cause, (b) managing her anxiety better to be able to participate in the senior housing leisure activities and outings, and (c) developing some friendships with people at her residence.

CONCLUSION

The CR for PTSD program is a 12- to 16-week individual program based on the principles of cognitive behavioral therapy, with 50- to 60-minute sessions usually delivered on a weekly basis. The primary eligibility criteria for participation in the program are that clients have PTSD, are interested in trying the program, have stable symptoms to the extent possible, are not presenting a significant threat to themselves, and are not currently in another treatment focusing on trauma. For individuals who have ongoing exposure to trauma (e.g., domestic violence), efforts should be taken to assure the person's safety and reduce their vulnerability to trauma to the extent possible before beginning this intervention.

The CR for PTSD program can be provided in any setting providing at least intermediate (e.g., 3–6 months) or long-term treatment to people with an SMI, such as at a community mental health center, in a longer stay hospital or prison, or in private practice. Traditionally, this program has been delivered in person; however, tips are provided for successful remote treatment as well.

Integration of the client's involvement and progress in the CR for PTSD program with other treatments they are receiving is critical, including such service providers as prescribers, case managers, other clinicians, and rehabilitation specialists. Therapists providing the CR program should have a good understanding of and experience with the major mental illnesses in the clients they treat (e.g., schizophrenia, bipolar disorder, major depression) and PTSD, including diagnostic criteria and symptoms, associated problems, and effective treatments; as well as some experience with cognitive behavioral therapy. Clinicians with less experience are encouraged to seek consultation or supervision from individuals adequately trained in the CR program, including the authors of this book.

5

Beginning Treatment

Engagement, Orientation, Wellness Planning, and Breathing Retraining

This chapter describes the first steps of initiating the Cognitive Restructuring (CR) for PTSD program after completing the assessment of PTSD. These steps encompass engaging the client in treatment, dealing with ambivalence about change, and then providing an orientation to the CR for PTSD program, which includes creating a Wellness Plan with the client for managing any potential symptom exacerbations or crises. Breathing Retraining is then taught as a skill for coping with anxiety and reducing PTSD overarousal symptoms.

THE ENGAGEMENT PROCESS

Following screening for PTSD and confirmation of eligibility described in Chapters 3 and 4 in this volume, the treatment engagement process begins. For many clients, engagement in the program is straightforward and flows naturally from the assessment of trauma and PTSD into discussion of the disorder and treatment options.

When the CR for PTSD program is being provided in a community mental health clinic that incorporates routine screening of trauma and PTSD of all clients and referral to the program is made by an intake clinician, primary therapist, or another provider, the client may have already received some information about their PTSD diagnosis as well as a description of the program (see Chapter 3, this volume, for screening methods and the Routine Screening of Trauma and PTSD section in Chapter 4, this volume). However, in other settings or private practice,

https://doi.org/10.1037/0000423-005

the CR for PTSD clinician may need to conduct the PTSD screening and provide some explanation to clients who screen positive for PTSD and appear eligible for the program.

Depending on the treatment setting and the client's previous interaction with the therapist who will provide the CR for PTSD program, the engagement process can occur as an initial brief session or can be embedded into the formal Session 1 of the intervention. The duration of the initial engagement components usually requires 20 to 30 minutes but may take longer, depending on the client's level of engagement and information processing abilities, as well as the number of questions and concerns they may have.

The process of engagement typically includes informing the client that they have PTSD (if this has not already occurred via the referring clinician), discussing their reaction to this diagnosis, providing an overview of the CR for PTSD intervention, and motivating the person to participate.

During this engagement portion, instilling motivation for treatment, offering hope and the expectation of recovery, and summarizing the nature and goals of the program are important components to set the stage for the client to be an active learner in the intervention and to be able to play a lead role in overcoming the impact of PTSD on their life.

Providing Information About PTSD

When a diagnosis of PTSD has been established via a reliable screening process (and/or via the process recommended within this program), the therapist should inform the client and provide some basic information about the disorder. The therapist's immediate goal is to help the client understand that the symptoms and difficulties they have experienced following the traumatic events are due to a common disorder or syndrome (PTSD). This normalizes the individual's reactions to traumatic events by letting them know that they are not alone. This information can reduce feelings of shame traumatized people often have about how they have coped with their experiences and instill hope that the disorder is well understood and treatable. For example, continuing the earlier case vignette of Edmundo:

THERAPIST: We've spent some time talking together about your traumatic (highly stressful) experiences and the ways they've affected you. Based on these discussions and our screening, it is clear that you have posttraumatic stress disorder: PTSD. PTSD is a common disorder that people have after exposure to traumatic events, such as experiencing childhood physical or sexual abuse, being assaulted or raped, being in a bad accident or natural disaster, or being in combat. Some of the most common symptoms of PTSD include intrusive images or memories of the experiences, difficulty sleeping, and avoiding things that remind you of the traumatic events.

Has anyone ever told you have PTSD before? Have you heard of PTSD?

EDMUNDO: Yeah, I know what it's called, and I thought maybe I had it. I wasn't sure. But I haven't really talked with anyone at this clinic about it before, and I don't know much about it. It's just like something I've kept to myself. Do you mean other people have these same sorts of things happen to them, and their lives get messed up as a result?

THERAPIST: Yes, exactly. These sorts of problems are actually quite common among people who have experienced traumatic events. About one in 10 people develop PTSD at some point in their lives, so you are definitely not alone in your experiences with this, Edmundo.

EDMUNDO: I didn't realize that. I used to think I was crazy because I would keep having those thoughts and pictures in my head coming back again and again of my brother and other stuff, and wondering why I hadn't been able to just move on by now.

THERAPIST: Absolutely. Thinking about your experiences that way is also really common—and does make things feel harder. And actually, unfortunately, it is also common for people to not have been given the opportunity to learn more about trauma and PTSD from mental health providers they've worked with in the past. So it is good we are here now. You're in the right place.

This amount of information about PTSD at the outset of the engagement session is sufficient for most clients, and the therapist can proceed to briefly explore how PTSD has affected the client's life. Some clients want to know more about PTSD, and the therapist should provide this information freely. If a client's desire for more information continues for more than 10 to 15 minutes, the therapist should inform them that they have many excellent and important questions and that these and other questions will be addressed in the upcoming sessions of the program, which the therapist can then proceed to describe, as delineated next.

Some clients may not resonate with the term "trauma" or "traumatic event", and so it may be preferable to use the expression "very stressful experience" or "difficult life experience" instead. While the goal is not to promote avoidance or minimization of the seriousness of these experiences, in some cases in these early sessions, it can decrease clients' fear and anxiety to avoid use of clinical labels and adopt their preferred language, which can, in turn, increase treatment engagement at this critical phase.

Brief Description of the CR for PTSD Program

The therapist next provides a brief introduction to the CR for PTSD program, explaining that it is a recovery-oriented program specifically designed to address PTSD, briefly describing its empirical support, and conveying hope that participation in the program will reduce or eliminate many of the client's symptoms and problems due to PTSD. The most critical information to provide at this early stage of engagement are the following:

- The program is time-limited (12–16 weeks).
- It focuses specifically on PTSD and related problems.
- Research on the program has shown that it has been helpful to other people with PTSD.
- The program works by providing information about PTSD and teaching strategies for coping with anxiety and other trauma-related negative feelings.

THERAPIST: Now that we've talked a little bit about PTSD in your life, I would like to describe this treatment program in some more detail so you can have a better sense of what it is like and what to expect. This program is a cognitive behavioral treatment (CBT) specifically designed for people with PTSD. We will meet in individual sessions, once per week, and for 12 to 16 weeks. As we go forward, we'll decide together how many sessions we'll end up having.

At last the aim of this program is to help people toward their personal recovery by overcoming the impact of trauma on their lives. This includes reducing or eliminating PTSD symptoms and also helping people manage their symptoms so they don't interfere with their lives as much. The focus of this program is on providing you with basic information about PTSD, teaching some really good strategies for dealing with anxiety and other distressing symptoms, and teaching you skills for dealing with thoughts and beliefs related to your traumatic experiences that cause problems or make you upset. We'll work directly on the trauma you noted on your screening as most distressing and track how the program is impacting your symptoms related to that event, and we'll also likely use the skills to help you with other traumatic events you've experienced in your life. How does that sound so far?

EDMUNDO: Sounds sort of good I think. Do you mean that this program can get rid of my problems from my past traumas?

THERAPIST: Some people who participate in this program have all of their PTSD symptoms completely eliminated. Most other people have experienced significant reductions in their PTSD symptoms and less interference from them in their daily lives. This can make a big difference for people who have experienced a lot of problems in life as a result of their PTSD, like you've shared with me.

EDMUNDO: So can you really make those bad memories go away? I've had them lots of years now, and they can be so intense, I don't even know how that would be to not have them.

THERAPIST: Well, nobody really knows how to make memories go away, but we do know how to make it easier for people to cope with the memories they have. The primary goal of this program is to help people live more fulfilling, enjoyable, and meaningful lives, despite the traumatic experiences they have had and their memories of those experiences. Even though this is something you have understandably struggled with, Edmundo, we do know that it is possible for people to live worthwhile and rewarding lives even when they have suffered much trauma over many years without making their memories go away completely. Those memories are part of you. This program will help you learn how to better cope with and live with those memories and at the same time move forward in your life in the ways that are important to you and help move you toward your ongoing recovery. This program is aimed at helping you do that.

Working With Ambivalence

Some individuals are ambivalent about participating in any treatment program for PTSD, which is normal, given the nature of PTSD avoidance symptoms. Clients have often struggled with their symptoms for years and have reached a precarious balance in their lives that they are afraid to upset. Some people lose hope for a better life and are reluctant to commit the effort to participating in a new program, especially those who have been involved in the mental health system for many years. Still others are skeptical that a short-term intervention could help them overcome the effects of trauma they have endured for so many years.

Ambivalence or skepticism is a normal part of the change process (Prochaska & DiClemente, 1984). All people are hesitant about making significant life changes, even for the better (e.g., getting married, taking a new job), because change involves dislodging a person from their usual routine and facing uncertainty, even when that routine has been highly distressing. Therefore, when encountering ambivalence about participating in the CR for PTSD program, efforts should focus on normalizing, understanding, and exploring the basis of the person's concerns rather than on pathologizing those concerns as "resistance."

First and foremost, it is important to acknowledge and empathize with the natural fear the client has about dealing with disturbing memories of past events. The therapist can validate these concerns, while also providing support and encouragement:

THERAPIST: I can completely understand how scary it is for you to think about confronting and dealing with your abusive experiences. These are memories that you've tried to keep tucked away for a long time, but they have somehow managed to keep intruding on your life. It's true that dealing with these experiences can be frightening. However, in this program we will focus on teaching you specific skills for coping with your anxious feelings and for emotionally processing your memories of traumatic experiences. I'll be here with you, supporting you every step of the way as you learn these skills and recover from your traumatic experiences. And we will be sure to go at a pace that is comfortable for you.

Another useful strategy for dealing with ambivalence, as needed, is to briefly help the client make a short list of the pros and cons of participating in the CR for PTSD program. When exploring the advantages of participation, attention should be given both to the potential benefits of reduced PTSD symptoms and distress, as well as to reduced interference with other parts of the client's life, such as social or romantic relationships, work or school, or parenting. Reference to the client's most severe symptoms, as reported on the screening assessment, can be a good launch point or reminder for such brief discussions. Directly querying clients about their concerns is usually straightforward. The most common concerns include worry about focusing on past traumatic experiences and having to recount traumatic experiences in detail, despair that renders the person hopeless about the future, and high levels of internal or environmental stress that make it difficult for the person to commit the effort to participating in the program.

The therapist should remind the client that the program is not an exposure-based approach to PTSD, meaning that they do not have to recount details of their traumatic experiences, and that it is entirely up to them how much they would like to share about it. The therapist can also explore how well the client's current efforts to cope with PTSD are working. Despite great efforts to avoid trauma-related stimuli, most people with PTSD are repeatedly triggered by situations in their daily lives that are only remotely related to their trauma, and they continue to be bombarded by memories of their traumatic experiences. Helping clients see the limited effectiveness of their current coping strategies can tip the balance in favor of participating in this program.

For some clients, the anguish and despair they experience make it impossible for them to conceive of a better future. Hopelessness is a common feature of depression, which is frequently compounded by the PTSD symptom of a foreshortened sense of future. In responding to such despair, the therapist needs to walk a fine line between validating the client's distraught feelings while not reinforcing their beliefs of hopelessness. The therapist can explain that when people feel depressed, they often have a bleak outlook on life and their future but that this outlook is often not accurate. The therapist can also point out that some of the skills taught in the CR for PTSD program have been shown to be very helpful in dealing with and overcoming feelings of depression as well as PTSD symptoms.

Clients with serious mental illness (SMI) and PTSD often face multiple stresses in their lives, many of which are not directly related to their PTSD, and it may be difficult to focus their energies on just one particular source of stress. For example, a person may have ongoing medical, financial, or housing challenges or may have other responsibilities, such as taking care of an elderly parent or a young child. The therapist should first explore whether the most pressing current problems or obstacles may be resolved in the near future. For example, if a person is experiencing housing insecurity, it may be preferable to postpone treatment until that situation has been resolved. If the stresses the client is facing appear unlikely to improve soon, the therapist can help the client explore whether participating in effective treatment for their PTSD might actually reduce the stress in the long run. For example, PTSD often interferes with employment (Lu, Waynor, et al., 2017; Mueser, Salyers, et al., 2004; Ng et al., 2016), and clients who are unable to work and are under great financial stress could explore whether this intervention might help them return to work and reduce this strain.

The goal of explaining the CR for PTSD program is not strictly to persuade clients to participate but rather to enable them to make an informed and self-determined decision about treatment. This could also involve discussing other potentially adjunctive treatment options, such as pharmacological treatment for PTSD (de Moraes Costa et al., 2020; Huang et al., 2020). If after weighing the advantages and disadvantages of the CR for PTSD program the client decides to not participate in it, the therapist should raise the option of trying the program at a later date. If the client indicates an interest in going forward, the program can begin with the Session 1 components as described next.

ORIENTATION TO THE CR FOR PTSD PROGRAM (SESSION 1)

The orientation process can usually be covered in a single treatment session (Session 1) and includes the following:

- providing a more detailed description about the CR for PTSD program and how it works;

- developing a Wellness Plan both to assure the client's safety and to minimize the chances of symptom exacerbations or crises interfering with completion of the program; and

- teaching Breathing Retraining, an easy-to-learn skill that can provide rapid in vivo relief from anxiety and other PTSD symptoms, which can facilitate program participation.

If more than 3 weeks have passed between the client's initial screening for PTSD and the first session, it is recommended that the PTSD Checklist–5 be administered again in the session, using the same index trauma used for the initial screening. As described in Chapter 3 in this volume, PTSD symptoms and depression should be routinely tracked every three sessions in the CR for PTSD program, with information from the assessments integrated into the treatment sessions. The review of the client's trauma history questionnaire (Difficult Life Events Inventory) does not need to be repeated. If depression symptoms are also being tracked (as is also recommended in Chapter 3, this volume), the depression inventory should be administered at the start of Session 1.

At the outset of this first session, the therapist should explain that each session in the program will begin with the client and therapist setting an agenda together as a way to introduce the client to the structure of therapy sessions and to reduce any anxiety that the client may be experiencing. It is common for clients to feel anxious when beginning treatment for PTSD, and collaboratively setting an agenda allows clients to know what to expect in the session and to be assured that they will be able to raise any concerns they would like to talk about. Agenda setting usually begins when the therapist briefly outlines the topics they would like to cover in the session corresponding to the appropriate session content, and then the client is asked whether they would like to bring up or add anything else to the agenda. Additional concerns raised by the client are then integrated into the session agenda as needed. The CR for PTSD Agenda-Setting Worksheet (see the online Appendix) can be used to create a written plan for the session. A portion of a sample agenda for Session 1, using the worksheet, is as follows:

Today's date: 9/12/23   Session no. (1–16):   1
Overall topic: Orientation, Wellness Plan, Breathing Retraining

Topics to cover (your therapist will likely have a list based on where you are in the CR intervention):

1. Review the CR for PTSD program, and answer any questions.
2. Briefly discuss common PTSD symptoms.
3. Develop and review a Wellness Plan.
4. Teach and practice Breathing Retraining skill.
5. Discuss an outside practice, and plan for what will happen between now and the next meeting.

Are there any other topics that you'd like to cover today that haven't already been listed out above? (Write down below any additional, specific topics that the client would like to talk about):

1. Will I continue to meet with my regular therapist during this CR for PTSD program?
2. _____

Following setting the agenda, the therapist provides a more detailed explanation of the program to set clear and positive expectations, which typically takes about 10 to 15 minutes of Session 1. When providing this information, the therapist can use the Orientation to the CR for PTSD Program handout (Brief Version), which provides a simple explanation of the program components. Alternatively, if the client seems interested in more detail about what to expect in each of the 12 to 16 sessions, the CR for PTSD Orientation and Session-by-Session Plan handout (Long Version) can be used instead. These handouts serve as a guide for the clinician in describing the CR for PTSD program and can reduce any anxiety clients may have about what will happen in the therapy sessions. It can be helpful to note that in the first session of this intervention, some clients may experience anticipatory worry associated with PTSD, have some understandable uncertainty about what to expect during the therapy sessions, and therefore may feel anxious about the nature and content of the upcoming sessions. Often a more detailed, written schedule, such as the CR for PTSD Orientation and Session-by-Session Plan handout (Long Version), can assuage that anxiety. For other clients, though, this may be information overload, and so therapists should use their clinical judgment about which handout version to use.

The therapist reviews the orientation information with the client, briefly elaborating on the different points and responding to any questions that arise along the way. When discussing the goals of this program, the therapist can integrate information about the client's specific PTSD symptoms and the problems they cause in day-to-day life as important foci of treatment. An example of how to discuss intervention logistics with a client is as follows:

THERAPIST: In the beginning, we'll meet once a week for a total of about 12 to 16 sessions. Toward the end of the program, we may want to space out our sessions to every other week. The CR for PTSD program is time-limited but involves teaching you specific skills that you will be able to continue to use as needed long after we stop meeting together. Later in the program, we will also meet with your case manager or primary therapist, who can support you in continuing to use these skills after our therapy ends.

The therapist's goal when describing the components of the CR for PTSD program is to inform the client about the nature of the program and the details of how it works. Clients may already have some familiarity with how the program works based on previous discussions with the therapist or referring clinician, but a brief review in the first session helps to ensure understanding. Prior to describing the details of the program, the therapist reviews any other treatment services the client will continue to receive.

THERAPIST: We will be working together on difficulties you are having related to your traumatic experiences. This program is aimed at helping you reduce your PTSD symptoms and their impact on your life. And I just want to mention again, in case you were feeling concerned about this, this particular treatment is *not* based on retelling the details of your experiences. There may be times when we talk about past upsetting events, but we will not have to discuss them in detail, and deciding how much you want to share will be up to you. Our focus together will instead be on the here and now to better understand how your past experiences are making life difficult for you and to learn some strategies to reduce that stress and distress.

There are three main things we will work on together in this program. First, I will teach you a technique for coping with anxiety: Breathing Retraining. This skill will help you reduce your anxiety, your physical tension, and other PTSD symptoms. We will focus on this skill today so that you can begin using it right away.

Second, you will learn about PTSD and other common symptoms that people experience. Being aware of and understanding your own PTSD symptoms are important steps toward learning how to cope with them and reduce them.

Third, I'll teach you a skill called cognitive restructuring, or CR for short. Traumatic experiences often lead to upsetting feelings like the ones we've talked about, and these emotions can be really difficult to handle. CR is a skill that can help you identify and challenge the unhelpful thoughts and beliefs that may be contributing to your upset feelings. You will learn how to use CR to help you to better understand and change unhelpful and inaccurate trauma-related thoughts about yourself and the world that contribute to your negative feelings and PTSD symptoms.

The Importance of Home Assignments

The therapist should explain the importance of home assignments in the first session and discuss them further as needed throughout the course of the program. After describing the Breathing Retraining and CR skills taught in the program, the therapist can note the importance of practicing these skills outside of therapy sessions in order to master them and alleviate PTSD symptoms. The therapist can then explain that at the end of each session the therapist and client will together come up with a home assignment for the client to practice specific skills over the following week. The therapist may find it helpful to briefly explain some of the differences between the CR for PTSD program and other non-CBT-based (and less structured) treatment approaches. In addition, it may be useful to point out that research shows the CR program clients who completed home assignments more regularly experienced greater improvements in their symptoms than those who completed them less often (Mueser et al., 2008). For example:

THERAPIST: The CR for PTSD program may be a little different from other types of therapy you have participated in. I will teach you some new skills for managing difficult feelings related to your stress and your traumatic experiences. Because learning is so important in this program, part of it also involves practicing the skills we covered in session when you are on your own, as a home assignment. In fact, practicing these skills on your own is just as important a part of the program as coming to the sessions. In a large study that was done with this program, it was found that although many people who participated experienced big improvements in their PTSD symptoms, those who completed home assignments more regularly and practiced their skills more got the greatest benefit. Since this is a time-limited therapy, I definitely want us to help you make the most of our time together, and so we'll want to be sure to keep up with that outside practice component. At the end of each session, we will work together to come up with something you can practice before the next session. How does that sound to you?

WELLNESS PLANNING

A crisis can be defined as anything unexpected that happens in the client's life that could threaten their clinical stability or ability to continue to participate in the CR for PTSD program. Trauma work can be emotionally challenging, and temporary increases in symptoms (or related problems) sometimes happen before improvements occur. Developing a crisis (or wellness) plan can prevent these symptom increases from becoming a crisis through systematic monitoring of the signs of an impending crisis and identifying of specific steps and strategies that can be used to contain and reduce these problematic signs or symptoms.

The most common symptoms or problems that can become a crisis include the reemergence or worsening of psychiatric symptoms (e.g., psychotic symptoms, depression), resumption of or increase in substance use, self-harming behavior (e.g., cutting), or suicidal thinking. Some of these symptom increases may come directly from more general stressors, medication changes, or other unexpected events. However, it is also common for situations related to the traumatic event itself to occur, which can understandably trigger the exacerbation of PTSD or other psychiatric symptoms and/or unhealthy behavioral reactions. These trauma-related situations may include trauma anniversaries (i.e., the annual marking of a loved one's suicide or one's sexual assault) or more jarring, unexpected events (such as a violent former partner's release from prison or one's child getting suspended from school for beating up a classmate), all of which can trigger an associated PTSD reaction.

When initiating a discussion of the Wellness Plan, the therapist begins by explaining that learning how to take care of one's day-to-day mental health is an important goal of the CR for PTSD program. One way of helping clients learn how to do this is to review past challenges they have had with their mental health symptoms and to develop a plan for preventing or responding to those problems in the future. Although this program is not expected to cause increases in symptoms or problems, developing such a plan can make both the client and the therapist feel more confident when working together in the program.

The client may already have a similar plan in place with their primary therapist or in their medical record or treatment plan, such as a Wellness Recovery Action Plan (Copeland, 2011) or a relapse prevention plan from the

Illness Management and Recovery Program (Gingerich & Mueser, 2011). In such cases, that plan can be reviewed and modified as needed. If no plan exists, the Wellness Plan Worksheet should be completed together, as illustrated next.

THERAPIST: Before we begin with Breathing Retraining as a skill for reducing anxious feelings, I'd like to spend a few minutes talking together about how we can help you to take better care of your own mental health and your overall recovery. As you know from your own experiences, when things are really bad and you are in a place in which your symptoms are really severe, you didn't get there overnight. Usually, what happens is a slow increase of symptoms over a few days or weeks. For example, you might start feeling more anxious or sad, start noticing that you don't feel like going places or that you're missing appointments, or start wanting or using alcohol or drugs (insert other symptom escalations that may be more appropriate to the client). It's important that we figure out your specific pattern because if you know what your own warning signs are, you can learn to notice them earlier and try to prevent them by getting some help sooner. This can actually help you prevent a mental health crisis, including a hospitalization, giving you more control over your day-to-day life.

I want us to think through together and write down all of the warning signs that you have experienced before a really challenging symptom time that you've had in your life. I like to think of this as a Wellness Plan. And I want to be clear that working on this does not mean that I think that participating in this program will cause an increase in symptoms or make things feel unmanageable for you or create a crisis in any way. This plan is more like a safety net or an insurance plan that will help us work together. Here is a worksheet for us to fill out that will guide us through the steps of figuring out what your own unique warning signs are, what to do if you notice them, and how to help avoid having things get worse.

The therapist takes out a Wellness Plan Worksheet and briefly reviews the items with the client:

THERAPIST: This is an important thing for us to do together because while most people participating in this program get significant and lasting improvements in their symptoms and functioning, from the first session onward, sometimes PTSD symptoms don't get better immediately. It can take time and effort to learn the skills before you finally experience relief from the symptoms of PTSD. This can be especially hard when you are dealing with thoughts and feelings related to traumatic events that you have tried to avoid thinking about for so many years. Therefore, having a plan for dealing with any increases in symptoms or problem behaviors, like the one we are doing now, can help assure your safety and help both of us feel confident and comfortable about your well-being as we work together in this program. How does this sound to you, and do you have any questions?

Sometimes it is helpful for other supportive people to be involved in monitoring and helping the client respond to any exacerbating of symptoms or triggering of PTSD or other crises. This can be especially crucial for clients whose first warning signs may involve the loss of insight, experiencing paranoid thoughts or hallucinations, depression, social withdrawal, or substance use problems. Potential supports include family members, friends, or a member of the person's treatment team, such as their primary therapist, prescriber, or case manager. In addition, it can be helpful to share (with the client's permission) a copy of the finalized Wellness Plan with other treatment team or family members, as applicable and appropriate.

Some clients can readily identify potential warning signs or crises but are reluctant to communicate their distress and get help from others. Some of this reluctance may stem from the mistrust that traumatized individuals often have about other people. Clients who have been involved in the mental health system for a long time may also be afraid that telling other people about their distressing feelings could lead to being hospitalized, especially if they are related to suicidal thoughts or psychotic symptoms like hearing voices or paranoia. The CR for PTSD program therapist should show understanding of these concerns and explain that developing a plan together that both client and therapist feel comfortable with can help prevent such a hospitalization. The therapist can also take responsibility for the need to develop a Wellness Plan by explaining that it is the therapist's duty to ensure the client's safety while participating in the program and that the plan will also maximize the ability of the client to complete and benefit from the program.

Breathing Retraining

Breathing Retraining is a widely taught skill in the treatment of anxiety disorders (Craske & Lewin, 1998; Foa & Rothbaum, 1998; Rygh & Sanderson, 2004). Breathing Retraining can directly reduce physiological overarousal, a defining symptom of PTSD, and serve as a tool for clients to use anytime they experience arousal symptoms or preemptively in times when they anticipate arousal due to an upcoming trigger. This skill also serves to reduce the exaggerated fight-or-flight response that people with PTSD often have to due to misinterpreting innocuous stimuli as potential threats when they are physiologically overaroused. In addition, Breathing Retraining can serve as a sleep aid for clients with insomnia, another common and very challenging symptom of PTSD, as well as a centering strategy to combat chronic rumination.

Relatedly, for clients who experience high levels of hypervigilance or paranoia, Breathing Retraining can serve as a head-clearing reset. In fact, when working with clients who have distressing paranoid or suspicious beliefs, it is recommended to frame the primary benefit of this skill as a way to "clear your head so you can think straight." This language and description tend to resonate more with and appeal to people with paranoia, as opposed to suggesting that they should use the skill to "relax" or "feel calmer," given that those with paranoia often strongly believe that they need to be on guard and should not relax when they feel threatened or in danger (see more about working with people with psychotic symptoms in Chapter 12, this volume).

By learning Breathing Retraining at the beginning of the CR for PTSD program, clients are able to start using it from the first session onward and to gain some immediate relief from the intense anxiety that often accompanies posttraumatic reactions. As clients learn Breathing Retraining, they can use it to reduce distress that occurs in and outside of sessions. The skill requires approximately 15 minutes to teach and can be taught at the end of the first session.

Teaching Breathing Retraining involves three basic steps. First, the therapist establishes the rationale for Breathing Retraining as a strategy for reducing anxiety and overarousal. Second, the therapist teaches the skill by actively demonstrating it and then engaging the client in practicing the skill in the session. Third, a plan is agreed upon for the client to practice the skill as a home assignment.

Rationale for Breathing Retraining

Before explaining how Breathing Retraining works, the therapist should ask the client about any experiences they have had using relaxation techniques. These experiences can often be built upon when explaining the purpose of Breathing Retraining. Here's an example of the therapist working with Leigh-Ann on Breathing Retraining:

THERAPIST: The first skill we're going to work on is called Breathing Retraining, or BRT for short, which may be easier to remember. When PTSD symptoms pop up unexpectedly, people often experience high levels of physical tension and anxiety. Breathing Retraining is a strategy for reducing the tension and anxious feelings you have in the moment so that you can feel a little calmer or can think straight if you start to feel stressed or triggered by symptoms. It can also be really helpful if you have difficulty falling asleep or getting back to sleep after waking in the middle of the night.

I'm going to teach you this skill today. We'll practice it together, and then we can make a plan for how you can practice it on your own. That way you will have a really effective skill right off the bat that you can begin using to deal with upsetting feelings, anxiety, or any other PTSD symptoms you might be having a hard time with.

LEIGH-ANN: I mean, I could definitely use that. I'm usually not really into this sort of thing, though. I'm not a real yoga or meditation person, you know.

THERAPIST: I totally understand your apprehension about this. That is completely normal. Before we start, though, I'm wondering whether you've ever used any relaxation techniques before. If so, what have you used, and have they helped?

LEIGH-ANN: Sometimes, when I'm feeling really tense, I like to listen to music. And I was in a group a few years ago where they taught this deep-breaths thing, but it seemed complicated, and it didn't really work for me. A coworker taught me a relaxing thing from her yoga class once at the bar, but as I said, it didn't really work or feel comfortable to me.

THERAPIST: Well, I'm glad to hear that you feel like you have one solid strategy for dealing with tension and anxiety—that you sometimes find it helpful to listen to music. That's definitely a good one. There are a lot of breathing techniques out there, and to be honest, some work better than others. I do think you might find Breathing Retraining helpful. It's a bit different than the breathing skills that people have usually been taught before. It's also a good one because you can use it anywhere and on the fly, even when other people are around.

Some clients report that they already know or use Breathing Retraining or that they have tried it and it was not effective. The therapist should acknowledge their experience and explore whether the client found the skill helpful and currently uses it to deal with anxiety and other distress. Although clients sometimes report that they know Breathing Retraining, they are often not familiar with the skill as taught in the CR for PTSD program. In addition, many clients have not had this skill taught effectively to them in the past, and they may not have practiced it sufficiently (or correctly), so that they were not able to successfully learn the skill and make it part of their repertoire of coping strategies. Therefore, it is important to review the skill with the client and practice it in session, even if the client reports being familiar with it or having had unsuccessful experiences with breathing techniques in the past.

The rationale for Breathing Retraining can be established by explaining that it is a skill for reducing the high flow of oxygen to the brain that occurs during periods of high tension and anxiety. When initially teaching and practicing this skill, review the Breathing Retraining Instructions handout with the client, as described in the following:

THERAPIST: When we're stressed out or upset, we often are given the advice, "Take a deep breath," right? But what tends to happen when we are distressed is that we often end up breathing in too much air and breathe too quickly. And this can get overwhelming and make us more anxious or panicked. Are you familiar with what it is called when a person takes in too much air too quickly in a repeated way and has a really anxious reaction?

LEIGH-ANN: Do you mean hyperventilating?

THERAPIST: Yes, exactly. When people feel upset, they often breathe more quickly, or hyperventilate. What's it like for you when you feel upset or anxious?

LEIGH-ANN: I guess I definitely breathe faster. I'm not sure I've noticed that, though. My muscles feel tense, and I sometimes clench my jaw and fists. My mind starts whirring.

THERAPIST: Yes, those are very common reactions to feeling anxious. The problem with breathing more quickly is that it increases the amount of oxygen in the brain, which can make you feel lightheaded, even more stimulated, and even more anxious.

LEIGH-ANN: That definitely happens to me. I begin to feel totally panicky.

THERAPIST: Exactly. Sometimes people try to take a deep breath to calm down. Have you ever tried that?

LEIGH-ANN: Yes. It sometimes helps a little but not much. And it's hard to keep up with it when I'm really upset or anxious.

THERAPIST: Right. The problem with taking a deep breath is that while it may slow down your breathing, you're still getting lots of oxygen to the brain, and that's responsible for those anxious feelings. So actually taking in more air from a deep breath doesn't tend to help. It tends to make things worse.

LEIGH-ANN: So what am I supposed to do? Stop breathing?

THERAPIST: No, you can definitely keep breathing! The idea is to slow down your breathing and also get rid of some extra air that you don't need. Instead of taking a deep breath, the idea is to instead take a normal breath and then exhale very slowly. While you exhale all the air, say a soothing word like "calm" or "peace" out loud. By taking normal breaths instead of deep breaths and exhaling slowly, you'll reduce the flow of oxygen to your brain, which will reduce your feelings of anxiety. Here, I'll show you how it looks and then we can try it together.

After this explanation, the therapist should next demonstrate the skill with the client observing. Then, the therapist and client should practice it together with the therapist leading by cueing the client when to inhale and exhale and for how long. Clients sometimes feel self-conscious or anxious during this initial process, which is understandable. The clinician should normalize these concerns and suggest ways to help the client feel more comfortable as needed. For example, some clients prefer to keep their eyes closed during the practice or even face away from the therapist. As long as the therapist is able to observe the client practicing the skill, it is fine to make these accommodations.

After providing any needed corrective feedback to the client's techniques, the therapist should encourage the client to practice the skill for a few minutes alongside the therapist. When the client has finished, the therapist should ask what the experience was like for the client and make minor modifications to the method to suit the client's preferences. For example, some clients like to include imagery of a pleasant scene into the Breathing Retraining. Some clients have difficulty pausing between breaths and feel that they're always trying to catch their breath. For these clients, the pause between breaths can be shortened or eliminated. Some clients like to combine tensing and releasing their muscles with the Breathing Retraining. It can also be suggested that clients try the skill at home while lying down rather than sitting. Other modifications may be related to the client's general comfort and/or their trauma history. For example, for some clients with a history of sexual abuse or assault, keeping eyes closed or lying down while practicing may not feel safe or comfortable.

When helping the client choose a personal soothing word, therapists should suggest that a one-syllable word be used (i.e., "calm" or "peace") rather than a two-syllable word, as the combination of making a long exhalation and saying a longer word aloud can be challenging. The clinician should encourage the client to use a short word whenever possible. In addition, the therapist should check with the client to make sure that the word they choose is actually one that is calming and relaxing and is not in any way arousing or activating. If unclear, ask the client directly why they chose a specific word, and brainstorm some alternatives if it seems that the chosen word is not healthy or useful for the purposes of this skill.

The first time Breathing Retraining is practiced in the session, the client may indicate that the skill feels awkward and/or that it does not significantly reduce anxiety in the moment. The therapist should normalize this reaction and explain that Breathing Retraining is a skill that requires practice in order to achieve proficiency. It is also helpful for the therapist to describe their own personal experience learning and mastering the skill:

LEIGH-ANN: I guess this is OK. It just feels weird.

THERAPIST: I completely get that, and you are right. It does definitely feel weird at first! I had the same reaction when I was first learning and practicing this skill. But I have to honestly tell you that the more I stuck with it and practiced it over time, the more natural, comfortable, and effective it felt. I personally use this skill in my life as needed, and it really works. It is a very powerful technique if you give it time to sink in.

The therapist should be sure to explain that with practice, many people find that Breathing Retraining is very useful for reducing their tension and anxiety and that they can use this skill anytime they want throughout the day.

It can be helpful to either start and/or end some or all of the CR for PTSD intervention sessions by leading the client (and eventually having the client lead the therapist) in some brief Breathing Retraining. In addition, this skill can be employed in the middle of any of the sessions as well. This can serve to center the client, buffer against any high levels of PTSD-triggered distress, and provide another opportunity for in-session practice of the skill.

SESSION 1 HOME ASSIGNMENT

At the end of the session, a home assignment to practice Breathing Retraining should be agreed upon with the client. The suggested between-session task for this session is to practice Breathing Retraining (5–10 minutes) once a day for the next week. Initially, Breathing Retraining should be practiced in a calm setting and at a time when the client is not distressed to facilitate learning the skill. The home assignment should address where and when this practice can take place (as well as brief troubleshooting around any obstacles to practicing the skill, as needed). As clients become more skilled at Breathing Retraining, they can begin using it to cope with stressful or upsetting situations. There are two different tracking sheets that the client can use for practicing in these two types of situations: (a) the Practice BRT Tracking Form 1: Nondistress Version, and (b) the BRT Tracking Form 2: Distress Version. In order to help the client remember the week's home assignment and to have a written record of outside practice throughout the course of the program, it can be helpful to use the Home Practice/Outside Practice Plan handout.

At the beginning of the next session, the therapist should review with the client the home assignment to practice the Breathing Retraining. They should problem-solve together any difficulties the client experienced using the skill as well as any obstacles that interfered with practicing the skill. If the client reports practicing the skill, the therapist should reinforce this, gather some more information about the client's experience with the practice, and plan for the following week to continue practicing the skill and (if the client is willing) to begin using it in more challenging situations. Although other topics and skills will be introduced in subsequent sessions, it is important to continue to encourage practice, use, and troubleshooting of the Breathing Retraining skill in an ongoing way to increase the likelihood that this technique will become incorporated into the client's repertoire of coping strategies over the course of program (and beyond).

CONCLUSION

The therapist's initial main role at the beginning of the CR for PTSD program is to engage the client, address any concerns and questions they have, motivate them to participate in the program, and prepare them for what is ahead. This can be accomplished in a single initial session in most cases or, depending on the treatment setting, as part of Session 1. From there, the therapist begins the Session 1 orientation to the CR for PTSD program.

Clients with SMI and PTSD are often sensitive to the stress of working on their traumatic experiences, and establishing a Wellness Plan to detect and respond to any increases in problematic symptoms or behaviors ensures the client's safety during the program and maximizes the chances of successful completion. Teaching Breathing Retraining provides clients with a skill they can immediately begin to use to reduce general distress, anxiety and other PTSD-related symptoms (including insomnia or sleep disturbances), and paranoia. These activities, which are usually accomplished in a single first session, set the stage for the subsequent sessions aimed at education about PTSD and, from there, cognitive restructuring.

6

Psychoeducation and Goal Setting

The three steps of providing an orientation to the Cognitive Restructuring (CR) for PTSD program, developing a Wellness Plan, and teaching Breathing Retraining (in the first session) are followed by delivering basic education about posttraumatic reactions, including the symptoms of PTSD, to educate clients and establish that PTSD is a common and treatable disorder. Providing this information can decrease the shame that people have when they believe their reactions to traumatic events reflect personal weaknesses and let them know they are not alone in experiencing PTSD symptoms. Learning more about PTSD and the fact that it is a treatable disorder can instill hope for change and harness motivation to actively participate in treatment. In this chapter, the components and content of the educational sessions are described, including tips for the provision of personalized and effective psychoeducation, as well as a structure and session timeframe for this portion of the intervention. In addition, strategies for collaborative and meaningful goal setting (which takes place as a capstone to the psychoeducational sessions) are detailed.

Following the brief introduction to psychoeducation provided in Session 1, we recommend two full sessions (Sessions 2 and 3) to teach and discuss the educational material, one focused on the core symptoms of PTSD and the second on associated problems. The therapist should strive to limit psychoeducation to two sessions even when working with clients who have significant cognitive impairments or severe symptoms (e.g., high levels of anxiety, distracting psychotic symptoms like voices) that require the material to be presented more slowly and reviewed more often. With such clients, the therapist should highlight the key points of the educational topics, help the client identify their most severe symptoms or problems based on information already gathered during the PTSD

https://doi.org/10.1037/0000423-006
Treatment of Posttraumatic Stress Disorder in Serious Mental Illness: The Cognitive Restructuring Program, by K. T. Mueser and J. D. Gottlieb

Checklist (PCL) assessments, and spend less time on other symptoms or problems. Additional sessions devoted to psychoeducation alone are unlikely to produce significant symptom relief, and the time is better spent teaching cognitive restructuring, the most critical ingredient of the CR for PTSD program. Additionally, clients continue to learn about their PTSD over the course of the program, even in the absence of more psychoeducational sessions.

At the end of Session 3, the therapist reviews with the client the impact of the traumatic events experienced, their PTSD symptoms, and associated problems on the client's life. The purpose of this review is to identify one or two areas of functioning that have been affected by PTSD that the client would like to improve over the course of participating in the program. In addition to playing a contributing role in the overall recovery process, the identification and solidification of such meaningful goals can further increase motivation to complete the program and can be a focus of collaborative work aimed at overcoming the effects of trauma. Work toward achieving these goals need not wait until PTSD symptoms have been reduced or eliminated but can occur simultaneously, with cognitive restructuring used to help clients deal with the negative feelings and perceived obstacles encountered when pursuing them.

PSYCHOEDUCATIONAL TEACHING TECHNIQUES

Psychoeducation—teaching people about their psychiatric illness and helping them relate this information to their own experiences—is a widely used therapeutic technique (Anderson et al., 1986; Ascher-Svanum & Krause, 1991). Psychoeducation involves helping clients understand and incorporate information about their psychiatric illness that has personal relevance and significance. The provision of skillful psychoeducation also serves two additional purposes:

1. Normalizing and objectifying the subjective: People with PTSD often feel as though their experiences and reactions to their traumas are highly unique, in the sense that the events they experienced are uncommon and that their psychological responses to these events are abnormal. As a result, they have emotions, thoughts, and actions reflecting the belief that "no one else has these problems and symptoms," which can be very alienating and maintain or exacerbate their PTSD symptoms. Psychoeducation teaches clients about the commonness of trauma, the frequency of PTSD as a common reaction to trauma, and the ways in which the specific symptoms often impact the daily lives of people with PTSD.

2. Undoing the fight-or-flight response: Similar to increased arousal, people with PTSD also have an exaggerated fight-or-flight response. This includes both physiological (e.g., heart racing as "preparation" for fight or flight), behavioral (e.g., bracing to avoid or flee a perceived threatening situation), and cognitive responses (e.g., thinking "I feel scared so I must be in danger"). As is the case with the Breathing Retraining skill, psychoeducation can help

clients decrease or undo this automatic response by helping them recognize it is a symptom of PTSD that often does not reflect that they are in actual danger.

Information about PTSD and associated problems is taught and discussed using two multitopic handouts containing worksheets that clients can utilize to identify specific symptoms or problems they have experienced. The therapist can give the relevant handout to the client at the beginning of the session, refer to it over the course of the session while paraphrasing and personalizing the material, and pause frequently for the client to write down their experiences, symptoms, or problems. The therapist can also take turns with the client reading the handout, discussing points, and exploring their relevance to the client's experiences. For clients who do not have good reading skills, the handout can be dispensed with during the session, and the therapist can instead teach some key concepts related to PTSD symptoms and discuss the client's personal experiences with these symptoms. Where possible, some simple key words can be written down on notecards to illustrate the main points.

Effective teaching about symptoms and problems follows a general pattern. The therapist describes a symptom or problem area, elicits the client's understanding and experience with that symptom, and has the client record their experience in the pertinent worksheet in the handout. While most of the time the psychoeducational component of this intervention goes smoothly and is well received by clients, some common challenges at times may arise. These, along with tips and suggested solutions, are summarized in Table 6.1.

COMMON REACTIONS TO TRAUMA I: PTSD SYMPTOMS (SESSION 2)

The therapist should be familiar with the client's primary PTSD symptoms (based on the initial PTSD assessments) prior to reviewing this material with the client. If major discrepancies appear between the client's report on the initial assessment and the discussion of symptoms in the psychoeducational session, the therapist should explore them. For example, some symptoms may have improved or worsened since the initial screening, or the client may have misunderstood a particular symptom during the assessment.

Psychoeducation

During Session 1, the therapist provides a brief overview of the components PTSD, primarily in the service of providing an introduction and orientation to the client (see Chapter 5, this volume). At the beginning of Session 2 (after developing the agenda for the current session and then reviewing the Breathing Retraining homework from the prior session), however, the therapist provides the client with the handout (Common Reactions to Trauma I: PTSD Symptoms) and begins a fuller discussion. When reviewing the different PTSD symptoms with the client, the therapist should pay particular attention to those symptoms linked to the criterion traumatic event(s) on which the diagnosis of PTSD

TABLE 6.1. Common Challenges and Solutions in CR for PTSD Psychoeducation Sessions

Challenge	Tips and solutions
Client becomes distressed when engaging in psychoeducational material due to intrusive reminders of traumatic events (i.e., emotional triggers).	• Initiate Breathing Retraining in the session. • Take a break outside the therapy room. • Skip over sections of psychoeducation, and hit only the highlights (the objective is for clients to learn the basics; they do not need every detail).
Client seems overwhelmed or does not understand all the material or concepts (due to educational/literacy level, cognitive impairment, and/or intrusive psychotic symptoms).	• Reduce and simplify worksheets. • Use and write down keywords and short phrases. • Skip over sections as noted above.
Client frequently veers into very detailed description of trauma and becomes distressed.	• Provide gentle but assertive redirection. • Balance hearing and validating the client's feelings with preventing unsystematic and upsetting exposure. • Initiate Breathing Retraining to assist in grounding and redirection.
Client gives limited responses to the therapist's questions and states that they already know about PTSD, despite clear evidence that they either have not received accurate information about PTSD or internalized the information.	• Check in about and gently correct any factual misconceptions. • Collaboratively negotiate about how much material to review and discuss. • Tie the material to the client's personal life (and goals) as much as possible.

Note. CR = cognitive restructuring; PTSD = posttraumatic stress disorder.

was based, while also exploring symptoms related to other traumatic events. Throughout these psychoeducation-based sessions, the therapist should be on the lookout for trauma-related thoughts and beliefs, which often emerge quite naturally during these discussions. These cognitions should be noted, either in the session with the client (e.g., "This sounds like just the sort of belief we might want to tackle together using the CR skills in our future sessions") or in written notes for the clinician to refer to later in the program using the Therapist Tracking Sheet for Client's Trauma-Related Cognitions in the Appendix.

The therapist's goal during psychoeducation is to gather helpful information about the client's experiences, giving the client the opportunity to share the basic nature of what happened and how it has impacted them, while making sure the client is comfortable and does not become overly distressed. This means that the clinician needs to take care to have this discussion without encouraging the client to describe— or veering into—the recounting of excessive details of the traumatic event(s). While some degree of discussion of traumatic events is common and therapeutic in the CR for PTSD program, extended focus on the events themselves is not part of the intervention (in contrast to prolonged exposure therapy). Clients may at times need to be reminded about this as the sessions progress, as during this session with Edmundo:

THERAPIST: I completely understand how what we are talking about brings up a lot and maybe a flood of upsetting memories. I'm here to help you with these, and what we do together in this program will help you cope better with this distress you are experiencing. I want to remind you that the purpose of this treatment is not to have you feel like you need to dredge up and recount lots of upsetting details. So we will work to understand how the trauma impacted you, but we'll also be careful to make sure that we do it in a way that keeps us in the present and isn't overwhelming to you. This will help keep us focused and help you learn more about your PTSD and ways to use our coping strategies with these symptoms. Does that sound OK to you?

To initiate the psychoeducation discussion in this session, the therapist introduces the topic to Edmundo:

THERAPIST: Today I want to give you some information about trauma and the ways clinicians and doctors determine whether someone has trauma symptoms. We can start by reading together some of these handouts that provide useful information about trauma and PTSD symptoms. We'll take some time to pause to discuss these topics so we can talk a bit about how these might line up with your own experience. We'll also begin to learn about some reactions that are common after experiencing a traumatic event. Today, we are going to start with what the specific symptoms of trauma and PTSD are for people in general and what those symptoms might be for you specifically.

Posttraumatic stress disorder (PTSD) is one diagnosis that can be used to describe some people's trauma symptoms. Some people who have experienced traumatic events may experience all of the symptoms of PTSD, whereas others may experience only some of them. During our last session, we talked a bit about PTSD and identified (some of) the traumatic event(s) that you've experienced and ways that has impacted your life. Do you remember us working on that last time?

EDMUNDO: Yeah, I do.

THERAPIST: You did a great job with those assessments and our discussion. Some of this you may already know from things you've read or conversations with other providers, but it is always good to review to make sure we are on the same page. Here's some background. The symptoms of PTSD can occur after the experience of any traumatic event. This could include experiencing physical or sexual abuse or assault, being in an accident or natural disaster, being in combat, or experiencing the sudden or unexpected death of a loved one, like your brother. Regardless of the specific event, the same types of symptoms can occur.

For PTSD to be diagnosed, the symptoms have to be present and severe for more than a month after the event occurred. There are four different groups of symptoms that are all part of having PTSD: (a) reexperiencing symptoms, (b) avoidance symptoms, (c) overarousal symptoms, and (d) negative changes in thoughts and mood. I'll explain each of these groups of symptoms, and we can talk about them some more. Any questions so far?

EDMUNDO: So does everybody who has had traumatic events develop PTSD? Like, are some people OK after having this stuff happen to them, but I'm just not OK for some reason?

THERAPIST: That's a very good question. No, not everyone develops PTSD. But we know that it's a pretty common response to trauma. About one in 10 people develops PTSD at some time in their lives, and the more trauma they have been exposed to and the more severe the trauma, the greater their chance of getting PTSD. And so given the kinds of things you have experienced, it does make sense that you would struggle with PTSD. It is not uncommon at all.

EDMUNDO: So I guess I'm not the only one you know of? Even other guys have it who weren't in combat or something like that?

THERAPIST: No, you are certainly not the only one, Edmundo. It's much more common than most people realize, and it is also more common than mental health professionals and researchers previously thought.

Let me tell you a little bit more about this, and then we can talk through it some more. Let's start with the first group of symptoms on the worksheet here: reexperiencing symptoms.

Reexperiencing Symptoms

Reexperiencing symptoms are among the most pervasive of all PTSD symptoms. Common reexperiencing symptoms are intrusive memories of the traumatic event, distress when exposed to reminders of the event, and nightmares. *Intrusive memories* are memories of a traumatic event that suddenly and unexpectedly come into the person's head (like a mental picture of the event), which can be both distressing and distracting, even when they last for only a second or two. Many clients mistake intrusive memories for flashbacks. The distinction can be made by explaining that unlike intrusive memories, flashbacks involve temporary loss of contact with the present reality and a momentary reexperiencing of the event as though it were occurring again. Flashbacks are rare compared to the other reexperiencing symptoms. Helping clients understand the difference between these two symptoms can help reduce catastrophizing about symptoms and fear of overwhelming distress and impairment, as the therapist does here with Leigh-Ann:

THERAPIST: The first type of PTSD symptoms involves reexperiencing the traumatic event. The most common way people reexperience trauma is by having thoughts or memories of the event just pop into their mind at odd times, like when they're doing regular things during the day. For example, a person could be waiting for the bus or doing dishes when out of the blue the memory pops into their mind, or they just start thinking about what happened to them for no apparent reason. Have you had intrusive thoughts or memories of your traumatic experiences?

LEIGH-ANN: Yeah, that happens a lot of the time. It's awful.

THERAPIST: What's that like for you?

LEIGH-ANN: Like you said, I'll be in the middle of doing something or maybe nothing at all, and suddenly the memory comes out of nowhere. It's weird and just stops me in my tracks most of the time.

THERAPIST: And what type of memory pops into your head? Is it just one memory or several different ones?

LEIGH-ANN: It's usually a memory related to when my friend's father was abusing me. Sometimes the memory is him opening the door to their bathroom late at night to find me. Sometimes the memory is him making me do stuff.

THERAPIST: And what's it like for you when those memories come up?

LEIGH-ANN: Oh, it's so awful. I totally freeze, and my body completely tenses up. I get superanxious, like I can't breathe all of a sudden, and I just try to put the thoughts out of my head. Which doesn't really work.

THERAPIST: Well, I want you to know that your reaction to those memories is a very common one. Most people find them really jarring and hard to shake when they happen. Let's take out our handout on PTSD symptoms, and you can write some notes about your experience with intrusive memories or thoughts.

Avoidance Symptoms

Avoidance symptoms are usually related to situations that trigger trauma-related thoughts or beliefs. Most clients are aware of some of their avoidance, but for some who experienced trauma early in their lives, it is so deeply ingrained into their habits and lifestyle that they are not aware they are avoiding thoughts, feelings, and situations that remind them of their traumatic experiences. This is particularly salient among clients with a history of interpersonal trauma (abuse, assault, domestic violence, etc.) who have over time gradually reduced their relationships and interactions with others and have become so chronically isolated that they end up living a life of almost complete solitude. Consider the following example with Leigh-Ann:

THERAPIST: The second set of PTSD symptoms is avoidance. People who have experienced trauma often try to avoid people, places, thoughts, and feelings that remind them of those events. It's easy to understand this, since people naturally avoid things that make them feel uncomfortable or anxious or afraid.

Let's talk about some of the specific ways people who have experienced trauma avoid things that remind them of those events. One way is that people may try to push thoughts out of their minds when a trauma-related thought pops into their head, such as trying to think of something else or trying distract themselves by listening to music or engaging in vigorous exercise. What things have you tried to do to get rid of thoughts about your trauma experiences?

LEIGH-ANN: Sometimes I just force myself to think of something different.

THERAPIST: And is that effective?

LEIGH-ANN: A little bit, sometimes. But it seems like thoughts and memories always come back, no matter how hard I try to escape them. And they get worse and worse and harder to ignore.

THERAPIST: Yes, that's a very common experience for people with PTSD. Is there anything else you've tried to do to avoid or get rid of those thoughts?

LEIGH-ANN: If I'm sort of doing OK, I'll play with my cat or turn on the TV, which takes my mind off things for a while. In my worst moments, I'll think about cutting myself or going out to track down some meth, even though I haven't used in a while now. It's still tempting.

THERAPIST: Those are some really good examples of how you try to avoid thoughts related to your trauma—some of which may feel healthier to you than others. I'm glad you are bringing all of them up though because one of our goals in this program is to help you increase your healthy and effective coping strategies and decrease the ones that might keep you stuck. Another kind of avoidance is avoiding activities or places that remind the person of their trauma.

Overarousal and Reactivity Symptoms

In contrast to reexperiencing and avoidance symptoms, overarousal symptoms often do not have an obvious relationship to the specific traumatic events experienced by the individual. However, these symptoms may be especially prominent in situations in which people are reminded of their traumatic experiences, as they are with Edmundo:

THERAPIST: The next set of PTSD symptoms involves physical arousal or tension. People who have experienced traumatic events often have difficulty sleeping, feel irritable or easily angered, and may be jumpy and have trouble concentrating. Do you ever have these overarousal symptoms?

EDMUNDO: Yes, like constantly it feels like that. My girlfriend tells me I'm like a time bomb. She never knows what's going to set me off.

THERAPIST: And what happens when you are set off?

EDMUNDO: It isn't pretty. Sometimes I yell at her or my kids, and then later I feel bad about it. When I know that I'm feeling that way, I just try to get away from everyone and isolate myself. There is no reason they should pay for what I've gone through. But then she feels like I'm ignoring her and the family.

THERAPIST: That sounds so hard. I can see you care a lot for your family and are trying to protect them. It can be difficult to know the best way to react when you are feeling really distressed.

EDMUNDO: Right.

THERAPIST: How about your sleep?

EDMUNDO: I'm up half the night. I just can't settle down and relax.

THERAPIST: And what effect does that have on you?

EDMUNDO: I'm exhausted most of the time, and that also puts me in a bad mood. Makes me want to crawl into a hole.

THERAPIST: I can understand how frustrating that must be. Some other common arousal symptoms include being easily startled and always feeling on guard or alert—like you're always looking over your shoulder to make sure you're safe.

Negative Changes in Thoughts and Mood

The fourth cluster of PTSD symptoms involves negative alternations in cognition and mood. These symptoms are related to having strong negative thoughts about oneself, others, or the world, inaccurate or distorted thinking about the cause or consequences of the traumatic event(s), or difficulties in remembering important aspects of the traumatic event. These alternations can lead the person to excessive self-blame and can cause chronic strong distressing feelings such as fear, guilt or shame, sadness/depression, and/or anger. Numbing symptoms are also part of this cluster, which include feeling detached from others, having difficulty experiencing positive emotions, or not enjoying previously fun activities. Discussion of this symptom cluster is especially important in the program, as it ties in closely with the type of CR work that will be done as the treatment progresses, which the therapist mentions to Edmundo during this exchange:

THERAPIST: The fourth set of symptoms is experiencing negative changes in thoughts and mood as a result of the trauma. People may feel that the world is completely unsafe or that they are bad people. They may also blame themselves for how the trauma happened or for how they responded to it, or they may just feel down or negative a lot of the time. Have you had any of these kinds of feelings or thoughts?

EDMUNDO: Honestly, I feel like I've been like that for a while now, ever since my brother died. Like, it was 'cause of me and all the stuff I got him into over the years in our neighborhood. And we had been in and out of contact, but the last time we talked we had an argument.

THERAPIST: It sounds like you might blame yourself for his death. Do I have that right? How are things with your mom? Are you able to feel close to her?

EDMUNDO: She says it's not my fault—that he made his own choices, that no one could have stopped him. She tries her best to console me, but I think she feels guilty too. When she cries and hugs me, I don't really feel anything, and then I feel bad about that. I just don't know how to be with people. The world is so f'd up.

THERAPIST: Yes, those are exactly the kinds of symptoms I'm talking about. You feel bad and detached from people you care about and guilty for all that's happened. Those symptoms are very common, especially after a traumatic event where someone close to you has died. You are not alone in having that kind of reaction. I know this has been very painful for you in your life, and I appreciate you sharing it with me. I can assure you that these are the types of feelings and thoughts we will be directly working on together in our future sessions.

Home Practice Assignments

By the end of the session, the therapist should be able to cover the prominent symptoms of PTSD in sufficient detail so that the client can identify which symptoms they have, most of which can be written down on the associated worksheets.

While a logical outside practice assignment between Sessions 2 and 3 might be to finalize or review the informational handouts and/or worksheets, we do not recommend this early on in the CR for PTSD program. It is often the case that this early discussion of the traumatic events in conjunction with the distressing PTSD symptoms can be emotionally triggering for clients in these psychoeducation sessions, especially because they have not yet learned the most powerful of the coping strategies in the program (cognitive restructuring). To prevent further triggering, distress, and potential avoidance or decreased motivation to continue in the program, it is suggested that clients not take home the handouts and worksheets following these psychoeducation sessions. Instead, the therapist can keep them in order to resume work together in the subsequent session. In cases where clients indicate they really would like to have the materials with them (to share with a supportive family member, partner, or friend, for example), then they should be encouraged to do so. This should involve some collaborative troubleshooting around how clients might manage any upsetting reactions they might experience by having this material in their personal space (e.g., they could enact elements from the Wellness Plan, put the materials out of sight, initiate Breathing Retraining in order to reduce emotional dysregulation, etc.).

For Sessions 2 and 3, it is instead recommended that the home assignment focus on Breathing Retraining practice. At this point, the goal should be for clients to practice this daily, and once therapist and client agree that the skill has been understood and properly learned, clients should begin to apply the skill in situations where they feel stressed or distressed or are experiencing anxiety or other PTSD symptoms. Clients should be encouraged to use the associated tracking sheets (Practice BRT Tracking Form 1: Nondistress Version; BRT Tracking Form 2: Distress Version) to continue to mark their progress and learn more about their patterns of distress.

COMMON REACTIONS TO TRAUMA II: ASSOCIATED PROBLEMS (SESSION 3)

Psychoeducation about common problems associated with PTSD uses the same basic approach as for PTSD symptoms, enabling clients to understand that many other problems they may be experiencing are common among trauma survivors with PTSD. Again, this serves to normalize those problems and instill hope that the program may improve them. This discussion also paves the way for a more focused discussion on how PTSD has affected the person's life and which meaningful areas of functioning the client would most like to see improved.

Psychoeducation

After reviewing the home assignment from the previous session with the client (Breathing Retraining practice and tracking), the focus of Session 3 can be introduced as follows:

THERAPIST: We talked last week about the four core symptoms of PTSD and
                  ways those have impacted you. Many people with PTSD also
                  experience other symptoms that interfere with their lives and
                  cause them distress apart from those four symptom clusters.
                  Today, we'll talk about some of these problems. First, people
                  with traumatic experiences typically have a range of different
                  upsetting feelings they are struggling with, such as depression,
                  guilt, and anger. Also, and this probably does not come as a
                  surprise, people with PTSD often have difficulties in their
                  relationships with other people. People sometimes use drugs
                  and alcohol to cope with their PTSD symptoms, which can
                  unfortunately lead to another set of problems and challenges.

Upsetting Feelings

When discussing common distressing feelings associated with PTSD, it can be
helpful to focus on "the big four" negative feelings (fear/anxiety, sadness/depres-
sion, guilt/shame, anger) as a way to help clients learn about the emotions they
experience. Here a therapist introduces the discussion of upsetting emotions:

THERAPIST: People who have PTSD often experience a range of distressing
                  feelings. The most intense negative emotions reported by
                  people who have had traumas include fear/anxiety, sadness/
                  depression, guilt/shame, and anger. These feelings are common
                  after experiencing a traumatic event. Let's discuss these four
                  distressing feelings in more detail.

The therapist should focus on the client's experience of these emotions in
daily living, whether or not they are clearly related to PTSD symptoms or the
traumatic event(s) itself. Fear and anxiety, both related to the traumatic event
and more generally, are (not surprisingly) very common in persons with PTSD.
Depression is the most common comorbid disorder in people with PTSD (Breslau
et al., 2000; Panagioti et al., 2012). The pervasive avoidance associated with
PTSD and the high level of arousal often make it difficult to enjoy activities
the person used to enjoy prior to the traumatic event(s). In addition, people may
feel sad when they look back on their lives and consider the losses related to their
traumatic experiences, such as the loss of innocence caused by childhood sexual
abuse, the loss or absence of love in a physically abusive environment, or the loss
of a loved one (O'Hare & Sherrer, 2011b). The therapist teaches and explores the
nature of Donata's co-occurring sadness and depression here:

THERAPIST: Other common reactions to trauma include sadness and
                  depression. After a trauma, people often feel less interested
                  in things they used to enjoy and have a hard time having
                  fun. People may feel hopeless or think about suicide. As we've
                  talked about earlier, it sounds like you've had some of those

kinds of hopeless thoughts. And you mentioned last week that you feel sad and depressed a lot of the time. What about being interested or uninterested in doing things?

DONATA: Yes, a lot.

THERAPIST: What's that like for you? Can you tell me a little more about it?

DONATA: I feel like there is no hope, you know? That I have no future. That there's no point in trying anything new or doing anything that's supposed to be fun.

THERAPIST: That must be very difficult to bear.

DONATA: I guess I am used to it, but it is. The voices say it too. Sometimes it seems like the hardest thing to do is to keep going on.

THERAPIST: I can understand how hard it must be for you. I've mentioned this before, but I want to say it again because it is important: I want you to know that I think that you're taking a very courageous and important step in dealing with your traumatic experiences by participating in this program for your PTSD. The skills that we will be focusing on can be helpful not only for your PTSD symptoms but also for your feelings of sadness and depression—and we'll be able to talk through a lot of that together to help you move forward.

Feelings of shame and guilt are common in trauma survivors, especially those with childhood sexual abuse (Feiring et al., 2002). It is important to identify these feelings as early as possible in treatment so that the therapist can normalize them to the client and also can be alert for opportunities when teaching cognitive restructuring to address and reexamine the beliefs underlying those feelings, as the therapist does here with Leigh-Ann:

THERAPIST: Another type of upsetting feeling people often experience after trauma is guilt or shame. People may blame themselves for what happened. Or they may think that they are weak and inadequate because they were not stronger in dealing with the trauma. Do you ever have feelings of guilt or shame about what happened to you?

LEIGH-ANN: I think about that a lot. I look back on the night I was raped—if you can call it that, I mean. I knew the guy. He was a neighbor, kind of a friend (so-called), and I saw him in the hallway of my apartment building when I was coming home from work late one night. The next thing I knew, he was forcing himself upon me. I tried to say no and push him off, but he wouldn't listen.

THERAPIST: Sometimes people find themselves blaming themselves when something like that happens. Do you find yourself doing that?

LEIGH-ANN: I shouldn't have had that third beer at the bar I worked at before I left. I should have been more forceful or fought more. I could have screamed.

THERAPIST: But you didn't.

LEIGH-ANN: No. I was afraid.

THERAPIST: Afraid of what?

LEIGH-ANN: That he was going to hurt me even more!

THERAPIST: That's very understandable. Your reaction is a very common one people have after being assaulted. They blame themselves for not acting differently. Is there anything else about this experience that you blame yourself for?

LEIGH-ANN: I think I should have been stronger in dealing with it after it happened. I could have reported him, but I didn't. I could have just learned my lesson and gotten on with my life, but I didn't. Instead, I just broke down and went into a depression—kind of fell off the grid of having a life. I just felt like between that and what happened to me with my friend's father a few years earlier, there was nothing I could do to fix myself.

THERAPIST: I understand. People often blame themselves for not coping with their traumatic experiences better. But just because you blame yourself, it doesn't mean that it is true and that you did something wrong. When we begin work on cognitive restructuring in the next sessions, you'll find that not all of the thoughts that lead to upsetting feelings—like self-blame or guilt—are totally accurate. And I'll be teaching you a skill for evaluating just how accurate those thoughts are and how to deal with them better.

Feelings of anger are also common in people with PTSD (Chemtob et al., 1997; Williamson et al., 2015). Sometimes anger is the dominant emotion and may consume the individual's thoughts about past traumatic experiences, as well as characterize how they respond to any perceived threats in their day-to-day lives. Clients may oscillate back and forth between anxious and angry feelings. For some individuals, the processing of traumatic experiences involves helping them deal with unresolved anger to move forward in their lives. Other clients may develop healthy and appropriate feelings of anger after their incorrect beliefs of responsibility for traumatic events have been challenged, and these feelings need to be dealt with. CR and Action Plan (Chapters 7–9, this volume) exercises and Payoff Matrix (Chapter 10, this volume) exercises can be directly applied to the processing and healthy coping with anger in later sessions.

Relationship Difficulties

People with PTSD can have relationship difficulties due to a wide range of factors, such as distrust of other people, problems with emotional and/or sexual intimacy because it triggers trauma-related memories, avoidance of people in general, or feelings such as anxiety, anger, shame, or depression. Discussing the effects of trauma on close relationships both normalizes these difficulties and identifies areas that clients are often strongly motivated to change (which can be connected to the goal-setting process that occurs at the end of Session 3).

Drugs and Alcohol

Drug and alcohol problems are common in people with PTSD (Goldstein et al., 2016; Lecomte et al., 2013), who often use substances to cope with or numb disturbing symptoms (Nishith et al., 2001), to serve as a sleep aid for insomnia, or to temporarily escape from the misery of their lives (Nishith et al., 2022). However, there are numerous negative consequences of substance use, including addiction and retraumatization (Gearon & Bellack, 1999; Mueser, Rosenberg, et al., 2002; Najavits & Hien, 2013).

While unhealthy substance use and addiction are common problems for people with PTSD and other serious psychiatric conditions, this is not the case for everyone. It is recommended that the therapist initiate at least a brief discussion about the client's current or past relationship with substances, but if it becomes clear that they have no history of or current problematic substance use, the therapist should feel free to move on to the next segment of the session. Where there is some clear history of associated substance problems, the discussion of substance use problems and PTSD can be initiated.

OTHER FUNCTIONAL DIFFICULTIES: WORK, SCHOOL, AND MANAGING PHYSICAL HEALTH

It is not unusual for people with PTSD to have a multitude of additional social, occupational functioning, and health challenges. Compared with persons with serious mental illness (SMI) alone, those who also have PTSD have higher rates of unemployment (Mueser, Salyers, et al., 2004; Ng et al., 2016; Russinova et al., 2018) and benefit less from evidence-based supported employment (Mueser, Essock, et al., 2004). Sometimes PTSD symptoms themselves (such as intrusive memories and avoidance) can interfere with getting or keeping a keeping a job or with successfully enrolling in and completing school. As an indirect result of PTSD, individuals may develop beliefs about their capabilities of performing work or school tasks successfully, of fitting in with other students or colleagues, or of dealing effectively with supervisors or professors.

People with PTSD also have more medical problems than those without PTSD (Pacella et al., 2013; Ryder et al., 2018), and this also holds true for persons with SMI (Calhoun et al., 2006; Mueser, Salyers, et al., 2004). Untreated PTSD can take a heavy toll on many areas of wellness. Similar to the manifestation of work and school problems, intrusive trauma-related thoughts and memories can be activated—in this case, as related to doctor visits and examinations—which can cause ongoing avoidance of medical appointments and therefore neglect of physical health needs and treatment. Furthermore, it can be a struggle for those with PTSD to consistently engage in a healthy lifestyle. Smoking, poor nutrition, sedentary behavior, and problematic substance use contribute to these problems.

Discussing these common areas of difficulty, using the worksheets for guidance, can be very validating for clients and can also serve to spark the potential creation of therapy goals to be collaboratively developed in the upcoming goal-setting segment of the session.

Associated Psychotic Symptoms

Although somewhat less common, hallucinations, paranoia, and delusions can also occur in people with PTSD who do not also have a psychotic disorder diagnosis (Braakman et al., 2009; Butler et al., 1996; Mueser & Butler, 1987; Shevlin et al., 2011). For example, a victim of a severe car accident may hear the voice of their deceased copassenger, or a rape survivor may develop paranoid thoughts about men watching her. These symptoms can lead to social isolation, suicide attempts, and/or odd or threatening reactive behavior. Psychotic symptoms, which are often associated with both societal and self-stigma, can be a source of considerable distress for the person experiencing them.

Some clients with a diagnosis of schizophrenia-spectrum disorder or mood disorder with psychotic features who have recently also been diagnosed with PTSD may wonder whether their initial diagnosis is incorrect or whether their psychotic symptoms and their associated consequences instead stem from their traumatic experiences and untreated PTSD. Further discussion of this topic and some strategies for addressing these concerns with clients are provided in Chapter 12 in this volume.

For individuals who have a long-standing psychotic disorder alongside PTSD, it is crucial to provide psychoeducation about hallucinations, delusions, and paranoia/suspiciousness and their linkages to the traumatic events that have been experienced. This can serve as an enormously validating and normalizing experience, as it greatly assists clients in making sense of how their earlier traumatic events may have contributed to or exacerbated their psychotic symptoms over time and impeded their overall functioning and goal attainment (Catone et al., 2015). Using the Hearing Voices and Other Distressing Experiences Worksheet as a guide, a discussion can be initiated similar to the therapist's with Donata as follows:

THERAPIST: I know that you had previously mentioned hearing some pretty frightening things going through your head over the years and that those have understandably caused you a lot of distress. What has that been like recently for you?

DONATA: Yeah, it's all the voices. Well, now really two people—screaming at me, telling me I am disgusting and that I shouldn't go out or come here or go on living even. I can't even think straight.

THERAPIST: I'm so glad you are sharing this with me, and I can tell it is something that has caused you so much pain and struggle. I don't know if anyone has ever talked to you about this, but for people who have had the kinds of experiences that you have had in your life, it is not that uncommon to hear things that others can't hear. And those voices can be extremely upsetting and scary.

DONATA: You mean that they are there because of what my family did to me when I was a kid and what happened in school growing up?

THERAPIST: Well, it's always hard to say what causes what for sure, but we do know that a lot of times people who have had these kinds of traumatic events often go on to hear voices later in their lives. And those voices can be incredibly distressing. Sometimes the voices even sound like the people who were involved in the traumatic event or say things related to the details of the trauma. Is that something you have noticed?

DONATA: If I think about it more, yeah, that makes sense. I don't know if I should tell you about them though so much. They say not to. But for a long time, one sounded like my older brother, and the other was this guy I went to school with. They say horrible things. I can't get them to leave me alone. It keeps me up all night sometimes.

THERAPIST: I know this is hard to talk about, and I totally understand that you may not feel like you can give more details. We can pause our discussion here and move to another topic and try some Breathing Retraining if that helps you feel more comfortable. What I can say is that it is not at all easy to live with that kind of thing all the time, and you certainly don't deserve to have to. Sometimes understanding that these voices may be connected to traumatic experiences can provide a little bit of relief. Also, as we move into our next sessions, where you'll learn the cognitive restructuring skill, we can also explore some ways to help you feel like you can make more sense of and cope better with the voices when they feel overwhelming. I hope that will be something that will provide further relief.

DONATA: Yeah, knowing a little more about how this is connected together might help. I guess I have to think about it more. But getting some relief would be good too.

OTHER TRAUMA-RELATED SYMPTOMS

Although psychoeducation for associated problems with PTSD focuses on the aforementioned topics, clients are often curious about other symptoms they have and whether these could also be related to their trauma. One common associated symptom is dissociation (Gershuny et al., 2003; Lewis-Fernández et al., 2002; Weinberg & Gil, 2016). People may feel temporarily disconnected from their bodies or the world around them and may "space out" during stressful times and not be aware of what's happening around them.

Difficulties in cognitive functioning are another common problem in people with PTSD (Brandes et al., 2002; Fan et al., 2008; Seow et al., 2016). These problems may be apparent in areas such as attention and concentration, memory, information processing, and planning. Distraction and preoccupation due to PTSD symptoms, such as intrusive trauma-related thoughts and exaggerated perceptions of danger, can make it difficult for people to perform important tasks such as work or school. For specific information on how to modify teaching strategies for clients with cognitive impairment, including those with cognitive impairment related to a schizophrenia-spectrum disorder, see Chapter 12 in this volume.

Wrapping Up Psychoeducation

Following the completion of the two sets of PTSD symptom descriptions and worksheets and the teaching about common associated symptoms, the therapist should help clients synthesize what they have learned during the psychoeducational sessions and what it means in terms of their own personal experiences. This enables clients to make better sense of their traumatic experiences, their PTSD symptoms, and ways those have impacted their lives. This discussion also serves to start the transition into the next phase of the intervention—cognitive restructuring—as the therapist goes through the How Trauma Affects Thoughts and Feelings worksheet with the client. Here, the specific types of distressing trauma-related thoughts and beliefs that clients have can be clearly delineated, further enhancing their understanding of how these cognitions are linked to their PTSD symptoms—as shown here with the therapist and Edmundo:

THERAPIST: Edmundo, you've done such an impressive job with me these past three sessions working to understand your experience with trauma and PTSD symptoms and ways that has impacted your life. We talked a good amount about how the gang and neighborhood violence throughout your childhood and adolescence and your brother's suicide have caused PTSD and the ways in which those events have led to some beliefs about the negative aspects of the world and some self-blame too. As we start to wrap up this segment of the program, I'd like us to summarize together some of the most important ways that your trauma and PTSD have impacted your thoughts and feelings. Getting this down on paper will really help us know specifically what to help you with as we start the cognitive restructuring portion of this intervention. Let's take a look at this worksheet, How Trauma Affects Thoughts and Feelings, together.

EDMUNDO: OK.

THERAPIST: The first part here asks about self-blame or self-criticism, which you and I have talked about a bit already. Let's get down on paper some of these types of thoughts that you find yourself thinking often. What should we write down?

EDMUNDO: Yeah, I have these all the time. You can write: "It's my fault my brother killed himself."

THERAPIST: Yes, I know that is one that you have on your mind almost constantly. During our last session, you had also mentioned something about how you view yourself for having gotten involved in the gang life in the first place.

EDMUNDO: Right—like, I'm a weak, screwed-up person for having been so susceptible to that lifestyle.

THERAPIST: OK, good, I've written that one down. Anything else that feels important? What about what you had said last week about doubting your ability to be a good father because of what you've gone through?

EDMUNDO: Yeah, "I'm damaged, and I'll never be able to be a good role model for my kids. I'm such a mess."

THERAPIST: Yes, from what you've said, I know that one causes you a lot of pain and is very related to what you experienced yourself growing up. We're getting a very useful list here. Really good work here, Edmundo.

For some clients, identifying specific PTSD-related thoughts comes easily, and they are readily able to conjure up these beliefs in these psychoeducational sessions. Other clients have a harder time recognizing particular thoughts they have regularly and may need the therapist's help in suggesting some common themes or actual specific thoughts that have been mentioned in these early sessions. The therapist may find it helpful to refer back to the Therapist Tracking Sheet for Client's Trauma-Related Cognitions to assist the client in identifying previously mentioned distressing thoughts that fit into the PTSD symptom categories in the written exercise. The finalized list of client thoughts on the How Trauma Affects Thoughts and Feelings handout should be saved for future use once the trauma-related CR sessions have been reached.

Exploring and Establishing Meaningful Personal Goals

Toward the end of the second psychoeducational session (Session 3) and before transitioning to the cognitive restructuring portion of the intervention (Session 4), the therapist should explore the client's functional goals for treatment in areas such as relationships, leisure activities, self-care, and role functioning. As previously noted, from the time that the client's PTSD has been confirmed, the therapist is on the lookout for understanding how traumatic experiences and PTSD have influenced their functioning and adjustment. Once the client understands the nature of PTSD and has had the opportunity to talk about and contemplate the effects of trauma and PTSD on their life, the time is ripe to explore areas of functioning that they would like to see improved as a result of treatment. Discussion about and establishment of meaningful personal goals as they pertain to PTSD treatment also serve to advance client's overall mental health recovery plan.

During the psychoeducational sessions, some clients talk openly about how their traumatic experiences and PTSD have affected their lives and interfered with attaining personal life goals. Other clients may talk more about their symptoms but are less clear about the effects of PTSD on their functioning or goals. Many clients with PTSD either do not appear to have functional goals, have trouble articulating them, or believe they could never achieve them as long as they have PTSD symptoms. For clients who want a better life but have felt stymied by their PTSD, it can be enlightening to be encouraged to talk about which areas of life they most want to improve and to be informed that progress toward these changes can be accomplished in this program while working on PTSD symptoms.

There are many opportunities to talk about the effects of trauma and PTSD on the client's functioning during the psychoeducational sessions, and it is quite natural for the therapist to inquire how those symptoms and problems have interfered with important aspects of daily living. Even if a client reports impaired functioning in a particular area, the therapist should not assume that improving in this area is an important personal goal but should inquire as to which areas of functioning the client most wants to change.

Sometimes clients are afraid to set personal goals and cannot imagine pursuing such goals as long as they have PTSD symptoms. It may be helpful to ask these clients to talk about how their lives would be different if they had not experienced their traumas and did not have PTSD. Getting people to imagine their lives without PTSD can begin the process of identifying areas they care most about changing. The purpose of this discussion is to identify the specific ways in which PTSD currently is a problem for the individual to harness motivation to continue to participate in treatment to better manage it (see Goal-Setting Worksheet for the CR for PTSD Program worksheet).

Once goals have been collaboratively identified and elaborated upon using the worksheet, the therapist should review them with the client and emphasize that the CR for PTSD program can help them make progress toward them. To initiate the exploration of goals, the therapist can ask a few probe questions to explore how PTSD has affected the person, based on the information gathered during these two psychoeducation sessions (as well as on the highly endorsed items from the completed PCL). A great deal of exploration is usually not necessary. Usually 5 to 10 minutes is sufficient, including work on the worksheet, as is shown here with Leigh-Ann:

THERAPIST: Let's spend a couple of minutes talking about how PTSD has affected you, based on some of what we discussed with these psychoeducational worksheets. One of the symptoms you described is having frequent memories of your abuse pop into your head. What's that like for you?

LEIGH-ANN: It's horrible. I hate it. I sometimes try to make them go away by cutting myself. But the relief is only temporary, and the memories keep coming back.

THERAPIST: That must be very difficult to cope with. How about your sleep? How do your difficulties sleeping affect you?

LEIGH-ANN: Well, I'm awake most of the night, and then I usually drift off when it's finally morning. I only get a few hours every night, and I always feel groggy—like a zombie.

THERAPIST: I completely understand, and that's such a common struggle for people who have had experiences similar to yours. How about avoiding things that remind you of your trauma that you had noted earlier? Can you share an example of that in your daily life?

LEIGH-ANN: I avoid most public places. I do my shopping very early in the morning because I don't like other people looking at me.

THERAPIST: That makes you feel uncomfortable?

LEIGH-ANN: Yes, especially when men look at me.

THERAPIST: That makes complete sense, given what you have experienced. I want you to know you are not alone in that. And how have your symptoms interfered with doing things that you'd like to do and enjoying life?

LEIGH-ANN: What life? I can't seem to hold down a job. I'm a nervous wreck. I'm super lonely. It's like I want female friends, but I just feel so anxious and distrustful of everyone, I can't even have anyone in my life, it feels like.

THERAPIST: I know how hard this has been for you, and I want to let you know that, together, we can help you with a lot of these things that have been so difficult for so long. The skills in this program can make a big difference in terms of helping people to feel like they can have their life back and move toward the things that are important to them, like having a better work life and starting to get closer to people.

Let's work together on getting some of these important goals down on paper. This is the Goal-Setting Worksheet for the CR for PTSD Program, and it will serve as a list of a few things that you'd like to see be different in your life in the areas that are most important to you. And we'll work on these things together throughout this intervention. But also, these goals that we create together here will help to contribute to your overall mental health recovery going forward. How does that sound?

In subsequent sessions, these goals should be followed up on and progress toward them reinforced and celebrated. This follow-through on goals maintains the thread of goal work over the course of the intervention and is an important strategy to maintain and increase the client's motivation to continue to address distressing PTSD symptoms. Obstacles to goal attainment (i.e., thoughts of self-doubt, physiological anxiety and avoidance around specific activities) should be addressed using the CR, Action Plan, and Breathing Retraining skills, as applicable.

Home Assignments

As the format and the material covered in the session on associated problems related to traumatic experiences are similar to what is covered in the previous session on PTSD, a comparable home assignment can be agreed upon. As mentioned earlier, the focus should ideally be on ongoing Breathing Retraining practice. At this point, it is suggested that clients start to try out initiating the skill during instances where they feel distress or other PTSD symptoms. The therapist should continue to encourage ongoing daily use of the skill and tracking of patterns and observations of the impact of Breathing Retraining on anxiety and other upsetting symptoms.

CONCLUSION

Providing information about PTSD and associated difficulties both normalizes clients' reactions to traumatic events and helps them develop a fuller understanding of how these experiences specifically have affected their lives. This knowledge can alleviate some of the self-blame that trauma survivors often have about their responses to trauma, while instilling hope that the CR for PTSD program may improve not only their PTSD symptoms but also other problems. This expectation is further reinforced at the end of the psychoeducational sessions by discussing and delineating meaningful and personalized functional goals the client would like to make progress toward in the context of the program (and as contributions to their overall mental health recovery plan). These sessions help solidify the therapeutic relationship with the client and serve as a foundation for beginning work in subsequent sessions on cognitive restructuring, the cornerstone of the CR for PTSD program.

7

Cognitive Restructuring I

The Thought–Feeling Model and Common Styles of Thinking

Cognitive restructuring (CR) is a broad set of strategies aimed at helping people change inaccurate thoughts or beliefs that lead to negative feelings and distress (Beck et al., 1979). The basic theory underlying the use of cognitive restructuring for posttraumatic reactions is that how people interpret and respond to traumatic events shapes their thoughts and beliefs about themselves, other people, and the world in general (Dalgleish, 2004; Ehlers & Clark, 2000; Ehlers et al., 2022). Trauma-related beliefs may develop soon after a traumatic event has occurred (e.g., "no situation is safe and I could be attacked at any time" after a violent robbery), gradually over a period of time during which multiple traumatization occurs (e.g., "men can't be trusted" over the course of childhood physical abuse and a subsequent assault in adulthood), or after a long period following traumatic events (e.g., "I am shameful and did 'bad' things because I didn't prevent myself from being sexually abused as a child"). These beliefs (or schemas) shape individuals' perceptions of the world, their associated emotional reactions (such as a heightened perception of threat leading to chronic feelings of anxiety), and their behavioral responses (such as avoidance or attempted numbing via substance use).

However, these trauma-related schemas are largely inaccurate and often destructive perspectives that cause a great deal of distress and exacerbate posttraumatic stress disorder (PTSD) and other psychiatric symptoms. In some cases, individuals cling to beliefs that may have been accurate in the past but no longer are (e.g., the belief that "the world is an unsafe place" for a child raised in a physically abusive environment). In other cases, the schemas are understandable but

https://doi.org/10.1037/0000423-007
Treatment of Posttraumatic Stress Disorder in Serious Mental Illness: The Cognitive Restructuring Program, by K. T. Mueser and J. D. Gottlieb

exaggerated beliefs based on a traumatic experience that shattered the person's assumptions about the world (e.g., inflated perceptions of danger in a person who was the victim of a violent crime). For still others, the beliefs are wholly inaccurate and were formed in the aftermath of trauma as part of the individual's attempts to understand and create meaning out of the experience (e.g., a woman's belief that she was responsible for her childhood sexual abuse because she experienced some sexual pleasure from the abuse and did not try to stop it).

Teaching individuals how to identify, investigate, and challenge trauma-related thoughts can correct these inaccurate beliefs and ameliorate the negative feelings associated with them. Cognitive Restructuring in the CR for PTSD program is taught to clients as a self-management skill for dealing with common negative emotions related to PTSD, such as anxiety, depression, guilt, or anger. The initial focus of cognitive restructuring is on helping clients learn how to use this skill to cope with any type of negative feelings they experience, in general. As clients become more skilled at cognitive restructuring, the focus gradually shifts to identifying and challenging core trauma-related beliefs that underlie their PTSD symptoms.

In this chapter, we provide guidelines for how to introduce the concept of cognitive restructuring to clients across Sessions 4 and 5, first presenting the Thought–Feeling model and then teaching and practicing the first level of CR: the Common Styles of Thinking (CST). These techniques are illustrated via therapist dialogues with the client Donata, and outside practice strategies are discussed.

"Cognitive Restructuring I" is aimed at teaching clients first about the relationship between thoughts and feelings (Thought–Feeling model) and then about ways to recognize, evaluate, and challenge CST, common logical errors that occur (such as jumping to conclusions) when people draw conclusions about specific events before there is sufficient evidence. These errors are often referred to in the cognitive behavioral therapy (CBT) theory and treatment literature as "dysfunctional" or "distorted" thinking. However, we have chosen to instead call them "common styles" for a few reasons: (a) to more generally normalize this type of thinking as something "that everyone does," regardless of whether they have a psychiatric diagnosis; (b) to increase the likelihood that clients will be more willing to acknowledge their own struggles with CSTs; and (c) to depathologize and destigmatize this experience specifically for those with serious mental illness, who are often told that their thoughts, feelings, behaviors, reactions, and so on are incorrect, flawed, or not based on reality. That said, when introducing the idea of CST in these sessions, it is nevertheless important to highlight that these patterns of thinking are in fact problematic and unhelpful and should be examined more closely, in that they often cause unnecessary or exaggerated distress that contributes to PTSD and other symptoms.

Beginning cognitive restructuring with a focus on the Thought–Feeling model and explicating the CST gives clients a tool they can immediately grasp and begin using to cope with their distressing feelings and challenge the thoughts associated with them.

"Cognitive Restructuring II" (Chapter 8, this volume) builds upon the CST by teaching the 5 Steps of Cognitive Restructuring (CR). The 5 Steps of CR is a user-friendly self-management method for identifying core thoughts and schemas that contribute to negative feelings and reactions and for systematically evaluating the evidence for and against those thoughts. The 5 Steps of CR method is a more powerful and comprehensive cognitive restructuring skill because it helps people pinpoint core beliefs related to their traumatic experiences, methodically evaluate and weigh their accuracy, and then potentially modify them accordingly. Prior to moving on to introducing and teaching the 5 Steps of CR, typically two to three sessions devoted to the CST skill (including the teaching of the Thought–Feeling model and CBT Triangle) are advised.

Cognitive Restructuring I: The First CR Session (Session 4)

We recommend that cognitive restructuring be started in the fourth session, after the client has learned and practiced Breathing Retraining (BRT) and has an understanding of the nature of PTSD symptoms and associated problems. CR can be started earlier if feasible but should not be delayed past the fourth session unless the client is in crisis (see more on timing in this section).

The typical agenda for Session 4 is as follows: (a) review the home assignment (BRT practice) and questions related to Session 3, (b) readminister the PTSD Checklist–5 (PCL-5; and the depression inventory if using) and discuss score(s) and any changes, (c) introduce the Thought–Feeling model, (d) introduce CST and review and practice it, and (e) plan home assignment to practice BRT and use the Common Styles of Thinking Worksheet.

Readministration of the PCL-5

As mentioned in previous chapters (see Chapters 3 and 5, this volume), routine monitoring of PTSD symptoms and depression should be conducted with all clients in the CR for PTSD program, starting with baseline screening for eligibility and including readministering the PCL at the beginning of every three sessions, starting with Session 1. Given the strong link between PTSD and depression, we also recommend (where possible) that clinicians administer a brief self-report depression inventory like the Beck Depression Inventory–II (Beck et al., 1996) with the same frequency as the PCL-5.

We recommend beginning the first cognitive restructuring session (Session 4) with this assessment. This provides a good indication of the level of distress experienced by the client at the beginning of cognitive restructuring, which can be used to evaluate the effectiveness of the client's ability to use the skill over subsequent sessions. The review of recent PTSD and depression symptoms can also prove useful for teaching cognitive restructuring in upcoming Sessions 5 and 6, where the therapist can then refer to specific highly endorsed items from the PCL or Beck Depression Inventory–II ratings to explore whether they reflect particular CST and/or could be used as examples in practicing the 5 Steps of CR.

When readministering the PCL-5 in all sessions of the program, it is important to remind clients of the specific index trauma that was identified during the screening process and ask them to keep in mind that particular incident while they complete the symptom checklist. This allows for consistency and continuity and serves as a way to effectively track progress toward reducing PTSD symptoms related to that specific distressing traumatic event.

Once the client has completed the assessment form(s), the therapist scores and then briefly reviews the results with them, including a short discussion about whether any changes in symptoms have occurred since the previous administration of the measures (e.g., in Session 1). Improvements in symptoms can be briefly explored (e.g., What does the client attribute these changes to? Has the use of Breathing Retraining reduced anxiety?). Further guidelines for how to discuss changes in assessment scores across different sessions of the CR for PTSD program are provided in Exhibit 7.1.

EXHIBIT 7.1

Discussing PCL-5 (and Other Assessment) Score Changes Across Intervention Sessions

Readministration notes

1. Be sure that the client is completing the PCL-5 based on the index trauma (perceived most distressing event) that had been previously evaluated during the screening process.

2. Once the measure(s) is completed, score it quickly, and have a brief discussion with the client about the score(s), comparing them to the screening score(s) and Session 1 scores.

3. Discuss any changes in the scores over time and the client's attributions about those changes.

4. Provide the following feedback, as applicable.

If client's scores have decreased

1. Ask the client what they attribute this decrease to, probing to ascertain whether certain intervention elements played a role thus far (i.e., learning that what they experienced for years actually has a name and is somewhat common; using Breathing Retraining to manage anxiety or other symptoms, etc.).

2. Praise the client's efforts in the program, and encourage continued review of psychoeducational materials and ongoing use of Breathing Retraining.

If client's scores have stayed the same

1. Normalize this, as it is very common for clients' symptoms not to change too much at this point in the intervention after only three sessions and prior to initiation of the powerful CR skills.

2. Praise the client's efforts in the program thus far, and encourage continued Breathing Retraining use as you move into this next CR phase.

(continues)

EXHIBIT 7.1

Discussing PCL-5 (and Other Assessment) Score Changes Across Intervention Sessions   (*Continued*)

If client's scores have increased

1. Normalize that it is not unusual for scores to increase and that there is no cause for alarm, given that the recent confrontation of trauma-related material in the psychoeducational sessions can bring PTSD symptoms more to the surface.

2. Ask the client what they might attribute this increase to, and initiate a brief discussion around this topic.

3. Note how positive changes sometimes don't start to happen until CR is underway. Gently correct any assumptions that increased scores at this phase are indicative that the program is "making things worse" or "not going to work."

4. Encourage the client to stick with Breathing Retraining practice and use, and remind the client of their newly established meaningful personal goals (from Session 3) to maintain treatment motivation.

5. If needed, refer to the Wellness Plan developed in Session 1, and/or consider creating a specific distress coping plan with the client and the treatment team if needed.

Note. PCL-5 = PTSD Checklist–5; CR = cognitive restructuring; PTSD = posttraumatic stress disorder.

After the client's symptom ratings have been discussed, the therapist and client review the home assignment from the previous week (daily Breathing Retraining practice and tracking, including during times when the client is triggered with PTSD symptoms or distressed in any manner). The therapist can also answer any remaining questions the client has about associated problems related to PTSD. The remainder of the session is devoted to introducing the rationale for cognitive restructuring, explaining the Thought–Feeling model (Understanding the Thought–Feeling Model With the CBT Triangle handout) and then teaching the client how to start to recognize and challenge the CST (Common Styles of Thinking Information Sheet). At the end of the session, a home assignment is developed with the client to practice using the CST via the Common Styles of Thinking Worksheet to cope with any negative feelings or stressful situations that occur during the upcoming week.

Introducing Cognitive Restructuring

The transition to this phase of the intervention can be introduced as follows:

THERAPIST: Up to this point in our time together, we have worked on two things to help you with your PTSD symptoms. First, you have learned Breathing Retraining as a way of dealing with anxiety and tension. Second, you have learned about the symptoms and associated problems of PTSD and ways they've affected your life the most. By understanding that your reactions to traumatic events are common ones that other people also have, we can begin to help you learn better ways of handling these problems and feeling less distressed. Today we are going to begin working on a skill called cognitive restructuring. We briefly talked about this skill in the beginning when I was describing this treatment to you, and now we are ready to start in on this phase of the program. *Cognitive restructuring*—which we can call CR for short—is a strategy for dealing with the upsetting feelings that often accompany traumatic reactions.

The Thought–Feeling Model

After laying the groundwork for cognitive restructuring, the therapist engages the client in a discussion of about how thoughts can influence feelings (the Thought–Feeling model). To aid in helping the client learn and understand this model, clinicians can use the Understanding the Thought–Feeling Model With the CBT Triangle handout, as, for example, in the following discussion with Donata:

THERAPIST: We've talked about how people with PTSD often experience a wide range of negative feelings. Some of the most common upsetting emotions include fear and anxiety, sadness and depression, guilt and shame, and anger. And we will definitely be working on those feelings together during your time in this program. But first, I'd like to talk with you about how all of our emotions—whether or not they are related to traumatic experiences—are actually linked to our thoughts and about how if we are feeling upset, chances are we are thinking a thought that is making us feel upset. Those upsetting thoughts and feelings often lead to us to react in a certain way in any given situation. This is called the Thought–Feeling model. I'd like to give you a general example about how this works. OK?

DONATA: Yeah, I guess that is OK. I definitely need help with my emotions and the things I think about.

THERAPIST: Yes, of course. We all do, really. The first step is understanding how the patterns work. So let's use an example of how our thinking affects our feelings in a situation—one that doesn't have to do with your personal experience this time so that you can get the gist. First, I'm going to show you this handout called Understanding the Thought–Feeling Model With the CBT Triangle. At the top here, there's a description of what we just talked about. And then below, you can see the triangle. Here's an example that we can fill in together.
    Pretend you were sleeping at night and were awakened by a sound of a scratching noise at your window. You think,

"There must be a burglar trying to break into my bedroom." How would you feel? And how would you react? What would you do if you were having that thought?

DONATA: I'd be afraid. I'd think he was going to hurt me. And I guess I might try to hide in the bathroom? I don't know.

THERAPIST: Right. It would only be natural to be afraid if you thought someone was trying to break into your apartment. Let's write that thought in the thought section here: "There's a burglar trying to break in." And let's write the feeling in the feeling section—"afraid or fearful." And in the behavior part, let's write, "Hide in the bathroom." See how those three areas are connected? If you have the thought that someone is trying to break in, it is totally understandable that you would then feel afraid and take action to hide and protect yourself.

But now, let's pretend that you were lying in bed and you heard that same scratching noise at your window. But this time you remembered that you let your cat out before you went to bed, and you think, "Oh, that must be the cat. She wants to come in." Now how would you feel? What would you do?

DONATA: Well, I haven't been able to have a cat in a long time, but if I did, I would feel maybe a little annoyed if she'd woken me up. Or maybe I'd be happy to see her and know that she's OK. I'd just get up and let her in.

THERAPIST: Right. If you thought that scratching sound was your cat at the window, you'd respond differently, maybe by being a bit annoyed or maybe by being glad to see her. Let's fill in this alternative thought and then feeling and behavior on the sheet as well. All of this is an example of how your specific thoughts determine how you feel and how you react, even if the identical event occurs—the scratching noise at the window at night. Until you look out the window and know what's there, you don't know whether it's your cat, a burglar, or something else. If you thought it was a burglar, you'd be afraid, but you would have a totally different reaction if you thought it was your cat. See what I mean?

DONATA: Yes, that makes sense to me. I always think the worst thing, though, 'cause the worst thing seems to happen a lot, I guess. That's, like, who I am.

THERAPIST: Thinking of the worst-case scenario is very common in people who have PTSD and who have had the kinds of traumatic experiences you have. We're going to talk more about that very thing in a few minutes, actually. First, though, here's another example to make sure we've gotten the hang of the idea of the Thought–Feeling model and CBT triangle. Let's imagine you are walking down the street and see someone you know walking with a few other people across the street. You say hello to her, but she doesn't say anything back. How would you feel if that happened?

DONATA: Well, I think I'd be hurt. Why shouldn't she say hello to me? I said hello to her.

THERAPIST: OK, that's good. Let's jot that down in the feeling section of the triangle. So you'd feel hurt. And why would you feel hurt? What would you be saying to yourself that would make you feel hurt?

DONATA: Maybe that she doesn't like me. Or she thinks she's better than me.

THERAPIST: Right. I'll write down those two thoughts in the thought section of the triangle here. So if you thought your friend didn't like you or was deliberately ignoring you, you'd feel hurt. That makes sense, right? Now, let's say that you noticed that when your friend didn't say hello to you, she was talking to the other people, and you thought, "She must not have heard me say hello." How would you feel then?

DONATA: I'd probably just shrug it off. I don't think I'd feel anything in particular.

THERAPIST: Would you feel hurt or offended?

DONATA: No, there wouldn't be any reason to, I guess.

THERAPIST: Right. If you didn't think your friend was deliberately ignoring you, you wouldn't feel bad about her not saying "Hello." I'll write that in here in the thought section too, so you can see the difference in how those different types of thoughts about the same exact situation can cause very different feelings. With one thought, you end up feeling upset, and with the other thought, you don't. This is an example of how thoughts determine your feelings. How people react in a situation depends on their thoughts about it. You'd feel bad if you thought your friend was ignoring you but not if you thought she hadn't heard you.

Discussing either of the aforementioned examples (hearing a cat scratching at a window or seeing a friend walking across the street) and illustrating these patterns on the Understanding the Thought–Feeling Model With the CBT Triangle handout are usually effective at helping the client understand the relationship between thoughts and feelings. If the client understands the first example, the therapist can move on to talking briefly about how life experiences shape thoughts and feelings. If the client has difficulty grasping the first example, the second one should also be used to illustrate the point.

In general, the more cognitively impaired the client is, the more important it is for the therapist to provide concrete examples of extreme and different thoughts in a particular situation and to discuss the different feelings associated with each thought in order illustrate how one's thoughts influence one's feelings in the situation. Using the written worksheet is key to assisting clients in understanding this concept and the ways it applies to them. This lays the groundwork for realizing that not all thoughts that a person has in a particular situation are equally accurate, which sets the stage for evaluating the accuracy of thoughts and the CST skill. For clients with more intact cognitive functioning, the therapist may elect to brainstorm with them a variety of different thoughts someone might have in a given situation (such as in the "walking down the street" scenario) and then consider the different feelings associated with each thought. Encouraging clients to consider different possible thoughts for a particular situation establishes that there are multiple perspectives for any particular situation and that different feelings are associated with those perspectives.

When the relationship between thoughts and feelings has been established, the therapist next explains how personal life experiences, including traumatic ones, can affect the way people perceive and think about situations they experience throughout their lives. It can be helpful to mention the previously completed How Trauma Affects Thoughts and Feelings handout (used in Session 4; see Chapter 6, this volume) to tie together these themes for the client. However, the therapist should keep in mind that the goal of the current session is to help the client gain initial understanding about the Thought–Feeling model and the CST. Therefore, it is important to avoid digressing into trauma-related material and/or the client's retelling of the event—both of which can get the client off track of learning and practicing this CR skill. Typically, a minute or two of "connecting the dots" between the Thought–Feeling model and the client's previously noted trauma-related thoughts and feelings is sufficient.

THERAPIST: So, given any situation that you experience, your feelings depend on what you think about that situation. What makes people think the way they do?

DONATA: I don't know. Most of the time I'm not even aware that I'm thinking. Or I just know it's bad thinking.

THERAPIST: That's a good point. Often the thoughts that we have in situations are automatic. You might not be aware that you're having these automatic thoughts, but you're having them nevertheless. One of the things that shape the thoughts we have, including our automatic thoughts, is our life experiences. Over the course of your lifetime, you've learned ways of understanding or thinking about things from your different experiences, including your traumatic experiences. Do you remember last session when we filled in that handout called How Trauma Affects Thoughts and Feelings and we talked about the ways in which the trauma you experienced has shaped your thoughts, beliefs, and feelings over time?

DONATA: You mean like what my parents did to me?

THERAPIST: Yes, exactly. Over time, those ways of thinking about yourself, other people, or the world grow stronger and develop into more strongly held beliefs. And these beliefs continue to shape the way you look at things. As you very smartly noted a minute ago, you may not even be always aware of what your beliefs are or how they influence your reactions to the world around you.

DONATA: Right. That's for sure.

THERAPIST: Every one of us has thoughts and beliefs that affect the way we look at the world. However, here's the thing: These beliefs are often not entirely true or true at all, even though people may take them for granted because they've thought that way for so long. This can often be the case when people have had traumatic experiences, which can lead to negative and unhelpful beliefs about themselves, other people, or the world. And of course these negative beliefs lead to the negative feelings that we've been talking about, such as anxiety, guilt, and depression. Those are exactly the sorts of things that we are going to learn more about now as I start to talk with you about something called the Common Styles of Thinking.

The Common Styles of Thinking

After the therapist has taught the Thought–Feeling model, illustrated it with the CBT Triangle in a collaborative discussion with the client, and briefly reviewed the connection with one or two examples of how the client's traumatic experiences have influenced their thoughts and associated feelings, the CST are introduced. The focus here is teaching CST as a strategy for examining the thoughts underlying negative feelings and changing them when they are inaccurate or unhelpful. The CST skill can be conceptualized as both a precursor to the next level of CR— the 5 Steps of CR—as well as a concrete and useful stand-alone skill. Note that any trauma-related beliefs that are identified via this initial discussion should be added to the Therapist Tracking Sheet for Client's Trauma-Related Cognitions for use in later sessions.

THERAPIST: So we know that thoughts and beliefs contribute to the feelings that we have in our everyday lives. We know that traumatic and other life experiences affect these thoughts and beliefs. And we know that the thoughts and beliefs we have are sometimes not accurate. Learning how to examine and challenge thoughts and beliefs that lead to distressing feelings is an important tool for helping you deal with those feelings and process your life experiences. Our work together from here will start to involve helping you learn how to identify and challenge thoughts and beliefs that lead to upsetting feelings.

I'd now like to teach you a helpful method for identifying when your thinking is leading to unpleasant feelings and for evaluating whether your thoughts are accurate or not. This method involves learning about the Common Styles of Thinking and the common inaccurate, unhelpful ways of thinking that lead to distressing feelings. Everyone engages in these CST sometimes, but some people with traumatic experiences are more prone to these styles of thinking than others. This method is helpful for managing any kind of stress or upset you may feel in life, not just things that are related directly to your traumatic experiences. As I'm teaching you this skill today, we'll first focus more on how to use it generally and less on how to apply it to your specific traumatic experiences, which will come later. How does that sound?

DONATA: Good. To be honest, backing off the stuff about my family and the abuse for the rest of the session might help me think better.

Using the Common Styles of Thinking Information Sheet, the therapist then briefly explains what each style is and why it is inaccurate and then helps the client identify examples of situations in which they may have engaged in that specific style. An example of introducing and discussing the CST is provided as follows:

THERAPIST: Let's spend a few minutes talking about what the Common Styles of Thinking are and why each one is inaccurate. The first style is all-or-nothing thinking. With this style of thinking, you look at a situation in absolute terms and believe that everything is either all one way or all the other way, with nothing is in the middle. For example, let's say a tech company worker named Bill tried to do a really good job on something, put a lot of solid effort into it, but made a few minor mistakes. If Bill believed that he was a failure because he didn't do a perfect job, that would be all-or-nothing thinking. How do you think Bill would feel if he put in a lot of effort but thought he was a failure because of a few minor mistakes?

DONATA: Pretty bad.

THERAPIST: That's right. So why would Bill's thinking that he's a failure in this situation be an example of all-or-nothing thinking? Why would that be inaccurate?

DONATA: Because he did a good job. Just because it wasn't perfect doesn't mean he didn't do a good job.

THERAPIST: Right. Doing a pretty good job or even an excellent job with a few minor mistakes is in-between doing a perfect job and being a failure at the job. In this situation, what might be a more accurate way for Bill to think about how he did?

DONATA: I don't know. He could maybe say, "I did a pretty good job. Nobody's perfect."

THERAPIST: And if you were Bill and had that other, more accurate thought that you just noted, how would you feel about your job performance instead?

DONATA: I think I'd feel pretty decent about it.

THERAPIST: Good. So you can see that catching and changing these CST can reduce upsetting feelings that are a result of inaccurate thinking. Can you think of an example of when you engaged in all-or-nothing thinking? Maybe something that happened this past week?

DONATA: No, because I don't consider myself a total failure, but I'm not perfect either.

THERAPIST: What about what you told me in our last session when we were talking about exercise and your doctor hoping you'd start a fitness program? And you said that you've thought that if you don't exercise every day, then what's the point? Do you think that could maybe be an example of all-or-nothing thinking?

DONATA: I don't know. But yeah, I see what you mean. Like, if I'm not perfect with exercising or doing exactly what the plan says, then it's not worth doing at all. When I think that way, then I don't end up doing anything at all, and I'm probably worse off. And I end up feeling like my weight gain from the meds is

	something I can never, ever change. Then I feel ashamed and don't want to go back to the doctor.
THERAPIST:	Right, exactly. If it's OK with you, I'm going to jot that down in the space here in the all-or-nothing section. So why might the thought "If I don't follow an exercise program 100%, it's not worth doing it at all" not be completely accurate?
DONATA:	Because maybe every little bit can help? Like, I was exaggerating before saying that "there's no point in trying if I can't do it all?"
THERAPIST:	Yes! That's exactly it. All-or-nothing thinking often involves distorting the truth, since the person sees only the extremes and doesn't recognize the in-betweens. And when you think of it differently and start to recognize the in-betweens of never exercising and perfectly following an exercise program, does that change how much shame you feel about not exercising and your belief that maybe you could exercise?
DONATA:	I guess if I thought that every little bit can help, then I'd feel less ashamed and a little more, like, hopeful or maybe like I could give it a try. More motivated?
THERAPIST:	Excellent. And I agree completely that having that new thought would very likely change your feelings about trying out some type of exercise program. This is a really good example of how all-or-nothing thinking works. It also is an example of how to look into a thought like this to see how and why it is not totally accurate and to start to be able to look at it differently. Really great job with this. Let's keep going to the other examples and see what we can come up with. The next Common Style of Thinking is catastrophizing. Catastrophizing is when you think or assume that the absolute worst thing—the worst-case scenario—is going to happen, no matter what. For example, a person who got into a bad car accident would think that every time they got into a car or onto a bus, they would probably be in another accident, even though that is actually very unlikely, from a statistical way of looking at it. Can you think of times when you have used catastrophizing, Donata—maybe even in this past week? Let's start with a basic example related to your daily life for now.

Given the packed agenda of Session 4 (including the readministration of the PCL-5 and subsequent discussion of symptom changes), there is usually not enough time for the therapist to review all of the CST categories on the worksheet and also develop a home assignment with the client at the end of the session. Thus, after going over several CSTs in the same fashion as described earlier, the therapist can save the rest and complete them in the next session (Session 5). The goals of this current session are to help acquaint the client with the idea of the CSTs, learn some examples of how others tend to use them, and understand the concept of how identifying a particular CST and thinking it through can help a person come up with a more accurate thought and therefore reduced distress. A secondary goal is to assist clients in starting to identify recent times in their own lives when they have had thoughts that fall into CST categories. Helping the client personalize the CST experience in session will set them up for practicing this strategy on their own during the upcoming week using the Common Styles of Thinking Worksheet.

Outside Practice/Home Assignment for Session 4

At the end of the session, the therapist develops an assignment with the client to practice recognizing CSTs related to distressing feelings. The Common Styles of Thinking Worksheet provides separate columns for clients to (a) briefly describe the upsetting situation, (b) write the negative feeling and thought they experienced, (c) identify the CST related to that thought, and (d) describe a more accurate way of looking at the situation.

The therapist should guide clients through at least one written worksheet example in session so that they know how to fill in the tracking form. It should be explained that having a negative or distressing feeling is the first signal that the person may be engaging in a CST. Any sign of stress, distress, or negative feeling should serve as a light bulb that the client should try using this skill with the accompanying worksheet as soon as possible. Given that this is usually the first time the client has been exposed to this type of CBT-based skill and the goal is to enhance comfort with and mastery of this CR strategy, they should be strongly encouraged to practice using it in situations in which they are experiencing relatively minor levels of negative feelings rather than initially trying to use the skill with very distressing or trauma-related situations. As such, therapists should instruct clients to try out the skill using situations that they find merely stressful, annoying, or irritating when first practicing the CST skill. Similarly, as the current focus is on familiarization with the Thought–Feeling model and recognizing CSTs as they come up in daily life, it should be noted that the last worksheet column (generating a new, more accurate thought) can be attempted but that clients should not worry if they cannot think of a more accurate thought as this section will be worked on more thoroughly in future sessions. It is suggested that clients be encouraged to try to complete one entry per day on the worksheet, based on any situations that cause them stress or negative feelings.

THERAPIST: Donata, you've done a great job today of coming up with examples of situations in which you may have engaged in a CST. You can see how the different Common Styles are inaccurate and how distressing feelings are associated with them. You've also seen how challenging and correcting the Common Styles of Thinking can reduce distress and improve mood. When people take a more balanced look at an upsetting situation by trying to catch and correct themselves when engaging in an inaccurate Common Style of Thinking, they usually don't feel as badly as before they examined their thinking.

Let's come up with a plan for you to continue this work on your own and for you to get some practice identifying Common Styles of Thinking in your day-to-day life. We'll do an example together with the worksheet, and then we'll talk about how to help you practice this each day this week prior to our next session.

THE FOLLOW-UP SESSION ON THE COMMON STYLES OF THINKING (SESSION 5)

The next session begins with a fairly detailed discussion of the home assignment to practice using the Common Styles of Thinking Worksheet. The therapist and client should review the completed worksheet together, and the therapist should ask any clarifying questions about the examples the client worked on, including whether the skill practice resulted in any reduction of distress.

As is the case with all home assignments in the CR for PTSD program, any efforts by clients to try the skill should be praised and discussed, even if they did not complete any written worksheets. In these cases, it can be helpful to use the worksheet in the moment to help clients re-create a few situations so that they have the experience of seeing how the process works on paper. If the client reported getting stuck during the week on any attempted examples, this provides a good opportunity for the therapist to guide the client through the example together in the session. This level of written review and collaborative practice helps the clinician to better understand the client's current comprehension of the CST skill as a way to gauge further teaching and practice of the CR skill in the session.

Continued CST Teaching

Assuming that all of the CSTs were not reviewed in the previous session, the remaining ones are taught and discussed in this session (Session 5). The bulk of the session is spent on additional teaching and practice recognizing and modifying the CST. At the end of the session, another home assignment is agreed upon for the following week. Some helpful tips to consider when continuing to teach the CST to the client are summarized in Exhibit 7.2.

EXHIBIT 7.2

Tips for Continued Teaching of the Common Styles of Thinking (CST) After Introduction in Session 4

- It is not necessary that the client understand or be able to accurately recognize all of the different types of CSTs, as there is significant overlap among their definitions (e.g., all-or-nothing thinking and overgeneralization).

- The primary goal is for the client to just get the gist of all the CSTs: "Not all of our thoughts are accurate, and if a thought falls into one or more of the CST categories, that means it may not be 100% accurate and is worth examining more closely."

- After reviewing the list of CSTs, it is sometimes helpful for the therapist to focus on 1–4 CSTs that most resonate with the client to reduce information overload and enhance understanding.

- If client has difficulty identifying examples of upsetting situations from their own life when learning CSTs, explore whether the client can think of a time when someone they know used a CST. Taking the immediate focus off the client and putting it on someone else can increase comprehension and eventually willingness to acknowledge using CSTs.

- The therapist can offer their own (nonoverly personal) examples of their own use of CSTs if helpful or if the client is reluctant or seems stuck.

Following is an example of the therapist continuing to facilitate the client's practice of recognizing and challenging CSTs:

THERAPIST: I can see from your home assignment sheet that last Thursday you caught yourself using a Common Style of Thinking when your case manager was late to come pick you up the other day. It looks like you did a great job getting started—recognizing that you were upset and using that as a cue to try out the skill. Excellent.

DONATA: Yeah, I got stuck, though. I was stressed.

THERAPIST: Totally understandable. This is still a new skill, so it is perfectly normal to get a little stuck. Why don't we walk through this example together? Let's review what you wrote here in the first column—the situation.

DONATA: OK. Vern was really late, more than 30 minutes and I panicked.

THERAPIST: OK, so we have that situation written in there. It sounds like your emotion was panic or anxiety? Is that right?

DONATA: Yeah, both.

THERAPIST: Yes, good. We've got both feelings down here now. So let's review the thought you wrote down here.

DONATA: I was sure somebody had attacked him or something terrible had happened. He's usually on time for me.

THERAPIST: If you were having that thought, it makes perfect sense that you were very anxious. That must have felt pretty frightening.

DONATA: It was. I always think something has happened if someone is late.

THERAPIST: So it sounds like you may have caught yourself using a Common Style of Thinking. Did you catch yourself in the moment, or did you recognize it later?

DONATA: A little of both, I guess. At the moment, I was so scared, and all sorts of things started going through my head about what must have happened to him. I was getting more and more panicked. But as I was thinking about what might have happened, I remembered our session last week talking about these Common Styles. I knew from that discussion that I often jump to conclusions and panic because of the abuse, or I think the worst is going to happen, even when it usually doesn't. So I kind of remembered all of this stuff we talked about here but didn't know what to do from there exactly.

THERAPIST: I'm so glad you thought of that in the moment and made that connection, even if it was hard to come up with the exact next steps or the specific Common Style of Thinking. And you were also right on point remembering that a lot of this panic is related to your past trauma. That is something we will definitely be addressing together and helping you with in future sessions. Let's work together on a particular situation. What do you think might be the Common Style of Thinking in this situation, based on your thought, "Something terrible has happened to my case manager because he is late to pick me up?" We can look at the Common Styles of Thinking Info Sheet together if that would help.

DONATA: Um, maybe catastrophizing or that other one—overestimation of risk? Not sure. There's a lot of these.

THERAPIST: Yes, you are right. There are several. And some do definitely overlap. I think either one of those—catastrophizing or overestimation of risk—would be a good fit. Tell me why you picked them.

DONATA: Well, catastrophizing because it's like coming to the worst possible reason right away. And then the other one because it's, like, just because he's late doesn't mean something as awful as him getting beat up happened, maybe?

THERAPIST: Yes, very good! And so if you realize that your thought is a Common Style of Thinking, what does that tell you about your thought that your case manager got beaten up?

DONATA: That it may be an exaggeration—or not totally true or accurate.

THERAPIST: Yes, exactly! So let's see if we can help you formulate a new way of looking at this situation for this last column of the worksheet—the more realistic thought. Were you able to think about it any differently at the time or now?

DONATA: Well, in the moment, I thought of all the reasons people have been late in the past, including Vern—even though he is usually on time—and that made me feel a little more relieved, I guess. That helped me clear my head a little. He ended up getting there about 40 minutes late. He said his other client had an emergency, so he had to make several urgent phone calls. He said he was sorry for not letting me know, but he was tied up on the phone, so I said it was OK.

THERAPIST: It sounds like you were able to think of a more realistic way of looking at the situation. That's so important. If we were to put that into a thought and write it on the worksheet here, how might we word it?

DONATA: Um, maybe something like, "It is maybe not the case that something terrible happened to my case manager. He has been late a few times in the past, and he has a busy job with lots of people he takes care of, so he has to run around a lot sometimes, which can make a person late."

THERAPIST: Yes, that sounds good. And when you review that new thought, how do you feel now? And how did recognizing your thinking style affect your feelings?

DONATA: Better, a little less panicked. More clear and calm. In that moment, even. But definitely now. Now I see it was unlikely that he was in danger or that something bad had happened to him.

THERAPIST: That's a really good example of how catching yourself using a Common Style of Thinking can be helpful and how thinking it through later on can help even more. Great job working through this one.

In the context of teaching the CST skill, the therapist should also explain and reiterate as needed that experiencing negative emotions is a sign that the person may be engaging in a CST but that not all unpleasant feelings are due to inaccurate thinking. Sometimes it is perfectly appropriate to have a distressing feeling in a situation. For example, if someone is riding in a car with a reckless driver, it would make sense to feel anxious. Therefore, the therapist helps clients see that the goal of identifying CSTs is to catch ourselves thinking inaccurate thoughts in situations that unnecessarily lead to high levels of distress. The therapist can then briefly mention that in future sessions clients will learn an additional skill related to solving real-life problems (Action Planning), with a focus on situations when their distress is caused by upsetting thoughts that are actually accurate (Chapters 8–9, this volume).

ADDITIONAL STRATEGIES FOR TEACHING THE COMMON STYLES OF THINKING

Several other teaching strategies are effective for helping clients learn how to recognize their upsetting thoughts and feelings, identify frequently used CSTs, and work toward modifying these inaccurate thought patterns to start to reduce general distress. These strategies are useful in both Sessions 5 and 6 and in later sessions as needed. Some common challenges emerge during the initial teaching of this CR skill that can be addressed using specific techniques, as described and illustrated next.

Helping Clients to Identify Thoughts and Feelings

In most cases, the CR for PTSD program will be a client's first real exposure to the concept of the Thought–Feeling model (and cognitive restructuring), and so many people will not have had the experience of systematically investigating their own thoughts and feelings and ways those are related. Understandably, clients sometimes mix up thoughts and feelings. Sometimes clients are able to identify upset feelings such as anger and fear but have difficulty tapping into and articulating the specific thoughts underlying those feelings. Other times, due to the emotional numbing that often occurs in PTSD, clients may have difficulty identifying the specific negative feelings they are having in an upsetting situation but be aware of what they are thinking. The Guide to Thoughts and Feelings Information Sheet handout can be used during these initial CR sessions to help clients make the connection between specific upsetting feelings and the types of thoughts that are typically associated with them, and the handout also can be used throughout the remainder of CR for PTSD program when clients have difficulty identifying their thoughts or feelings in a distressing situation, including during the subsequent teaching of the 5 Steps of CR. This handout can be introduced as follows:

THERAPIST: In order to deal with upsetting emotions, we need to pinpoint our thoughts or beliefs that resulted in the upsetting feeling. One clue to what we are thinking about is the nature of the upsetting feeling. This sheet—the Guide to Thoughts and Feelings handout—summarizes the thoughts associated with common distressing feelings.

For example, feelings of anxiety or fear are related to thoughts of being threatened. Feelings of guilt and shame are related to thoughts or beliefs of having done something wrong. Depression or sadness is related to thoughts of having lost something. Feeling angry is related to thoughts of having been wronged by someone else.

Once these concepts have been introduced in the Guide to Thoughts and Feelings Information Sheet, the therapist can use the handout in an ongoing way to help the client identify specific upsetting thoughts and feelings for exploration with the CST skill:

THERAPIST: So we've identified the stressful situation you found yourself in at the grocery store last week when it was very crowded and you noticed the voices [hallucinations] starting to say mean things to you. What's the next thing we do here: identify your upsetting feeling and then your thought, right?

DONATA: Yeah, the voices started in on me. I was starting to panic and freak out. I got superanxious. But I don't know what I was thinking at the time. I was just so overwhelmed, you know?

THERAPIST: I totally understand. We had talked about how when the voices act up, it's hard to focus. Sometimes it's hard to know what thoughts you are having. That's very common. Let's break down things together a little bit to see if we can help you with what you were thinking that was so upsetting at the time. So, you know that you were feeling panicky and anxious. It sounds like you were feeling afraid, based on what you've shared with me before, right? Now that you've pinpointed your feelings here, let's have a look at the Guide to Thoughts and Feelings and consider the questions next to the feelings of anxiety/fear. Did you think that harm might come to you [pointing to the handout and reading from it]?

DONATA: Yeah, the voices were telling me so—that I would be in danger.

THERAPIST: OK, so the main thought that led to feeling anxious was thinking that something bad was going to happen. What did you think might happen?"

DONATA: Well, the voices were the ones saying it, and then that got me thinking, "I'm not safe here. I can't handle this."

THERAPIST: So let's get that thought down on paper: "I'm not safe here. I can't handle this." It makes perfect sense that having a thought like that would make you incredibly anxious in the moment, right? Very good job identifying that here with me. Now that we are clear on the thought, let's see if we think it is a CST.

The Guide to Thoughts and Feelings Information Sheet can also be used to help the client distinguish between feelings (anxiety, guilt, depression) and thoughts ("I'm no good"). Encourage the client to use the words "I feel ..." when talking about feelings and "I think ..." when talking about thoughts. Normalize the fact that it takes practice to separate thoughts and feelings but that learning how to do so will pay off in terms of overcoming distress.

Shaping the Client's Ability to Identify More Accurate Thoughts

After a CST has been identified, a new and more balanced thought is sought, when possible. As previously noted, it may be difficult for clients to develop new and more accurate thoughts given their lack of experience and practice with CR, but developing such thoughts is a an important component of the CST skill. By developing a more accurate and more believable thought to replace the inaccurate, distressing thought (a CST), individuals gain some relief from their distress through a reduction in their negative feelings. This reduction in distress is the primary reinforcement for the client using the CST skill (i.e., negative reinforcement) and therefore the major motivation for practicing the skill and gaining mastery over it. Thus, it is important for the therapist to help clients come up with a new and more accurate thought in situations in which they have recognized their upsetting thought is a CST.

When initially teaching the CST skill, after the client has recognized that a distressing thought is a CST and is therefore inaccurate, the therapist can use Socratic questioning to help the client come up with a more accurate thought for the situation. This can include discussing reasons why the distressing thought is inaccurate, which can naturally lead to identifying more accurate (and less distressing) thoughts. If the client experiences significant difficulty early on identifying new and more accurate thoughts, even after such questioning, the therapist can suggest some alternative thoughts and inquire whether the client thinks they are more accurate and more believable. Sometimes actively helping clients come up with more accurate thoughts by offering examples helps them get the idea of how the process works and facilitates learning how to do it on their own.

When a new thought is developed, it is critical that the client believes that this thought is more accurate than the old one it is replacing. Clients often come up with new thoughts that are only slightly more accurate than the old ones but that still appear to the therapist to be inaccurate or exaggerated. However, rather than having a lengthy debate about the overall accuracy of the new thought, the therapist should instead focus on reinforcing the client for modifying the original thought even if the change is small and should draw attention to the benefits of the change in terms of reduced distress related to the new thought even if the benefit is slight at this point. This shapes the client's ability to identify and modify these thinking patterns through modest changes in the accuracy of their thinking (and semantics/language of the new thought itself) and therefore contributes to associated reductions in distress. Each time clients successfully correct their thinking and experience some relief in distress, however minor, they are reinforced for using the skill and more likely to use it again in the future.

For example, the client in the earlier dialogue may have initially believed "Something terrible has happened to my case manager because he is late to pick me up," and after some consideration, she may have been able to recognize this thought as catastrophizing (and/or overestimation of risk). However, even after recognizing that her initial thought was not completely accurate, she might have still believed that it was very possible that her case manager had been harmed in some way, leading to the new, "more accurate" thought that "There is a good chance that my case manager is in danger, but there might be some other reason he has not come to pick me up yet." Although technically this new thought is still most likely inaccurate, if it reduced at least some of the client's distress and panic, it would serve as a positive step in the right direction toward teaching the client how to modify CST-based thoughts. In addition, a slightly modified and more accurate thought can also function as an interim version that, with further guidance from the clinician, can eventually lead the client to an even more accurate thought, such as, "He is probably not in danger. He has been a late a few times before."

Focusing on (and reinforcing) small changes to inaccurate thinking avoids problems that often occur when the therapist tries to convince the client to make more dramatic changes in thinking, for two reasons. First, clients are more likely to own small changes in their thinking than larger changes that occur after a major debate with the therapist; that is, they are more likely to think that they are responsible for making these small changes themselves, which both makes the new thoughts more believable to them and reinforces their self-efficacy in using the skill. Second, therapists cannot win every debate they have about the complete accuracy of clients' thoughts, so when they are unsuccessful at convincing the client to make a major change in a belief, they lose the opportunity to demonstrate the utility of the CST skill through making more minor changes in inaccurate thinking (and therefore more modest reductions in accompanying levels of distress). These strategies are equally helpful in later sessions, as the therapist assists the client in evoking, challenging, and modifying long-held trauma-related and core beliefs (see Chapter 9, this volume).

MOVING ON TO TEACHING THE 5 STEPS OF COGNITIVE RESTRUCTURING

Typically, after about two sessions (Sessions 4 and 5) of working on the Common Styles of Thinking, the therapist can go forward to introduce and teach the 5 Steps of CR (in Session 6). In deciding when to proceed to the 5 Steps of CR, the therapist should evaluate a few variables, based on the client's progress with the CSTs. It is appropriate to transition to introducing and teaching the 5 Steps when the client has accomplished the following:

1. Demonstrated the ability to connect a current upsetting feeling with a specific thought;

2. Shown that they can identify and categorize their thoughts as CSTs (even if they don't always choose the specific CST that the therapist would identify);

3. Articulated understanding that if one of their thoughts falls into a CST category, the thought may not be 100% accurate and is worth looking into; and

4. Demonstrated some capacity to use the CST skill on their own in session and, ideally, independently via written home assignments between sessions (or plausible verbal report).

After two sessions of CST work (Sessions 4 and 5), if the client still does not sufficiently grasp the basic concept or is unable to use it to some extent on their own, a third session (Session 6) should be devoted to the CST skill, focusing on the written in vivo practice of identifying recently used CSTs related to stressful or upsetting feelings or situations that have occurred. After that additional session, regardless of the client's full grasp of the skill, the therapist should move on to teaching the 5 Steps of CR. Some clients find the 5 Steps of CR an easier skill to learn than the CST skill, as the 5 Steps tend to progress more linearly and allow for a more thorough, concrete examination of evidence for and against one's thought (see Chapter 8, this volume).

CONCLUSION

Cognitive restructuring is the main skill taught to clients in the CR for PTSD program for managing upsetting feelings and for identifying and correcting distressing thoughts, including trauma-related beliefs that underlie posttraumatic reactions. The introduction to cognitive restructuring involves first teaching clients the Thought–Feeling model and the CBT Triangle, which shows that thoughts and beliefs influence feelings and that recognizing and modifying inaccurate distressing thoughts can reduce those upsetting emotions and reactions. The CST skill is then introduced both as a stand-alone skill and as a precursor to more comprehensive CR work that takes place in future sessions. The purpose of the CST skill is to (a) normalize (and destigmatize) the ways in which people often distort information when they interpret different situations (particularly those with a trauma history and PTSD), leading to ongoing distress and problems; and (b) help clients learn the first steps needed to modify inaccurate thinking and therefore upsetting emotions and symptoms.

Teaching clients how to recognize and to change CSTs begins the active process of introducing CR as a self-management skill for dealing with any and all negative feelings. Helping clients practice the CST skill in Sessions 4 and 5 and developing home assignments to use the skill on their own can begin to provide relief from the severe distress experienced by many trauma survivors. The most fundamental goal of introducing CR in this way is for clients to begin recognizing that thoughts underlie their feelings and that not all of those thoughts are completely accurate. Helping the client to understand these two points and to begin recognizing their own use of CSTs in their day-to-day life are crucial steps toward learning CR as a self-management skill for dealing with distress directly related to PTSD symptoms in future sessions.

8

Cognitive Restructuring II

The 5 Steps of Cognitive Restructuring and Action Plans

Teaching clients how to recognize and challenge Common Styles of Thinking (CST; Chapter 7, this volume) provides them with a first-step, preparatory cognitive restructuring (CR) tool that can be used immediately to deal with any upsetting feelings. Many clients experience some relief within just one or two sessions of learning how to use the CST skill and continue to benefit with further practice in later sessions and on their own. However, despite these advantages, the CST skill (given its brevity and introductory nature) also has limitations as an approach to cognitive restructuring that make it less potent on its own at identifying and changing beliefs underlying many distressing feelings, including trauma-related beliefs underlying PTSD symptoms.

First, while the CST skill is effective at initially helping people identify thoughts underlying distressing feelings and recognize when these thoughts are inaccurate, it is common to have difficulty replacing those thoughts with more accurate ones since the skill does not teach people *how* to evaluate the accuracy of their thoughts. The CST skill relies primarily on people getting the gist of how common but inaccurate ways of thinking in different situations can lead to distressing feelings, which can enable them to recognize when their thoughts may be inaccurate and to consider alternative and more accurate ones. While it is useful for clients to have the general ability to recognize when their thinking may be inaccurate, teaching them specific skills for evaluating the accuracy of their thoughts becomes more important when it comes to identifying alternative and more accurate thoughts and selecting which new thought is most accurate.

https://doi.org/10.1037/0000423-008

Treatment of Posttraumatic Stress Disorder in Serious Mental Illness: The Cognitive Restructuring Program, by K. T. Mueser and J. D. Gottlieb

A second limitation of the CST skill is that although it can be effective at reducing distress in a wide range of situations, because of its brief nature it is less helpful for identifying and addressing the underlying trauma-related schemas or beliefs that lead to PTSD symptoms. While using the CST skill may reduce negative feelings such as depression, anxiety, and guilt, which can also impact PTSD symptoms, clients can get greater benefit from CR that more explicitly targets trauma-related thoughts and beliefs. This can be accomplished by teaching clients how to explore their more general upsetting thoughts in order to identify deeper, underlying, and/or core beliefs. *Core beliefs* are basic, global, and deeply held beliefs about oneself, other people, and the world as a whole. Common (negative) core beliefs—for example, "I'm completely worthless," "People only want to hurt you in life," and "The world is a totally dangerous place"—generally develop over time as a result of life experiences. These types of beliefs, not surprisingly, are often highly influenced by past traumatic events (see Chapter 9, this volume, for more on working with core beliefs).

A third limitation of the CST skill is that it is effective primarily in situations in which distressing feelings arise from inaccurate, maladaptive thought processes. While it is very useful at the outset to help clients identify these patterns, the CST skill does not provide guidance for dealing with upsetting situations that do not appear to be the result of inaccurate thinking. For example, someone who received an eviction notice from their landlord might quite reasonably be upset, and dealing with the situation effectively would require more than just examining and potentially changing some of their thoughts about receiving the notice. Learning effective strategies for responding to situations in which there is a genuine threat to the person's safety or well-being is especially important for preventing ongoing interpersonal victimization.

The 5 Steps of CR skill builds upon the CST skill while also overcoming its limitations as just described. The 5 Steps of CR is a step-by-step skill for identifying and examining the thoughts and beliefs underlying distressing feelings and then either correcting those thoughts when they are inaccurate or making a plan to remedy the stressful situation when the thoughts are accurate. The 5 Steps of CR include the following: (a) describe the upsetting situation, (b) identify the negative feeling experienced in the situation, (c) identify the most distressing thought or belief related to that feeling, (d) evaluate the thought by considering all the evidence supporting it and all the evidence against it, and (e) take action by either changing an inaccurate thought to make it more accurate or developing a detailed plan to deal with the situation.

In this chapter, we describe the transition from teaching and practicing the CST skill to introducing the more comprehensive 5 Steps of CR. Included here are guidelines for when and how to initiate the 5 Steps (and the associated Action Plan skill), strategies for how to teach each component, and tips for how to enhance initial and ongoing client understanding and practice of the 5 Steps both in session with the therapist and outside the sessions.

INTRODUCING THE 5 STEPS OF CR

The 5 Steps of CR skill (see the 5 Steps of CR worksheet) is typically introduced in Session 6, usually one to two sessions after introducing, teaching, and practicing the CST skill. (In some exceptions to this timeframe, a third CST-focused session is indicated; see Chapter 7, this volume, for details.) The 5 Steps should be introduced toward the beginning of a session, following the agenda setting and the review of the home assignment on using the CST skill, to provide sufficient time for client and therapist to work through an entire example of the steps together. It is important for clients to experience some reduction in distress during the session to demonstrate the utility of the skill. This can harness their motivation to learn and practice it in future sessions and eventually to apply it to highly distressing trauma-related beliefs.

THERAPIST: Today we're going to continue working on cognitive restructuring. For the last several sessions, we've talked about how your thoughts are connected to your feelings. We have also talked about how your life experiences, including traumatic ones, affect your thoughts and feelings. We've practiced the Common Styles of Thinking (CST) skill, and you've put in a lot of good effort and made progress in learning how to recognize and change your own CSTs that lead to distress. So now you know what it's like to get relief from examining your thinking when you feel upset. That's been our goal so far, and you've done a great job.

Today, we are going to continue working on understanding how your thinking influences your feelings by focusing on another related skill for dealing with distress. This skill builds on the CST skill and is called the 5 Steps of Cognitive Restructuring or the 5 Steps of CR. Let's go through the steps together to see how they work. We can work on a recent situation in which you experienced some distress.

For the first demonstration and practice of the 5 Steps of CR, the therapist should try to select a situation in which the client experienced strong negative feelings that both the clinician and potentially the client recognize were clearly out of proportion, suggesting the presence of inaccurate thoughts or beliefs that can be readily disputed and successfully changed at the end of the demonstration. Although the 5 Steps of CR can also be used to help the client deal with distress due to problematic life situations rather than inaccurate cognitions, focusing initially on negative feelings related to inaccurate thoughts builds more directly on the CST skill the client has just learned, making it easier for them to grasp the 5 Steps skill and achieve the similar predictable benefit of rapid relief from their negative feelings following the change in the upsetting thought. As with teaching the CST skill, ensuring that the client gets immediate relief from a distressing thought when the therapist is first teaching the 5 Steps of CR reinforces the client's use of the skill, increasing their motivation to practice it on their own for home assignments and onward.

The therapist has several options for selecting a first practice example. If the client recently completed a home assignment to practice the CST skill, the therapist can select an example from the client's worksheet and use it to demonstrate the 5 Steps of CR, knowing in advance that the client ended up identifying their thought as a CST and therefore as inaccurate. For example, if the client indicated on a home practice worksheet that they felt anxious when their supervisor said he wanted to talk with them but were then relieved to recognize that their feelings were due to catastrophizing thoughts, the therapist could use that situation to demonstrate the 5 Steps of CR.

Another option is for the therapist to focus on a time in a recent session when the client described a situation that resulted in upsetting feelings where their reaction appeared to be out of proportion to the situation itself, again suggesting the presence of inaccurate thoughts that could be corrected when demonstrating the 5 Steps of CR.

Yet another strategy the therapist can use is to identify a situation from the client's attempts to use the CST skill at home where they began the skill but did not finish it or got stuck somewhere trying to use it. While using one of these situations may be less of a "sure bet" in terms of clear inaccuracy of thinking compared with the previous scenarios, it has the benefit of providing more assurance that the client is still distressed about the situation, providing an opportunity for the therapist to skillfully guide them through the 5 Steps of CR skill and demonstrate its utility for reducing distress in the moment.

If none of these options produce a straightforward situation to show how the 5 Steps of CR work, the therapist can spend a few minutes exploring with the client any stressful or upsetting events that occurred since the previous session, and a first practice example can be formulated from there.

When initially teaching and working through the 5 Steps of CR with the client, the thought that is chosen in Step 3 and examined throughout the rest of the steps should ideally be expressed in the strongest possible manner and as specifically as possible, assuming that the client in fact believes it is true (which is usually the case, hence the frequent use of CSTs and increased distress related to these types of thoughts). The more extreme and specific the thought, the easier it is to weigh the evidence for and against it and to effectively dispute it. Here are two examples of this with non-trauma-related thoughts:

- To increase specificity, instead of examining the thought "I'm a terrible student," try examining the thought "I'm a terrible student because I did poorly on this test and I'll probably flunk my class."

- To increase extremeness, instead of examining the thought "I am uncomfortable around others, and so people don't show me respect," try examining the thought "I am always uncomfortable around people, and so no one ever shows me any respect at all."

The following example shows increasing specificity and extremeness of a trauma-related thought (for 5 Step work in later sessions, see Chapter 9, this volume):

- To increase extremeness and specificity, instead of examining the thought "I'm a bad person," try examining the thought "I'm a very bad person because I allowed myself to be sexually abused as a child when I could have stopped it."

When selecting an initial situation to demonstrate the 5 Steps of CR, it is also preferable to choose one in which the client reports primarily feeling afraid/anxious, sad/depressed, or guilty/shameful (or a combination thereof) rather than angry. Clients tend to be more open to considering evidence against thoughts related to distressing feelings such as fear, depression, and guilt rather than anger, which is a more complicated emotion to address for a variety of reasons. Working initially on distressing feelings other than anger maximizes the chances that using the 5 Steps of CR will result in changing the underlying thoughts, leading to relief from the distressing feeling. Guidelines for using the 5 Steps and other strategies for addressing anger are provided in Chapters 9 and 10 in this volume.

An example of how to introduce the 5 Steps of CR (with Leigh-Ann) is provided in the following:

Step 1: Identify the Upsetting Situation

THERAPIST: The first step is to describe the situation in which you feel upset. In Step 1, you write down the upsetting situation, just like you did on the Common Styles of Thinking (CST) Worksheet. Let's use a distressing situation you recently experienced to work through an example of the 5 Steps of CR. You noted in your CST home assignment for last week that you felt anxious and uneasy when you thought about starting your new job in the restaurant. Is that something that you are still worried about? How about if we work on that example, Leigh-Ann?

LEIGH-ANN: OK. Yeah, that's really on my mind a lot.

THERAPIST: Yes, you and I have talked about that a bit in the past few sessions. That means it is a good example to work on today! So in Step 1, we write down the upsetting situation. It is helpful to just stick to the facts of the situation because there will be lots of time and space to put down your thoughts and feelings about it later in the worksheet. For this situation, how about if I write down "Thinking about the new hosting job that I start next week?"

LEIGH-ANN: Sure, sounds good to me. I just am overwhelmed thinking about this job, although I definitely need it and am glad I landed it. I just don't know.

THERAPIST: That's not uncommon at all—to feel overwhelmed when thinking about starting something new, especially given some of your past experiences. We'll look into that feeling and your thought in these upcoming steps.

Step 2: Identify the Upsetting Feeling

THERAPIST: Now in Step 2, we want to identify the upsetting feeling that you are having related to this situation. On this worksheet, you'll see four groups of feelings: anxiety/fear, depression, guilt/shame, and anger. There may be other ones, but these tend to be the major types of emotions that occur in most upsetting situations. Sometimes a person feels more than one emotion in a situation, and that's OK. We want to try focus on the strongest or most upsetting feelings. What was your strongest feeling when you were thinking about starting your new job?

LEIGH-ANN: Anxious. I was feeling very worried and nervous.

THERAPIST: OK, let's go with anxiety for this example. Good job here.

Encourage the client to stick with one of the "big four" feelings when learning the 5 Steps of CR, if possible. These are common feelings associated with PTSD that can lead to high levels of distress. When the client reports several different feelings in a situation, it can be helpful to briefly explore these emotions before deciding which one to focus on and to encourage the client to focus on a feeling other than anger (as previously discussed). The therapist can first ask the client to talk a little about what each feeling was and then ask the client to consider which one is most distressing and focus on that feeling for remainder of the 5 Steps of CR. Alternatively, the client can temporarily choose more than one upsetting feeling in Step 2 and then, after identifying the most upsetting thought in Step 3, return to Step 2 and select the feeling most strongly related to that thought, if they are able to choose the predominant one.

It is important to not belabor a discussion about differentiating between feelings, however. The goal of this introduction to the 5 Steps of CR is to teach how the skill can be used to deal with any distressing feelings the person experiences, and a thorough examination of the upsetting thought is the key ingredient to the effectiveness of the skill. In some cases, clients may struggle to identify a specific upsetting feeling, either because they are extremely distressed or feeling emotionally numbed. When this occurs, it is best to back away from attempting to have the client choose a particular feeling and instead agree to work together in more general terms on their emotional experience of distress (or "upset," "stressed," "emotional," "overwhelmed," etc.), which can be easily written next to Step 2 on the worksheet.

Step 3: Identify Thoughts Underlying the Feeling(s)

THERAPIST: In Step 3, you want to identify your thoughts about the situation. In order to deal with upsetting emotions, we need to pinpoint our thoughts or beliefs that resulted in the upsetting feeling. If we need help pinpointing what our thought might be related to our feeling at any point when practicing the 5 Steps, we can use the Guide to Thoughts and Feelings Information Sheet, just as we did when working with the CST skill.

The therapist can continue to explain Step 3 along the following lines:

THERAPIST: Okay, let's talk about what thoughts you are having in this situation. You are thinking a lot about starting your new hosting job and feeling very anxious. What kind of thoughts have been going through your mind that make you feel anxious or worried?

LEIGH-ANN: I'm not sure. A lot of things really—like something bad is going to happen, or it'll be a disaster.

THERAPIST: OK, good! That's two thoughts you've identified: "Something bad is going to happen," and "It's going to be a disaster." I'm going to jot down both of those here. It's helpful to have a short list of thoughts first, and then we can take a closer look. Can you say what bad thing you think is going to happen?

LEIGH-ANN: Yeah—like, I will make a big mistake right away, and they'll just fire me. Or that one of the line cooks or bartenders will hit on me or something. That's happened in other restaurant jobs I've had.

THERAPIST: OK, so let's write down: "I will make a big mistake right away, and they'll just fire me," and "One of the line cooks or bartenders will hit on me." Let me ask you, what about that second thought makes you feel upset or anxious?

LEIGH-ANN: I don't know. It's happened before, and it gets uncomfortable or awkward. I can't deal with that this time.

THERAPIST: I see. So would it be correct if I wrote down that one for this thought: "One of the line cooks or bartenders will hit on me, which will be too uncomfortable for me to deal with"?

LEIGH-ANN: Yes, that's right.

THERAPIST: OK, good. So we've got a few important thoughts here. Do any other thoughts come to mind when you think about this situation?

LEIGH-ANN: No, I think that's about it.

THERAPIST: You've done a really good job of identifying several possible thoughts that are leading you to feel anxious in that situation. When we're upset, it is common to have more than one upsetting thought at a time. Sometimes identifying one thought can lead to another even more important thought related to the situation. When this happens, the best thing to do is to write down all the different thoughts you are having, just as we have written down all the thoughts you had related to starting your new job. Once you have done that, you can go through those thoughts and choose the one that is most distressing to you at the moment—the one that is getting to you the most right now. Examining this particular thought more closely is the best way of dealing with your distress in this situation and getting some relief. Just to be clear, it's not that the other thoughts aren't important, but we can work with only one thought at a time with the 5 Steps, otherwise it gets too confusing and doesn't work as well. But later on, if you find the other thoughts on the list are still bothering you, you can always do a new 5 Steps using one of those thoughts too.

In this situation, you identified several thoughts related to this new job—that "something bad might happen" and that "it will be a disaster." And then more specifically, we were able to identify these thoughts: "I will make a big mistake right away, and they'll just fire me," and also "One of the line cooks or bartenders will hit on me, which will be too uncomfortable for me to deal with." When you consider each of these thoughts, which one is most distressing in this moment?

LEIGH-ANN: They all worry me, I guess. But right now, since I'm starting next week, I think it's the one about making a big mistake and getting fired right away.

THERAPIST: OK, so that's the thought we'll work on. [The therapist circles that thought on the worksheet.] And just as a reminder, we can always work on some of these other thoughts later on if they continue to upset you. Does that sound OK to you?

LEIGH-ANN: Yeah, that's good. I hear what you mean about the others. But I'm more concerned about making a mistake since I start next week. I don't want to get too stressed out.

THERAPIST: That makes perfect sense, and I completely agree with you. Just so we are on the same page, the thought we are going to work on that is most distressing to you is "I will make a big mistake right away, and they'll just fire me." And when you think that thought, you feel anxious. Do I have that right?

LEIGH-ANN: Yes, that's it. I feel that way just thinking about this right now.

THERAPIST: That's totally understandable. And because you are still anxious about it, that's a good cue for you to know to try this skill. That's what the 5 Steps of CR is for—to work on any distress you are feeling in the moment.

At the end of Step 3, after the client has identified the most distressing thought they have about the situation, they are prompted to make a preliminary evaluation of whether they think this thought might be a CST, based on the CST skill they have just learned (as described in Chapter 7, this volume). If the client thinks their thought does reflect one or more specific CSTs, those CST categories are each circled on the worksheet. If the client indicates that their thought reflects one specific CST, the therapist should briefly inquire why the client chose that particular CST. Getting the client to articulate specifically why they think their thought may be inaccurate at the end of this step facilitates doing the next step (Step 4), when they evaluate the evidence for and against their thought. Once the client has explained why their thought might be a CST, the therapist should prompt the client by asking, "So now that we've identified your thought as a CST, what does that tell you about the thought?" This should reinforce the idea for the client that if their thought is a CST, that typically means that it is likely not 100% accurate and should be investigated further, increasing motivation and rationale to continue with the 5 Steps process. If the client is unsure whether the thought reflects a CST or is confident that it does not, the therapist can explain that they will be examining the thought more closely together in the next step to figure it out.

THERAPIST: Before we begin with Step 4, let's look at the thought you are working on to see whether it might reflect a Common Style of Thinking. If you think that the thought is related to any CST, you can circle the specific ones on the worksheet. When you consider the thought "I will make a big mistake right away, and they'll just fire me," do you think that it might reflect a Common Style of Thinking?

LEIGH-ANN: Probably. Catastrophizing?

THERAPIST: Good. Let's circle that one on the worksheet. Why do you think this thought might be an example of catastrophizing?

LEIGH-ANN: I've had some really bad things happen to me, and so I guess I'm always worried that bad stuff is always going to happen. Like, my mind always goes to the worst possible thing or outcome.

THERAPIST: Yes, that makes sense. That's a good point, given your past experiences. Are there any other Common Styles of Thinking that your thought might reflect?

LEIGH-ANN: Emotional reasoning?

THERAPIST: OK. [The therapist circles this on the worksheet.] Why might your thought reflect emotional reasoning?

LEIGH-ANN: I'm often nervous when I think about doing new things or having to prove myself.

THERAPIST: And when you feel that way, nervous, does that then make you think something bad is going to happen?

LEIGH-ANN: Yes.

THERAPIST: That's a good example of emotional reasoning: Feeling a certain way makes you believe that your worrisome thought must therefore be true. Are there any other Common Styles of Thinking that this thought might reflect?

LEIGH-ANN: Not that I can think of.

THERAPIST: OK. And just to remind ourselves: If we identify our thought as a CST (or two), what does that tell us about our thought?

LEIGH-ANN: Um, that it may not be totally true or right? And we should think about it more?

THERAPIST: Yes exactly! It may not be 100% accurate, and it is worth looking into further—with the rest of the 5 Steps skill. Now let's go onto the next step of evaluating the evidence.

Step 4: Evaluate the Thought

THERAPIST: Once you have identified the thought most strongly related to your upsetting feeling and note whether it is a CST, the fourth step is to closely examine the evidence that supports and also that does not support the thought. In the first part of this step, the goal is to think of all the evidence that does support your thought. Then after that, the goal is to think of all the evidence that doesn't support it.

Before we start doing that, let's talk a little about what evidence is and what good evidence is. *Good evidence* is evidence that is based on facts that have been collected in a systematic way and are as objective as possible. Coming up with good evidence takes practice, and I am here to guide you through doing this. In general, the way that we do this is to pretend that we are scientists or jurors in a court of law and to gather evidence for and against the thought. What do you think is special about how scientists evaluate evidence when they're trying to understand the results of an experiment or how jurors examine the evidence in a court case when they're trying to determine whether someone is innocent or guilty of a crime?

LEIGH-ANN: They try to look at all the evidence?

THERAPIST: That's right. Scientists and jurors look at all the available evidence, not just some of the evidence. And when they examine the evidence, do they look at all of it the same way, or do they look at some evidence more closely than other types of evidence?

LEIGH-ANN: I guess some evidence is more important than other evidence. I don't really know.

THERAPIST: You are right. And what type of evidence is most important and most helpful when determining whether something is true?

LEIGH-ANN: Evidence that is, like, clear or real?

THERAPIST: Exactly. The most important evidence to focus on when looking at the accuracy of a thought is evidence that is clear or real, as you said. Another way to describe this is evidence that is objective. By objective, I mean evidence that is based on facts and not just on what someone thinks, feels, or believes is true. Why do you think it's important to focus on objective evidence when evaluating an upsetting thought?

LEIGH-ANN: So you can really know whether the thought is true or not? So your feelings don't always get in the way of messing things up?

THERAPIST: Absolutely. By acting like a scientist or member of a jury and by focusing on the most objective evidence or facts available, we can be confident that our judgments about the accuracy of a thought are as correct as possible. And that's important because sometimes we believe that something is true simply because we've believed it for so long, even though there is little or no objective evidence to support it and the belief turns out to be dead wrong. During this Step 4, we'll work hard together to come up with as much evidence for the thought as we can and as much evidence against the thought as possible. We'll first consider all the evidence we can think of, including both good and bad evidence. Then later, we'll closely examine the evidence we came up with, focusing on the most objective evidence, to determine whether the thought is accurate and helpful. How does that sound?

LEIGH-ANN: OK. Sounds sort of complicated.

THERAPIST: When people are first learning this skill, it can feel that way a bit—because you are not used to breaking down your thoughts like this! I will be here to help guide you, and you'll get lots of practice on this, so that over time, you'll get more familiar and comfortable with this process.

Now that we've talked about the reason for coming up with evidence for and against the thought, let's go back to your job situation. You are thinking about starting your new hosting job, and you feel anxious. The thought that is making you the most anxious is that you'll make a mistake and get fired early in the job. Let's first think of all of the evidence that we can that might support your concern. What evidence can you think of that supports the thought that "I will make a big mistake right away, and they'll just fire me"?

LEIGH-ANN: Well, I've been fired from other jobs in the past.

THERAPIST: For making mistakes?

LEIGH-ANN: Yes.

THERAPIST: OK, that's a good start. Let's write that down on the worksheet in the section under "Things that do support my thought." What other evidence can you think of that could support your thought that you'll make a big mistake right away and get fired?

LEIGH-ANN: I don't know. Those managers can be real jerks.

THERAPIST: I understand. When coming up with evidence for and against a particular thought, it can be helpful to be as specific as possible. Can you be more specific about how the managers can be jerks?

LEIGH-ANN: Yeah. I've found they are moody and sort of on a power trip, and they get mad and then just fire people on the spot. That kind of a thing.

THERAPIST: OK, got it. So we'll write that down as evidence that supports your thought. What other evidence can you think of that supports your thought that you'll make a big mistake right away and get fired?

LEIGH-ANN: I can't think of any.

Prompt the client to come up with evidence supporting their thought, using other questions if needed and recording all examples on the worksheet, including evidence that is not objective. Once the evidence supporting the thought has been generated, the therapist summarizes it and then elicits evidence against the thought. In general, people have more difficulty coming up with evidence against their thoughts due to the *confirmation bias*, a normal human tendency to selectively attend to evidence supporting one's thinking and to ignore evidence that does not (Stanovich, 2019; Wason, 1960).

The therapist may be tempted to directly provide evidence to refute the client's thought. However, this can backfire when the client minimizes, discounts, or counters the therapist's evidence rather than accepting it. In addition, the goal of the 5 Steps of CR is to teach clients to develop and evaluate the evidence themselves in order to enable them to use the skill on their own without the help of a therapist.

Rather than directly providing counterevidence, the therapist should help the client explore the evidence against the thought in a collaborative fashion by asking questions using the Socratic method combined with a "Colombo style," without appearing to be invested in proving that the thought is wrong. This Colombo style is effectively utilized in situations where there appears to be a conspicuous contradiction in what the client says (e.g., the client describes a common and understandable reaction to a life-threatening event such as an assault but harshly criticizes their own reaction to the same event). Rather than directly pointing out these discrepancies, the therapist instead expresses genuine curiosity or puzzlement and asks the client to "help them understand."

There are several ways of helping clients consider evidence against a thought. The client can be asked to think of whether there is any evidence that might indicate that the thought is not completely accurate. For example, if the thought or belief is very strongly worded in categorical terms (e.g., "No boss can ever be trusted," "I always mess up everything at work"), any exceptions to it can serve as evidence against the thought (e.g., a single trustworthy boss, one example of a work success). If the client indicated that their thought might reflect a specific CST in Step 3 and therefore might be inaccurate, they can be prompted to review the reasons they gave for selecting the CST, which can then be included as evidence against the thought. Evidence against a thought can also be generated by asking questions such as whether there is another way of looking at the situation, what someone else might think if the same thing happened to them, and whether or not the thought is helpful. More strategies for developing and evaluating evidence can be found in the Tips for Finding Good Evidence Information Sheet, which can serve both as a guide for the clinician's Socratic questioning and also as a checklist for the client to use alongside the 5 Steps of CR worksheet as needed.

THERAPIST: OK, let's summarize the evidence so far. One piece of evidence is that you have been fired before for making mistakes on the job. And another piece of evidence is that you have experienced some restaurant managers as moody and on a power trip and have seen them fire employees on the spot. Is that correct?

LEIGH-ANN: Yes.

THERAPIST: Good. Now that we have identified evidence supporting the thought that you will make a big mistake right away and they'll just fire you, let's think of all the evidence we can that doesn't support that thought or that suggests the thought may be inaccurate. In other words, what evidence can you think of that you won't make a big mistake right away that will cause you to be fired?

LEIGH-ANN: I don't know. I just think about some of what's happened before with some of my other jobs and how it took me so long to find this new one. I'm already stressed.

THERAPIST: I understand. Our minds often go right to the negative parts of our past experiences—to jobs where it didn't work out, that kind of thing, especially because you have looked for work for so many months recently and this job feels important to you. Let me help you by asking a few questions. You mentioned that you had been fired from past jobs for making mistakes. When you think back, how many times did that happen to you?

LEIGH-ANN: I guess only twice, really.

THERAPIST: OK, that's important to know, right? So it sounds like there have been other jobs that you actually haven't been fired from, right?

LEIGH-ANN: Yeah, I haven't been fired from at least a few jobs. Sometimes I quit on my own because I didn't like it or I was having a hard time or I was moving away—but I wasn't fired.

THERAPIST: That's important evidence to note as well. Let's write that down here too. When you were fired from that particular job back then, what was going on in your life at the time?

LEIGH-ANN: Well, to be honest, for one of those jobs, I was in the time of my life where I was drinking a lot. I had started that job at the bar where I used to live, but I went in high a few shifts or called in sick, and one time I just didn't show up. That was bad.

THERAPIST: Ah, I see. So drinking back then really impacted your ability to do your job the way you needed to. Is that right? What would you say is different about that time in your life compared with now?

LEIGH-ANN: Well, for one, I haven't drank that way in, like, in 2 years, so I wouldn't be drunk or hungover this time.

THERAPIST: Right, that's an important point for sure. So it seems like we have two good pieces of evidence that do not support your thought that "I will make a big mistake right away, and they'll just fire me." The first piece of evidence is that one time you were fired because you weren't able to fulfill your job duties because you were drinking a lot. Let's note that under the column of evidence not supporting the thought. And the second piece of evidence is that you are in a very different space now in your life in that you are not drinking, so the chances of you getting fired for being drunk or hungover and not coming in for your shifts or doing your job reasonably are pretty low, right?

LEIGH-ANN: Pretty slim, I guess, actually. I'm definitely more on the ball in life now—at least as far as not being a drunken mess.

THERAPIST: Yes, there's a major difference between what you are able to do now and what you could do then, and you have good evidence for that difference from your current life. That's really important. Let's think of some more evidence that doesn't support the thought. You mentioned earlier that you have been fired twice. One of the times related to your being intoxicated on the job, but what about the other time? Was that firing related to a mistake you made too?

LEIGH-ANN: Actually, I guess it wasn't. The other place was this little family restaurant, and they weren't doing well. The owner decided he had to get rid of the host staff and have his wife do that job instead to save the place money. He was actually pretty nice about the whole thing, and he said it wasn't about anything personal related to me.

THERAPIST: So that means that there has only been one situation where you were fired for making a mistake. And the other situation was more of a layoff and didn't have anything to do with your abilities or a mistake you made? If so, we should put that information down in the section here for evidence that doesn't support your thought, right?

LEIGH-ANN: Yes, that's right.

THERAPIST: Let's see if there is any more evidence you can think of against that thought. You had said earlier that you have experienced bosses and managers to be jerks or on power trips, which you thought was evidence that you might be fired early in this new job. But has that been the case with every manager you've interacted with? What about the one you just described from the family restaurant?

LEIGH-ANN: Well, yes, he wasn't horrible. He actually gave me about a month's notice before they let me go, and he said he felt really bad about it.

THERAPIST: Good, let's also make note of that on the worksheet. Should I write down this: "Not all managers are jerks who fire you on the spot. The manager at the family restaurant was kind and didn't do that"?

LEIGH-ANN: Yes, that's right.

THERAPIST: Here's another thing to consider that we talked about earlier. You had decided that your thought "I will make a big mistake right away, and they'll just fire me" was in fact a CST—emotional reasoning. It sounds as though that would be a piece of evidence against your thought, right? Have there been other times that you have been nervous about a situation but nothing bad has happened?

LEIGH-ANN: Yeah, a lot, I guess. I'm almost always anxious when I'm starting something new and around a bunch of people that I don't know, other people. But bad things don't happen always in those situations.

THERAPIST: Good, that's another piece of evidence against your anxiety from the thought that "I will make a big mistake right away, and they'll just fire me." In other words, just because you feel anxious, it doesn't mean something bad is going to happen. You have proof from other times in your life that this is not the case.

Step 5: Take Action!

The last step of the 5 Steps of CR skill involves reviewing all of the evidence for and against the thought and then taking action based on whether or not the thought is accurate. If the evidence does not support the thought, then an alternative, more accurate one is developed.

An important note is that people with posttraumatic reactions frequently overestimate the probability that a low-occurrence traumatic event (e.g., being raped or assaulted by a stranger, being in an accident or a disaster; Foa & Rothbaum, 1998) will happen again or believe that because they experienced traumatic events early in their lives (e.g., childhood sexual or physical abuse), they will always be vulnerable to victimization throughout their adult lives (Briere, 1992). Individuals with PTSD also often experience guilt and shame about not stopping or somehow being complicit with their victimization when they look back with the full knowledge of what they now know much later in their lives (Street et al., 2005). For those with PTSD and serious mental illness, the tendency to overestimate these probabilities (and experience exaggerated accompanying emotions of fear or guilt) trickles down to distressing everyday experiences as well, and is not limited to more overtly trauma-related situations. Thus, it is important to initially teach the 5 Steps of CR as a way to manage any upsetting situation and to assist the client in more accurately evaluating these overestimations of risk in multiple facets of their lives. These initial examples also serve to set the stage for later sessions when trauma-related and core beliefs are systematically examined.

Continuing with the example, the therapist uses the Socratic method to prompt the client to consider the evidence for and against their thought:

THERAPIST: The last step of the 5 Steps of CR involves weighing the evidence and taking action. Once you have gathered all the evidence for and against your thought, you have to look at the evidence closely and make a decision about whether or not the thought is accurate. When looking at the evidence, it is important to focus on the strongest and most objective evidence—evidence that is concrete, specific, and not based only on feelings or impressions. Why do you think that evidence based on facts is better and more convincing than evidence based on feelings?

LEIGH-ANN: Because anyone out there can see the facts, but only I can feel my feelings, so my feelings may not be telling me the right things?

THERAPIST: Right! We know that the thoughts we have related to our feelings aren't always accurate. For example, do you remember which Common Style of Thinking is associated with the thought that "I feel afraid, and therefore I must be in danger?"

LEIGH-ANN: Yes, the one about emotions taking over—emotional reasoning, like we talked about.

THERAPIST: That's exactly right. Just because you feel afraid doesn't mean you're in danger. And as it is related to your 5 Steps with today's example, just because you feel anxious or have been anxious in the past, that doesn't mean that something bad is going to happen with your new job. That's why evidence based on feelings is not as strong as evidence based on facts. Another way of determining whether evidence is strong and objective is to ask, "Could I convince someone else that this thought is true based on the evidence?" Why do you think asking whether someone else could be convinced by the evidence is a good way of determining how strong the evidence is?

LEIGH-ANN: I guess it depends on who that other person is, but another person can be more objective than I can be about a situation I am in the middle of?

THERAPIST: Right again! It's easier for people to see the facts of a situation that they aren't directly involved in and don't have strong feelings about.

After briefly discussing how to weigh the evidence, the therapist finishes the introduction to the last step of the 5 Steps of CR:

THERAPIST: After examining all of the evidence and focusing on the strongest and most objective evidence, it's time to decide overall whether or not the evidence supports your thought. As we have discussed, the thoughts behind upsetting feelings are often inaccurate and are not supported by the evidence. When the evidence does not support your thinking, it's time to develop a new, more accurate thought to replace the old one. This new thought should be supported by the evidence you have come up with. Sometimes some evidence does support your thought, but you realize that there also is good evidence against it. That means that your original thought is not completely accurate. Even in these situations, it is important to come up with a new thought that is more accurate than your old one.

If the evidence does support your thought, then it's time to develop an Action Plan to deal with the situation. Why do you think it's important to come up with a plan for dealing with an upsetting situation in which your concerns are supported by the facts?

LEIGH-ANN: So that the situation doesn't continue to be a problem? To deal with it.

THERAPIST: Right. That way you can try to resolve the distressing situation and make a plan that will help you.

After the last step of the skill has been described, the therapist returns to the example:

THERAPIST: Let's continue with the situation about your job that has made you feel anxious. Now we'll go over the specific evidence for and against your thought that "I will make a big mistake right away, and they'll just fire me." Let's consider the evidence about making mistakes and getting fired in the past. Is that specific evidence about what might happen at this particular new restaurant you will be working at?

LEIGH-ANN: It's sort of specific in that it actually happened—but not at all of my jobs and, I guess, only once really, like we talked about. And also not about this specific restaurant I'm starting my job at.

THERAPIST: Right. So would you consider it strong evidence or not?

LEIGH-ANN: I guess not.

THERAPIST: How about the evidence that all managers are jerks and fire people on a whim? Is that strong?

LEIGH-ANN:	It makes me anxious still, but I guess it's not very specific because the other family restaurant owner wasn't a jerk and didn't do that to me. And also there are some managers who probably aren't jerks anyway.
THERAPIST:	Right, you may have a general belief that managers have those negative qualities, but based on your own personal experiences that we just talked about, not all managers have them. And so that doesn't provide very strong evidence that your new manager will act in this negative way toward you and that you'll lose your job right away. Would you agree with that?
LEIGH-ANN:	Yes.
THERAPIST:	The other related piece of evidence supporting the thought was that "I feel anxious about this, so that means something bad will happen." You've already identified that as a Common Style of Thinking—emotional reasoning—so we know that's not very strong evidence, because it's based on feelings and not facts. Right?
LEIGH-ANN:	Right.
THERAPIST:	OK, now let's look at the evidence against the thought that "I will make a big mistake right away, and they'll just fire me." How about the evidence that you were fired from only one job and that firing was related to how your alcohol use was affecting your ability to do your work?
LEIGH-ANN:	Well, it's true, and it's specific. The drinking and how it made me late and call out sick and be hungover was what made me lose my job probably.
THERAPIST:	Right, so that is good evidence. And how about the evidence that "I haven't drank like that for 2 years, and so I can think straight when at work these days." How's that?
LEIGH-ANN:	That's also true.
THERAPIST:	And how about the evidence that you have felt anxious in lots of situations and bad things have not ended up happening?
LEIGH-ANN:	I know that's true, but it doesn't stop me from feeling anxious around strangers or new coworkers that I don't know yet.
THERAPIST:	Right, just because you feel anxious, it doesn't mean something bad is going to happen, but that also doesn't mean that you will stop feeling anxious right away either. That is not unusual. OK, so now let's look at all of the evidence together and decide something. Is your thought that "I will make a big mistake right away, and they'll just fire me" supported by the evidence?

LEIGH-ANN: No, I guess its not.

THERAPIST: OK. So, let's check off on the worksheet that the thought is not supported by the evidence. Now let's try to come up with a more accurate thought for that situation. Considering all of the evidence against the thought that you'll make a mistake in your new job and get fired immediately, what's a more accurate thought in that situation?

LEIGH-ANN: That I'm definitely not going to screw it up and get fired right away? I'm not sure.

THERAPIST: OK. Now when you look at this situation and look at the evidence, how accurate and believable does it seem to tell yourself, "I'm definitely not going to screw it up and get fired right away"?

LEIGH-ANN: Well, I know it's more accurate, but it doesn't quite seem totally realistic because I still feel anxious and a little worried about it.

THERAPIST: I understand. So maybe we can come up with a more accurate thought that also acknowledges that you still feel a bit uncomfortable. How about something like this: "Even though I still feel somewhat anxious about what might happen at this new job, it is unlikely that I will make a big mistake and get fired right away." How does that sound to you—more realistic?

LEIGH-ANN: That sounds better to me.

THERAPIST: OK, let's write down that new thought. Let's compare your feelings related to your old, upsetting thought in this situation with your new, more accurate thought. How did you feel when you thought that "I will make a big mistake right away, and they'll just fire me?"

LEIGH-ANN: Very anxious. Super worried. A little nauseous too.

THERAPIST: OK. Now that we have examined the thought, determined that it is inaccurate, and come up with a more accurate one, how do you feel when you think about this situation: "Even though I still feel somewhat anxious about what might happen at this new job, it is unlikely that I will make a big mistake and get fired right away?"

LEIGH-ANN: Better. I no longer feel as vulnerable and as freaked out. I'm definitely less anxious than before.

THERAPIST: Great. This shows how using the 5 Steps of CR can help you carefully examine the evidence supporting upsetting thoughts and how changing these thoughts to more accurate ones can help reduce your upsetting feelings.

Session 5 Home Assignment

At the end of the session, the therapist develops a home assignment with the client to practice the 5 Steps of CR, using the worksheet to record their efforts:

THERAPIST: For your home assignment, I would like us to talk through a plan to get you started on practicing the 5 Steps of CR on your own over the next week. This skill can be used to deal with any situation that is upsetting or stressful to you. If you find yourself feeling bad in some way, that's your cue to use the 5 Steps of CR and to start looking into what you are thinking that is making you stressed or upset. Remember, if you have any trouble identifying your upsetting thought or feeling, you can use the Guide to Thoughts and Feelings Information Sheet to help you figure it out.

The goal is for you to get as much practice as possible using the 5 Steps of CR in this upcoming week. We could make a plan for you to try out using this skill and the worksheet to deal with at least one upsetting situation each day. This is a very new skill to you, so even if you get stuck on one of the steps, that's OK. Just do your best, and when we get together again next week, we can work together on any steps you got stuck on. How's that sound?

LEIGH-ANN: I'm not sure I can do it every day, but I am willing to try it.

THERAPIST: Well, let's come up with a plan that feels comfortable to you. Do you think you could try one entry every other day until we meet again?

LEIGH-ANN: Yeah, I could probably do that.

THERAPIST: OK, great. Let's start there. One other thing to keep in mind, Leigh-Ann, is that it is easiest to learn and get comfortable with the 5 Steps on your own when you stick to situations that aren't really heavy. Try to focus on the situations that are more along the lines of feeling stressed, irritated, or annoyed rather than situations that are really upsetting. That way you will have an easier time staying focused on practicing the skill. We will definitely get to the more challenging and distressing sorts of situations and thoughts, including those that are related to your trauma. But we will work on those together at first, so I can help you learn to address them with this skill before you try them on your own.

LEIGH-ANN: That's a relief because I am not sure I can handle really tough stuff on my own yet. It's overwhelming.

Given that most clients who participate in this intervention experience no shortage of daily stressful events, the plan for outside practice ideally would have the client practice the 5 Steps of CR each day, using the worksheet. It can be helpful to carve out some time to discuss a few potential scenarios where the client might anticipate encountering stress in the upcoming week and therefore consider practicing the 5 Steps of CR in order to manage their distress within those particular situations. This allows an opportunity for the client to become more aware of optimal times to use this new skill and also increases the likelihood that the client will carve out time to practice the 5 Steps.

Review: The Introductory 5 Steps of CR Session

As with each session in this intervention, the introductory session for the 5 Steps of CR should conclude with a review. The review can also be helpful for eliciting any comments or observations the client has about the session, such as what was interesting or helpful. An example of concluding the introductory session follows:

THERAPIST: OK, let's review what we have covered today. You learned a new cognitive restructuring skill—the 5 Steps of CR. These steps included describing the situation, identifying the upsetting feeling, identifying the thought underlying that feeling, examining the evidence for and against the thought, and then taking action, either by coming up with a new, more accurate thought or by developing a plan to deal with the situation. You saw that carefully examining the evidence related to upsetting thoughts can lead to more accurate thoughts and less distressing feelings. Learning how to use the 5 Steps of CR can be especially helpful when people have had upsetting, traumatic events in their lives, since these experiences have often shaped their thoughts and beliefs, which upon close examination are often not accurate or helpful. Cognitive restructuring is a skill that takes practice to get better at, and you are already on your way. You did a great job with this first example. Do you have any questions I can answer for you?

DEVELOPING ACTION PLANS

Everyone experiences problems in their lives, and negative feelings are often an important clue that something is wrong and that corrective action is needed. Although many thoughts associated with distressing feelings are inaccurate, not all are inaccurate, and it is important to help people identify concrete steps toward resolving situations that lead to valid negative feelings. To take an extreme example, if someone smelled smoke from the next room and opened the door to find a fire there, they would probably be afraid and think, "I'm in danger!" Instead of altering this thought, one would want to come up with a practical way to handle this emergency situation.

People with a trauma history often need help learning practical ways to deal with upsetting situations and problems. Anxiety, avoidance, and denial are common responses in trauma survivors to threatening situations that can contribute to revictimization (Arata, 2002). Teaching clients how to take decisive, well-planned action when faced with real-life problems can provide them with a useful skill for overcoming challenges and regaining control over their lives. This type of problem solving plays an integral role as part of the 5 Steps of CR, as described next.

In Step 5, after reviewing the evidence for and against the thought, if the client concludes that the evidence supports the thought, then an Action Plan is formulated. An *Action Plan* is a brief, structured approach to using specific problem-solving skills to develop practical strategies to address a distressing situation or problem. The separate Action Plan Worksheet should be used to facilitate detailed planning on how to deal with the problem situation.

Effective Action Plans generally include the following four steps: (a) a clear goal, (b) a list of possible strategies for achieving the goal, (c) a specific plan for implementing the selected strategies, and (d) a timeline to follow up on the plan.

The purpose of the goal statement is to specify the aim of the Action Plan. For example, Donata felt anxious about an impending move to a new apartment and concluded that the evidence supported her thought that "I'm going to have trouble adjusting to my new apartment." Some possible goals of her Action Plan could include "To learn more about my new neighborhood," "To feel more comfortable about moving into my new apartment," and "To prepare for my move so I'll be ready when it comes."

For the second step, it can be helpful to begin by brainstorming strategies for achieving the goal before evaluating each one. This can lead to identifying several possible solutions to choose from, including some unusual and creative ones. Next, each solution is evaluated, and the best one (or ones) is selected for implementation. Potentially effective strategies for dealing with the problem situation can come from anyone or anywhere (e.g., client, therapist, significant other, books, the internet). The client may have past experiences using some effective strategies to handle similar challenges, which can be applied to the problem situation at hand.

The next step of planning how to implement the chosen strategy involves determining the steps necessary to achieve the desired goal. Effective implementation plans should take into consideration several questions, including these: Do I need to get more information about what to do? Do I need help? When will I implement the plan? How could I prevent or deal with possible obstacles? Once the core elements of the plan have been determined, the steps for implementing it can be established.

The final component of the Action Plan is to specify a timeline to follow up on the plan. This facilitates troubleshooting potential obstacles to implementing the plan or developing additional strategies for achieving the goal, if needed. In addition to setting a follow-up time, when the plan involves interactions with people that the client feels anxious about or lacks experience with, it can be helpful for the therapist to engage the client in some role plays to practice handling the situation and to provide positive feedback and suggestions for improvement after each role play.

Typically, following through on an Action Plan that was developed during a session should be included in the home assignment collaboratively agreed upon at the end of the session, along with daily practice of the 5 Steps of CR. At the beginning of the next session, the therapist should follow up with the client on how the plan went.

An example of teaching a client (Donata) how to develop an Action Plan follows:

THERAPIST: Donata, you've finished evaluating whether the evidence supports your thought that "I'm going to have trouble adjusting to my new apartment," and you've decided that, overall, the evidence does support your concern.

DONATA: Right.

THERAPIST: OK. So when you decide that your evidence supports your thought, then the fifth step of the 5 Steps is to create an Action Plan to deal with that stressful situation. Creating an Action Plan means figuring out how to deal with a situation and how to either solve a problem or cope with a problem. What happens to most problems or upsetting feelings when you just try to ignore them?

DONATA: They don't really go away?

THERAPIST: Right. Or they get worse. Developing an Action Plan is like, as the expression goes, "facing the music." It means tackling the problem directly and either trying to solve it completely, if possible, or reducing it so it's not so much of a problem anymore. How does that sound?

DONATA: Good. I need that.

THERAPIST: OK, let's work on it together. I have another worksheet here that can help you develop an Action Plan that we'll use together, the Action Plan Worksheet. The first step is to define the goal of the plan. In other words, what would you like to accomplish in terms of dealing with the problem situation? You decided that the evidence supports your thought that you're going to have trouble adjusting to your new apartment, which is in a new part of town. What would you like to accomplish in your Action Plan to deal with this problem?

DONATA: I'd like to stop worrying about it so much. I'm thinking about it constantly. It really overwhelms me.

THERAPIST: OK. So one possible way of defining the goal of the Action Plan would be "to stop worrying so much about moving into my new apartment." If you were to stop worrying about your move but not forget about the fact that you are moving, how would you feel about the move?

DONATA: More comfortable, I guess.

THERAPIST: All right. So another way you could define your goal would be "to feel comfortable about my upcoming move." Right?

DONATA: Yes, that would be good.

THERAPIST: When you feel anxious and worry about your move, what do you worry about? What gets in the way of feeling comfortable about it?

DONATA: They said the staff will come check on me and help me, I guess, but there's just so much I don't know.

THERAPIST: Like what?

DONATA: Like where I'll shop for food. The closest pharmacy.

THERAPIST: Anything else?

DONATA: How to get to the clinic here. How to get to my art group.

THERAPIST: I see. Do you think if you figured out the answers to some of these concerns sooner rather than later that you'd feel more comfortable about the move?

DONATA: Yes, I think so. I've just been getting so nervous and then trying to not think about it. But maybe that's bad?

THERAPIST: It's not bad. It's actually really common to want to avoid thinking about something that is coming up that we are worried about. But that's the exact reason we need to tackle it with a plan! So another way of defining the goal of the Action Plan might be for you "to learn more about my new neighborhood." Would you agree?

DONATA: Yes.

THERAPIST: Good. We've come up with three possible goals: "to stop worrying about moving into my new apartment," "to feel comfortable about my upcoming move," and "to learn more about my new neighborhood." Of these three goals, which one best describes what you'd like to accomplish with your Action Plan?

DONATA: I think learning more about the new neighborhood would be helpful for now.

THERAPIST: OK. Let's write that down and go to the next step of the plan.

Timing and Frequency of Action Plan Development and Practice

Action Plans should be introduced and taught as soon as possible within the first few 5 Steps of CR sessions so that clients become familiar with this strategy early on. Ideally, the therapist should guide the client through at least one complete Action Plan related to a distressing situation at some point during Session 6, 7, or 8. In many cases, the need for an Action Plan will come up naturally as a client at some point decides in Step 5 that the evidence does, in fact, support their upsetting thought and that they therefore need a strategy to address the distressing situation they are experiencing.

In some cases, an early opportunity for Action Plan practice may not spontaneously emerge if the client consistently recognizes their distressing thoughts as inaccurate and modifies them in Step 5. In this situation, the therapist should be sure to introduce the Action Plan as a way to develop and practice a concurrent coping plan that is relevant to a situation the client is working on in the session. This plan can be something as basic as "how to remember my new, more accurate thought in my daily life" with such strategies as writing the thought in various places in the home or as a phone note, keeping the successfully completed 5 Steps of CR worksheet nearby, saying the new thought out loud each morning, and so on. (More details on this sort of Action Plan pertaining to internalizing a new thought related to one's trauma are provided in Chapter 9, this volume.)

Sometimes both developing a more accurate thought and creating an Action Plan in Step 5 are appropriate. In other words, the client may conclude that the evidence does not support their upsetting thought, come up with a new and more accurate thought, but still find this new thought is somewhat distressing. An Action Plan can then be developed to address the situation associated with the new, more accurate thought. An example of this strategy is provided in the vignette with Edmundo on page 184 of this chapter.

Common Distressing Situations Calling for Action Plans

There are several types of challenging situations that call for the development of an Action Plan, and one of the most common is coping with disruptive symptoms (e.g., depression, anxiety, auditory hallucinations, panic attacks, etc.). Collaboratively creating an Action Plan with some new coping strategies can both teach the client the basics of how to use this skill and provide a quick relief for distressing feelings at this stage of the program. Clients may also be struggling with acute PTSD symptoms and associated challenges (e.g., avoidance of important tasks or appointments, chronic insomnia, excessive drinking, etc.) that are interfering with their daily life. Especially in these initial CR sessions, before the shift to directly addressing trauma-related thoughts and beliefs, the skill of developing Action Plans provides a great opportunity for the therapist to help the client develop and implement effective coping strategies for dealing with these sorts of PTSD-related symptoms. (For further details on the development of trauma- and PTSD-focused Action Plans, see Chapter 9, this volume.)

Another common situation for clients to use the Action Plan skill is when there is a need for more information about a distressing situation. Sometimes there is insufficient evidence or information available to permit drawing a definitive conclusion about the accuracy of a thought. In these circumstances, an Action Plan can be made to obtain more information about the situation, which is then used later to further reevaluate the accuracy of the thought and either modify it or plan a subsequent course of action.

Exhibit 8.1 provides a summary of common situations in which therapists can assist clients in Action Plan development. (See also Chapter 9, this volume, for trauma-focused Action Plans.)

EXHIBIT 8.1

Common Situations Benefitting From Action Plans

- Needing more information about a concern
    - "Does my case manager dislike me because she cancelled three appointments?"
    - "Will I have to move to a new apartment at the end of my current lease?"
    - "Is my abusive former husband definitely moving back into my town?"
- Solving a real-life problem
    - The client wants to attend a family reunion, but the brother who assaulted her will be there.
    - The client gets anxious with panic symptoms when entering the grocery store.
    - The client is dealing with a difficult coworker at a new job.
- Coping with distress related to PTSD or other symptoms after inaccurate thinking has been addressed
    - Having trouble getting to sleep or having nightmares
    - Experiencing increased anxiety/distress when exposed to reminders of trauma
    - Hearing voices louder when trying to take an exam
- Exploring options or developing strategies for dealing with persistent angry feelings and/or behaviors
    - Experiencing rage frequently
    - Having angry outbursts at work
    - Getting so angry and distracted at home that the evening is lost
- Addressing obstacles to achieving goals
    - Finding places to meet new people in order to make new friends
    - Coping with anxiety about driving because driving is a reminder of an accident
    - Being tempted to overuse alcohol at social events as a result of past addiction

Note. PTSD = posttraumatic stress disorder.

The following scenario with Edmundo illustrates the ways in which a detailed Action Plan can reduce distress and avoidance. It pertains to obtaining needed information and doing problem solving in a situation that continues to feel stressful even after a client's upsetting thought has been effectively modified to a more accurate one:

> With the help of a vocational rehabilitation program at his community mental health center, Edmundo had recently obtained a part-time job working for a food delivery service. Two days before his weekly CR for PTSD session, he received a letter that his Social Security Disability Income (SSDI) would be reduced because of his new job. Edmundo was very distraught over this because he had met with a benefits counselor before taking the job, who had informed him that his SSDI would not change as a result of his new job. Edmundo was concerned because he now believed that he would not be able to pay off his debt and contribute to his household, given his previous accident, which had been his primary motivation for getting the job.
>
> Edmundo went through the 5 Steps of CR and evaluated the thought that "I'll never ever be able to get out of debt now and won't be able to contribute to my family," which was accompanied by strong feelings of anxiety, depression, and shame. He concluded that the evidence did not fully support the thought, which he changed to "It is very possibly a mistake, but I am still concerned that my SSDI check will be reduced. Even though I probably won't be in debt forever because I am now making smart choices, it may be harder to lower my debt as fast as I want to, but I am still contributing to my family anyway." Because Edmundo's new thought was still associated with some stress and he had a specific problem that needed to be solved, he developed an Action Plan to deal with the situation.
>
> He decided that the goal of this plan was to "Find out more information about whether my SSDI check will be reduced." After brainstorming several possible options for accomplishing this goal, Edmundo decided to set up meetings the following week with his vocational counselor and his case manager but to wait until after these meetings to find out whether he would also need to contact his local Social Security office. Edmundo learned from his meeting with his vocational counselor that the letter was a mistake. This counselor helped him contact his representative at the Social Security office, and in two weeks the problem was sorted out.

Figure 8.1 shows the 5 Steps of CR worksheet completed for Edmundo for this situation, and Exhibit 8.2 shows Edmundo's Action Plan.

A similar strategy would potentially be effective for the case example regarding Leigh-Ann's anxiety about starting her new hosting job at the restaurant. While she was able to change her thought to something more accurate about the situation, she still noted some anticipatory distress. A specific Action Plan including strategies for how to manage her anxiety when she started work (i.e., Breathing Retraining, reminding herself of her new more accurate and helpful thought, having a specific self-reward for completing her first day of work, etc.) could provide additional relief and increase the chances of having a successful new job experience.

TEACHING THE 5 STEPS OF CR IN SUBSEQUENT SESSIONS

After the introduction to the 5 Steps of CR, the remaining sessions are devoted to helping clients learn how to use the skill to deal with their negative feelings and eventually to address trauma-related beliefs and schemas that underlie their

FIGURE 8.1. Example of the 5 Steps of CR Worksheet for Edmundo Addressing Non-Trauma-Based Belief

1. Situation

Ask yourself, "What happened that made me upset?" Write down a brief description of the situation, including just the facts.

Situation: I received a letter this week that said my SSDI money would be cut down because of my new part-time job.

2. Feeling

Circle your strongest feeling. If you have more than one, that's ok. (If none of these fit, you can write one in.)

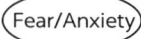 Fear/Anxiety   Sadness/Depression   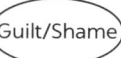 Guilt/Shame   Anger

3. Thought

Ask yourself, "What am I thinking that is leading me to feel this way?" You can use your Guide to Thoughts and Feelings Information Sheet to identify thoughts related to the feeling(s) circled above. You may have more than one thought related to the feeling(s). Write down your thoughts below, but then choose ONE thought to work on. Choose the thought that is most distressing to you right now, and circle that thought.

Thoughts: They are trying to screw me over.

I am an idiot and can't figure anything out with this government finance stuff.

I'll never ever be able to get out of debt now and won't be able to contribute to my family.

Is this thought a Common Style of Thinking? If yes, circle the style:

All-or-nothing   Mind reading   Overgeneralizing

Must/should/never   Catastrophizing   Emotional
reasoning

Overestimation of risk   Self-blame   Mental filter

Write the thought you chose from Step 3 here:

Upsetting thought: I'll never ever be able to get out of debt now and won't be able to contribute to my family.

4. Evaluate Your Thought

Now ask yourself: "What evidence do I have for and against this thought?" First, write down all the evidence that DOES support your thought. Then write down all the evidence that DOES NOT support your thought. You can use your Tips for Finding Good Evidence Information Sheet to help come up with evidence that DOES NOT support your thought.

Things that DO support my thought:

The letter said my monthly amount would be less.

I've heard about other people where this same thing has happened if they got a job.

I've been in debt for many years.

If I don't get all the SSDI money, I can't pay down the credit card the way I had planned.

My partner has had to pick up a lot of financial slack for the family.

(continues)

FIGURE 8.1. Example of the 5 Steps of CR Worksheet for Edmundo Addressing Non-Trauma-Based Belief (*Continued*)

Things that DO NOT support my thought:

> That benefits counselor at my job told me that SSDI wouldn't reduce my monthly amount.

> Some of the other people that I know who had their benefits taken away had gotten full-time jobs and mine is only part-time.

> My voc counselor told me a little while ago that the SSDI office had made a bunch of errors in checks they sent to her clients and other information they sent out, so maybe that's what happened.

> I got into debt because of bad choices I made and an irresponsible life-style, but I have been living very different since then, and I am spending a lot less and more responsible.

> Getting out of debt takes time no matter what.

> I have been contributing to the family somewhat financially still but also in other ways like taking care of the kids if my partner has to work overtime.

5. Take Action!

Now, ask yourself, "Do things mostly support my thought, or do things mostly NOT support my thought?"

☐ No, the evidence does not support my thought.

> If the evidence does NOT support your thought, come up with a new thought that is supported by the evidence. These thoughts are usually more balanced and accurate (and helpful). Write your new, more helpful thought in the space below. Remember, when you think of this upsetting situation in the future or when a similar situation happens, replace your unhelpful automatic thought with this new and more accurate thought.

> My new thought: It is very possible it is a mistake, but I am still concerned that my SSDI check will be reduced. Even though I probably won't be in debt forever because I am now making smart choices, it may be harder to lower my debt as fast as I want to, but I am still contributing to my family anyway.

I will make an Action Plan too so I can figure out what to do next to see if this letter is a mistake.

☐ YES, the evidence does support my thought.

> If the evidence DOES support your thought, decide what you need to do next in order to deal with the situation. Ask yourself, "Do I need to get more information about what to do? Do I need to get some help? Do I need to take steps to make sure I am safe?" Complete the Action Plan Worksheet to help you answer these questions and create a solid plan to deal with the situation.

Note. In some cases, you may decide that the evidence does not support your upsetting thought and change it to a more accurate and helpful one. If so, you may also find it helpful to make an Action Plan to deal with that situation. Thus, in some situations, you may find that doing both things—coming up with a new and more accurate thought AND ALSO creating an Action Plan—can be very helpful. CR = cognitive restructuring; SSDI = Social Security Disability Income.

PTSD symptoms. Each session begins with a review of the home assignment in which the therapist and client discuss efforts to use the 5 Steps of CR and the therapist helps the client with steps on which they got stuck. When the client reports using the 5 Steps of CR on their own, the therapist should be sure to explore whether they experienced relief from using the skill. Any reduction in distress, however small, should be highlighted. If the client describes using the

EXHIBIT 8.2

Example of a "Problem-to-Solve" Action Plan Completed by Edmundo

Instructions: Follow the steps below to develop a helpful Action Plan.

1. Define the goal: What situation requires action?

   Think about what change you would like to see in this situation. Be as specific as possible.

   To find out more information about whether my SSDI check will be reduced.

2. Brainstorm possible strategies: What can you do to change the situation?

   Using your creative problem-solving skills to think of all the possible things you could do to reduce your distress or address the problem in this situation. When you have made a list of different strategies, think carefully about each one, and place a star (*) next to the best one or ones.

   - Call up the SSDI 1-800 number right after this session, and get someone on the phone asap.
   - Keep trying to find out the information online from the SSDI website like I have all week. Maybe I'll find something helpful?
   - Call my case manager after today's session, and try to set up a meeting for next week to get help and support.**
   - Call my voc counselor after today's meeting, and try to set up a meeting with her too.**
   - Use BRT as needed to help when I get angry and anxious about all of this.**

3. Plan on how to put into practice the strategy (or strategies) you chose: What steps can you take to make this happen?

   Consider these questions:

   What information do you need to have?

   Do you need to get some help?

   Who can support you in taking this action?

   What obstacles or challenges could interfere with the plan?

   How could you prevent or deal with these obstacles or challenges?

   Then write down the plan below. Be specific about the actions you will take.

   I will call my case manager and voc counselor right away. But I will NOT contact the SSDI office until I talk with my case manager and voc counselor since they will hopefully help me figure out what to do as a next step. I will also stop trying to find info online because that has made things more confusing and frustrating.

4. Set a time or a situation to follow up your plan: When and how are you going to take this action?

Ask yourself: When do you want to begin your plan? Is there a specific situation or type of situation where you want to use your plan? When is that situation likely to come up again next?

I will call my case manager and voc counselor right after my CR for PTSD session, and hopefully they can meet with me early next week. In the meantime, I will use BRT if and when I start to get angry and anxious about this situation.

Note. SSDI = Social Security Disability Income; BRT = Breathing Retraining; CR = cognitive restructuring; PTSD = posttraumatic stress disorder.

5 Steps of CR but not experiencing any relief, the therapist should praise the client for trying the skill and then review the situation to determine whether additional work together may lead to a reduction in distress (see Chapter 10, this volume, for more details on this strategy).

Following home practice review, the remainder of the session is spent using the 5 Steps of CR to address other negative feelings the client may have experienced during the week. Again, the focus in these initial 5 Steps sessions (i.e., Sessions 6 and 7) is to aid the client in the following aspects of using the 5 Steps of CR skill: (a) understanding when to use the 5 Steps (any distress); (b) understanding the different steps and moving through them successfully to the end; (c) developing and scrutinizing evidence; (d) identifying more accurate thoughts when the upsetting thought is found to be inaccurate; and (e) developing clear, detailed, and relevant Action Plans when the upsetting thought is found to be accurate.

After the client has been introduced to the 5 Steps of CR, the therapist has walked them through a few examples in Sessions 5 and 6 (and Session 7 as well, as needed), and the client has attempted to use the skill for home practice, the focus can then start to shift to teaching the client how to use the skill more on their own during the session rather than having the therapist continue to lead them through the steps. This involves gradually handing over the role of completing the worksheet to the client, asking questions to prompt the identification of each step and its purpose (e.g., "OK, so what's the first step of CR? Why is it important to describe the situation?" "Now that you've identified your upset feeling, what's next?"), and assuming the role of a coach rather than a leader in helping the client learn how to use the skill. It is also important to reinforce the client for using the steps correctly, both by providing positive feedback and drawing attention to reductions in distress that usually occur when the 5 Steps of CR are completed. The more involved clients are in keeping track of the 5 Steps of CR, providing evidence for and against their thoughts, and developing new thoughts or Action Plans based on the evidence, the more able they will be to use the skill on their own to deal with upsetting feelings. This increased skill and comfort will help enormously as they move to the next phase of the intervention, where specific trauma-related and core beliefs are addressed (see Chapter 9, this volume).

ADDITIONAL STRATEGIES FOR TEACHING THE 5 STEPS OF CR

There are some additional helpful strategies to assist clients in learning each of the 5 Steps of CR, as described next.

Step 1: Describing the Situation ("Just the Facts")

The cue for clients to use the 5 Steps of CR is that they are experiencing any upsetting feeling whatsoever. When a distressing feeling seems to come out of nowhere, clients are sometimes confused about what to write under "situation" on the 5 Steps of CR worksheet. The therapist can explain that a brief description should be given about what the client was doing or the situation in which the upsetting feeling occurred (e.g., "I was eating breakfast when I had a memory of my stepfather abusing me"). Thus, while the situation can be an actual event (e.g., "My sister hung up on me during an argument yesterday"), it can also be a specific memory, image, or period of time thinking about something distressing (e.g., "Waiting for the bus last night and thinking about the day the car accident took place")—all of which are appropriate situations to use for the 5 Steps.

When the therapist is teaching the client to describe the situation, it is helpful to prompt them to keep the description brief and "stick to just the facts" (e.g., "My sister hung up on me yesterday" versus "My sister hung up on me yesterday because she has no respect for me"). They can be reminded that there will be plenty of time and space to explore their feelings and thoughts related to the situation throughout the rest of the steps.

Step 2: Identify the Strongest Emotion ("Any Distressing Feeling")

In some cases, clients do not feel that any of the emotions listed on the worksheet resonate with how they feel in the current situation, or clients are unsure what they are feeling. When this occurs, it can be useful to spend a few minutes with the Guide to Thoughts and Feelings to help them identify the feeling experienced. Nevertheless, it is crucial to not become bogged down spending too much time trying to pinpoint an exact emotion. It is sufficient for the client to acknowledge something more general such as "upset," "stressed," or "overwhelmed." In addition, the feelings the client is experiencing often become clearer after they identify the most distressing thought. Identifying any distressing feelings in Step 2 is sufficient to go on to Step 3 (identifying the thoughts underlying those feelings). When a more specific feeling becomes evident, the therapist and client can go back to Step 2 and fill in the feeling.

Step 3: Identify the Most Distressing Thought (Developing a "Workable Thought" for CR Practice)

Sometimes, the client is able to identify an upsetting thought related to a distressing feeling in a situation, but the thought is not expressed in a way that can be effectively evaluated using the rest of the 5 Steps of CR (Steps 3–5) and therefore is not workable for effective CR practice. A *workable thought* for CR is one that is a very clear conjecture or believed statement that is potentially subject to falsification. In addition, a workable thought is one that is phrased as a full, clear statement about something explicitly related to the client where the distress it causes is obvious. During 5 Steps practice, when a client identifies an unworkable thought (one that does not meet the above criteria), it is important that the clinician help them adjust the thought statement before moving onto Step 4. Without attending to this, the 5 Steps of CR are less effective at helping the clients change inaccurate and upsetting beliefs, which can be frustrating for both therapist and client. Some specific distinguishing characteristics between workable and unworkable thoughts are detailed in Table 8.1.

TABLE 8.1. Changing Unworkable Thoughts Into Workable Thoughts in Step 3 for Effective 5 Steps of CR Practice

Unworkable thought	Therapeutic strategy: Ask the client	Workable thought
Phrased as a question	"Can you answer your own question?"	Phrased as a statement
"Why do bad things always happen to me?"		"Bad things happen to me constantly because I am being punished for not reporting the assault."
"Will I be able to survive this court hearing?"		"I definitely won't be able to survive this court hearing at all."
Primarily a feeling/ emotion	"And what thought ran through your head just now to cause that feeling?"	Does not exclusively use feeling words
"I am so sad and depressed."		"I never do anything meaningful or important during the week."
Entirely about someone else	"And how does that impact YOU?"	About the client or, if it involves someone else, clearly includes an impact on client
"My sister treats everyone like a servant."	"What does that say about YOU?"	"My sister treats everyone like a servant, and it's obvious she fully disrespects me."
Not directly linked to trauma (where applicable)	"I wonder if that thought is trauma-related. Let's talk about that a bit"	Obvious why it is trauma-related
"All male bosses are complete jerks."	"How might it be trauma related?"	"Because I was sexually assaulted by my old boss, all male bosses are complete jerks."
Not entirely clear why upsetting	"And what's upsetting about that to you?"	Obvious why it causes distress
"I shouldn't go outside on the weekends."		"I shouldn't go outside on weekends since that's when I was mugged before."
Not a full statement	"Let's try to finish that sentence."	A clear and complete statement
"Full of bad luck, never getting a break"	"Can you expand the details on that a bit?"	"I have never had good luck or gotten a break in life."

There are several approaches that can be used to change unworkable thoughts in Step 3 to workable ones. Typically, this involves asking the client a few follow-up questions to clarify the nature of the unworkable thought and then helping them reword it accordingly. From there, the therapist can guide the client to the CST section at the bottom of Step 3 on the 5 Steps of CR worksheet and then proceed through the remainder of the steps. Table 8.1 also illustrates specific techniques for changing unworkable thoughts into more workable ones. (For more strategies to assist clients in transforming vague and general thoughts in Step 3 into more specific, trauma-related ones for fruitful evaluation, see Chapter 9, this volume.)

Step 4: Examining the Evidence ("Tips" Handout)

Teaching clients how to critically examine their upsetting thoughts is perhaps the most crucial step of the 5 Steps of CR. Evaluating the evidence is most effectively accomplished when the therapist asks the client questions to generate all the evidence supporting the thought (including weak evidence) and evidence against the thought, and both therapist and client carefully examine all of the evidence together while focusing on evidence that is most objective (i.e., most scientific or most compelling in a court of law). This avoids the problem of debating the quality of each piece of evidence when it is generated, while emphasizing the importance of giving greatest weight to the strongest types of evidence.

Teaching clients how to ask specific questions can help them learn how to generate evidence against their thoughts. Using the Tips for Finding Good Evidence Information Sheet can help clients to start to learn some of these strategies when using the skill on their own. Following are some useful questions the therapist can pose in session:

- "What is another way of looking at the situation?"
- "What is another possible explanation for what happened?"
- "Are there any examples that would suggest the thought isn't completely true?"
- "What would someone else think about the situation?"
- "Is this thought helpful to me?"
- "Is my thought based on how I feel rather than what happened?"
- "Am I setting for myself an unrealistic and unobtainable standard?"

Step 5: Making a Decision and Taking Action ("Believable" Thoughts)

In this step, clients sometimes come up with more accurate thoughts but still find these new thoughts not very "believable." The therapist should encourage the client to talk about the evidence against the thought in order to prompt a more realistic appraisal of the situation and to ensure that the new thought is believed more strongly than the old one. Sometimes the new thought may not feel believable, even though the client knows it to be true. In this case, the therapist can point out that this odd feeling reflects the newness of the client's thought but does not challenge its validity. The strange feeling people sometimes experience when they first challenge and change long-held beliefs can be normalized by explaining that their old thoughts and beliefs have been reinforced over many years and that it takes time and practice to replace them with new and more accurate thoughts, which will eventually feel just as believable. The therapist, via an

Action Plan, can also help clients devise a way of reminding themselves of the new thought when the old one keeps cropping up, as described in the previous section.

Another strategy for developing highly believable new thoughts is to teach the client to incorporate some of the evidence both for and against the old thought into the new thought. This serves to make the new thought feel more balanced but also more accurate and generally less distressing, based on the newly acknowledged facts from Step 4. For example, in the previous client–therapist dialogue with Leigh-Ann about her new hosting job, after exploring the evidence, Leigh-Ann decided that her upsetting thought ("I will make a big mistake, and they will just fire me right away") was inaccurate, so she initially modified it to "I'm definitely not going to screw up and get fired right away." However, she didn't find this new thought highly believable and still felt anxious. With the therapist's help, she modified her new thought further to "Even though I still feel somewhat anxious about what might happen at this new job, it is unlikely that I will make a big mistake and get fired right away." While this newer thought ended up being more believable, an additional modification could have been made if needed, such as this: "I have had some unfortunate work situations and met some unsavory managers, but my life is different enough now that I probably won't get fired right away even if this manager isn't that great." This example illustrates that coming up with a new thought that the client finds both believable and less upsetting can sometimes take some discussion. However, this trial-and-error approach is incorporated into the 5 Steps skill and can prove to be very useful to the client in terms of resolving distress and doubt.

BRIEF TIPS AND REMINDERS FOR ENHANCING LEARNING AND UPTAKE OF THE 5 STEPS OF CR

The following tips are useful for teaching and honing clients' ability to use the 5 Steps of CR on their own:

1. *Teach cognitive restructuring as a skill for dealing with negative feelings rather than as a tool for changing clients' thoughts and feelings.*
   Teaching clients the 5 Steps of CR as a skill fosters self-reliance and self-efficacy and avoids creating unnecessary dependency on the therapist for challenging and correcting thinking patterns that lead to distress. This is especially important when it comes to evaluating the evidence for and against the client's upsetting thought. Prompting clients to generate their own evidence—using the aforementioned Socratic questioning and Columbo style, rather than directly providing it for them—engages and invests them more in the task, leading to more convincing conclusions, including new and more accurate thoughts. In addition, focusing on skill development instead of changing the client's mind avoids the problem of *psychological reactance* (i.e., strongly resisting others' attempts to control one's behavior; Brehm, 1966) during the evaluation of evidence, which can paradoxically increase the client's conviction in a thought or belief rather than decrease it.

2. *Prompt the client to begin using the 5 Steps of CR as soon as possible after any negative feeling has been noticed or problem situation identified.*

   The more help and practice clients get using the 5 Steps of CR, both in session with the therapist and out of session on their own, the better the learning and outcomes. To maximize the time devoted to teaching cognitive restructuring in session, the therapist should initiate the 5 Steps right away after an unpleasant feeling or problem situation has been identified. For example, if the client indicates at the beginning of a session that they are feeling upset about a recent argument they had with their partner, the therapist should briefly empathize with the client, explore whether they would like to work on the problem together, and then begin the 5 Steps of CR by taking out a worksheet rather than just talking about the problem for the next 15–30 minutes.

3. *Steer away from overtly trauma-related situations or trauma-based core thoughts in introductory 5 Steps of CR teaching sessions.*

   While some clients naturally avoid mentioning trauma-related material at this point (in large part due to the nature of PTSD symptoms), others, because they are very aware that they are involved in a trauma intervention and these distressing experiences are understandably moving to the forefront their minds, may bring up trauma-related memories or situations in these early sessions. While it may be tempting to use the 5 Steps of CR skill to delve into and address these trauma-related situations with the client, it is recommended to hold off until the client has gained more understanding and has had solo practice using the 5 Steps in more general upsetting or stressful situations. This will greatly enhance their learning, mastery, and comfort with the skill, which will be much needed once more affectively-laden trauma-based topics and beliefs are addressed in later CR sessions (see Chapter 9, this volume). Thus, in these early stages of learning CR, an important balance exists between helping the client gain initial competence in the skill without becoming overwhelmed by trauma-related affect and not reinforcing avoidance of acknowledgment of the trauma and its impact in the person's life.

   In these situations, the clinician can do the following: (a) praise the client for bringing up the trauma-related material, (b) reinforce how they are "certainly on the right track" connecting these events to their current everyday distress, (c) provide a rationale for holding off on delving into the trauma material at this time in the favor of gaining initial mastery of the 5 Steps skill, and (d) make a collaborative plan to move into working on this trauma-related topic in an upcoming session (usually in a few weeks, around Session 7 or so). The clinician should continue to note trauma-related beliefs on their Therapist Tracking Sheet for Client's Trauma-Related Cognitions in order to remember these specific thoughts for later use and to demonstrate to the client that these important beliefs will be revisited and worked on in future sessions.

4. *Avoid getting bogged down during the 5 Steps of CR and failing to get through all the steps in a single session.*

   To ensure that clients are encouraged and reinforced for using cognitive restructuring when they feel upset, they must repeatedly experience relief when they use the skill in sessions with the therapist. This can occur only if the therapist makes a point of getting through all 5 Steps within a session and avoids doing some steps in one session and completing the rest in the next session. Working through all the steps at one time also makes the overall skill easier for clients to comprehend and eventually to use on their own.

5. *When teaching the 5 Steps of CR, pause frequently to review what has been discussed so far.*

   Frequent pauses to review progress (and prompt the client to assist in the review) when working on the 5 Steps of CR is a powerful teaching technique because it helps the client grasp the overall continuity and logic of the approach. Frequently reviewing what has been covered can also help correct any misunderstandings that may have occurred along the way. For example, after completing the second of the 5 Steps of CR with Donata, the therapist reviewed what had been discussed so far:

   THERAPIST: Let's pause for a moment to review what we have done so far in the 5 Steps of CR. In Step 1, you first identified that the situation in which you felt upset was when you went into the grocery store and saw how crowded it was. Then what did we do in the second step here?

   DONATA: I said my feelings that were upsetting?

   THERAPIST: Yes, exactly! In the second step, you identified several distressing feelings you had, including feeling embarrassed, nervous, anxious, afraid, and confused. Now let's begin the third step of cognitive restructuring, which involves identifying the thought underlying that feeling. What was the thought that you had decided was the most distressing of the four thoughts you came up with here in Step 3?

6. *Reinforce small gains in the client's ability to use the 5 Steps of CR.*

   It takes time and effort to learn cognitive restructuring, and gains often occur slowly over time and with much practice. The therapist should generously reinforce any and all efforts by the client to learn and practice the 5 Steps and provide specific reinforcement for small, incremental improvements in the client's skill understanding and effective use. Therapists need to be attuned to seemingly minor but significant gains in the client's ability to use the 5 Steps of CR and provide positive feedback accordingly (e.g., "You did a great job in generating a lot of evidence for and against your thought"). Similarly, clients may experience only modest reductions in distress from cognitive restructuring at first, but these improvements should be highlighted and used to encourage them that their relief will grow with continued practice of the skill.

7. *Encourage the client to embrace the 5 Steps of CR as a "self-management skill" as soon as possible.*

   Because the goal of teaching the 5 Steps of CR is for clients to use the skill in their day-to-day lives, the therapist should be on the alert for opportunities as early as possible to encourage the client to independently practice and use the skill. Once the client understands what the basic steps are and how the skill works, the therapist can begin to gradually help the client shift into taking more of the lead in walking through the skill and recording the steps on the worksheet with the therapist providing reminders and coaching as needed.

In addition to having the client complete the 5 Steps of CR worksheets for home assignments right after the first session introducing the 5 Steps, the therapist can also use specific language when referring to CR that promotes a sense of adoption of the skill by the client. For example, the therapist can inquire, "How is your cognitive restructuring working for you?" or "I'm interested in finding out from you in what ways you find the 5 Steps skill most helpful?" The therapist should encourage the client to make whatever adaptations they want in order to make the 5 Steps of CR work most effectively for them, as needed (see Chapter 10, this volume).

CONCLUSION

The 5 Steps of CR skill is a more advanced cognitive restructuring skill that incorporates the CST skill and serves to more comprehensively and powerfully address general distress and get to the root of beliefs underlying PTSD symptoms. This skill encompasses the following five steps: (a) describe the upsetting situation; (b) identify the distressing feeling; (c) pinpoint the associated thought and the CST; (d) evaluate the evidence that supports and does not support the thought; and (e) take action, either by modifying the thought for something more accurate or developing a problem-solving-based Action Plan to address the situation.

Teaching the client how to use the 5 Steps of CR to deal with distress builds on the CST skill in three important ways. First, the client is taught strategies for identifying thoughts related to their upsetting feelings and for pinpointing the way(s) in which these thoughts may be inaccurate and worth exploring (via identifying the appropriate CSTs). Modifying these more general beliefs initially will be critical to effectively evaluating and challenging schemas about traumatic experiences in the service of providing long-term relief from posttraumatic symptoms and distress. Second, the client is taught how to systematically evaluate evidence for and against those thoughts and how to weigh evidence based on its objectivity. Teaching the client how to distinguish between strong and weak evidence when evaluating the accuracy of the beliefs enables them to more critically examine the truthfulness and helpfulness their thoughts and ultimately change long-held and previously unchallenged trauma-related cognitions. Third, the client is taught to either change their thought (if the weight of evidence is against it) or to create an Action Plan for dealing with the upsetting situation (if the weight of evidence supports the thought). This final part of the 5 Steps of CR is crucial because it recognizes that not all distressing feelings are due to inaccurate thought processes, and it prompts clients to formulate a plan for dealing with genuinely problematic situations. In this manner, the client experiences distress reduction regardless of their choice in Step 5, an important and unique component of the 5 Steps of CR skill. This experience can provide immediate relief from distress and therefore reinforce the client's ongoing practice and use of the skill, particularly as the program shifts toward applying it to directly addressing trauma-related thoughts and beliefs.

9

Cognitive Restructuring III

Working With Trauma-Related Thoughts, Core Beliefs, and Persistent PTSD Symptoms

Helping clients identify and change distressing trauma-related thoughts and beliefs is a fundamental goal of the Cognitive Restructuring (CR) for posttraumatic stress disorder (PTSD) program. When and how these thoughts and beliefs are identified and addressed with the 5 Steps of CR vary from one client to the next. For some clients, the Step 3 ("Identify the Upsetting Thought") techniques (described in Chapter 8, this volume) for pinpointing the most distressing thought(s) quickly lead to upsetting trauma-related beliefs and core schemas, which can then be addressed in the remaining steps of the skill. For other clients, the relationship among traumatic experiences, upsetting feelings, thoughts, and functioning is less clear. Therefore, the therapist needs to use additional strategies to assist the client in eliciting these patterns in order to uncover the trauma-related schemas to address in CR. When teaching the 5 Steps of CR, the initial focus is on helping the client learn how to use the skill to deal with any negative feelings, typically of a more general (and non-trauma-focused) sort. Over time, as clients become more adept at using cognitive restructuring, the relationship between those feelings (and associated upsetting thoughts) and their traumatic experiences often becomes more apparent to the client and therapist and naturally becomes a focus of cognitive restructuring. Typically, the specific trauma-related content is associated with the identified index trauma, and the CR is focused there. However, because underlying trauma-related beliefs are often broad-based and generalized ("It is my fault that all these terrible things have happened to me"), other traumatic events that the

https://doi.org/10.1037/0000423-009
Treatment of Posttraumatic Stress Disorder in Serious Mental Illness: The Cognitive Restructuring Program, by K. T. Mueser and J. D. Gottlieb

client has experienced can sometimes also be addressed within the context of the intervention timetable.

Sometimes the relationship between distressing feelings and trauma-related beliefs seems apparent to the therapist but not to the client, who may even actively avoid making the connection. Alternatively, sometimes the impact of trauma-related beliefs on negative feelings may continue to be unclear to both the client and therapist.

In all of these aforementioned scenarios, the therapist has a number of options for bringing trauma-related thoughts and core beliefs into focus to address through cognitive restructuring. These techniques and strategies as well as a discussion of timing for initiating trauma-related cognitive restructuring are explicated next.

WHEN TO BEGIN TRAUMA-RELATED CR

It is strongly recommended that trauma-related CR be initiated by Session 9 so that there is sufficient time remaining in the program for clients to have the opportunity to address important trauma-related and core beliefs as effectively as possible. If this transition has not occurred by Session 9, then the therapist should use the results of the readministration of the PTSD Checklist (PCL) in Session 10 to identify the currently most severe PTSD symptoms the client experiences and to initiate the 5 Steps of CR based on one of those items (see additional details later in this chapter in the Drawing Upon Symptom Assessments section).

The exact timetable for when the therapist should initiate work on trauma-related thoughts and beliefs varies depending on each client, with many being ready to begin trauma-focused CR earlier than Session 9 but some others not. In general, prior to delving into trauma-based cognitions, the client should have a clear understanding of the rationale for and mechanics of the 5 Steps of CR, have had some practice using it, and have experienced some reinforcing reduction in distress following use of the skill. In other words, some mastery of the skill is important for the client to be able to handle the transition into more emotionally laden trauma material and for the skill to be effective at reducing PTSD-related distress. Some specific criteria to consider when deciding when to initiate trauma-based CR include the following:

- Has the client mastered the use of the 5 Steps in session (even if some prompting or coaching from the therapist is still needed)?
- Has the client used the 5 Steps successfully on their own for home assignments (the more the better)?
- Has the client consistently attended sessions around the time of the desired transition to trauma-related CR?
- To what extent has trauma-related material spontaneously emerged in CR work so far? (Evaluate frequent vs. nonexistent vs. avoidant.)

While the last item in the checklist does not have to be frequent to begin working on trauma-related material, it can make the transition easier if the client has already made some important connections between recent distressing situations and their trauma history. If the client seems to be actively or passively avoiding any mention of trauma material or consequences of PTSD, then it can be useful for the therapist to consider helping the client initiate a 5 Steps of CR exercise around the thoughts that may be underlying this avoidance (i.e., "If I delve into things related to the trauma, I won't be able to handle it and will fall apart"). (For details on this strategy, see Chapter 10, this volume.) Although addressing these fears with the 5 Steps is suggested for clients who seem to be avoiding the process, it is recommended that at least a brief discussion take place with all clients regarding their attitudes about transitioning into trauma-related CR prior to initiation of this phase of therapy.

Even if trauma-related material has not yet spontaneously emerged in sessions and clients do not appear to be avoiding the topic, they may still be ready and willing to begin trauma-focused CR. Furthermore, even if the aforementioned criteria are not met, it is still safe and effective to begin trauma-related CR work in Session 9 or (at the latest) Session 10. In these cases, the therapist should be aware that the client may need more help using the 5 Steps of CR to address trauma-related thoughts and beliefs.

HOW TO INITIATE THE TRANSITION INTO TRAUMA-RELATED CR

While trauma-related themes and core beliefs often emerge naturally as the sessions progress, sometimes the therapist needs to take a lead in eliciting this type of material. The clinician can use a broad range of strategies to bring trauma-related thoughts and beliefs into focus to address with the 5 Steps of CR. These strategies are discussed next.

Directly Inquiring About Everyday Stressful Situations and Linking to Traumatic Experiences

One effective technique is to simply ask whether a particular stressful situation may be related to the client's traumatic experiences. The therapist can ask a general question, inviting the client to consider this possibility, which the therapist does in the following example with Edmundo:

THERAPIST: Edmundo, I'm so glad that you added something to our agenda for our Session 7 today. You mentioned that you wanted to talk about how stressed you felt this week after not hearing back about that temp job you applied for. This is a really good stressful experience to address with the 5 Steps of CR. We started doing that together just now, and so let's review for a minute where we are. In Step 1, you identified that the stressful situation was that it's been 3 weeks since you applied for the temp contractor job, and you haven't heard back yet. In Step 2, you said that your strongest upsetting feeling was depression. In Step 3, you identified the thought "I'm no good" as the most distressing thought contributing to your depression. Do I have that right?

EDMUNDO: Yeah, that's right.

THERAPIST: Do you think that your thought that "I'm no good" could be related to your experiences growing up with your family and in your neighborhood with what you went through in the gang?

EDMUNDO: I guess so.

THERAPIST: Let's talk about how they might be related. You had said that as a child you didn't experience much love and positive attention, which, as we talked about, probably contributed to your getting involved in gangs when you were a teenager. How do you think growing up in that family environment could have affected the way you think about yourself now as an adult?

EDMUNDO: Well, they were telling me a lot that I'm no good.

THERAPIST: Could you explain a little more? Who was telling you that?

EDMUNDO: Mostly my dad, even when I was little—like I was a drain on the family. And then some of the gang guys when I first got started. And so I've always thought about that—because my family told me I was no good and then the guys out on the streets too. I believed them, and I still do, I guess. It's like what my other therapist said—"low-self-esteem coming from childhood."

THERAPIST: Did your dad actually say that you were no good, or was that the impression you got from how he treated you? And what about in the gang?

EDMUNDO: Yeah—both. My father used to punish me pretty harshly, and he sometimes said it, literally. And the same thing when I would get beaten up in the neighborhood. But mostly, I think it's because my parents never treated me like I was worth anything.

THERAPIST: I see. So it sounds like when you didn't hear about the job, you told yourself, "I'm no good," which was repeating something that you've believed about yourself for a long time and is directly related to how your family treated you when you were a kid?

EDMUNDO: Jeez, yeah. I think that's right. I'm not sure I ever really knew that.

THERAPIST: It makes a lot of sense though, doesn't it? Maybe we could look at that more closely. Let's make your thought in Step 3 a little more specific, now that we have talked through and better understand what has led up to it. How does that sound?

EDMUNDO: Yeah, OK. It does make sense.

THERAPIST: What might be a thought that captures your current situation about how you think about yourself—something like, "I'm no good because?"

EDMUNDO: Because my family treated me bad and told me I was a drain on the family.

THERAPIST: Yes, that's such a powerful and distressing belief, and it makes perfect sense that if you have held that belief for so long, it would impact so much of your everyday life. How about we work together on looking into the accuracy of that thought with the rest of the 5 Steps?

EDMUNDO: OK, yeah. That's probably a good idea.

Reviewing Trauma-Related Patterns and Beliefs From Prior Sessions

Sometimes specific themes become apparent across multiple situations addressed in prior CR sessions, and the relationship between these themes and the client's traumatic experiences can be explored. For instance, through discussions during the earlier psychoeducational sessions and CR exercises, the therapist may have noticed that the client has a pattern of interpersonal relationship struggles with different people in their life (family, friendships, work colleagues) that appears to be related to their difficulty trusting other people. The clinician can share their observation of this theme and ask the client if and how it might be related to their past traumatic event. From there, they can explore associated trauma-related beliefs (e.g., "Men will only hurt you and cannot be trusted at all") and proceed from there to examine one such belief with the 5 Steps. The therapist can use probe questions to help the client identify and explore the theme. An example is provided in the following exchange with Leigh-Ann:

THERAPIST: Let's spend a few more minutes talking about the situation you described in your home assignment that happened last week when you decided to try out that recovery group meet-up at the park.

LEIGH-ANN: OK. I remember that I felt really nervous because this guy I don't know came up to me after the presentation and tried to start a conversation.

THERAPIST: Yes, and I can see from the worksheet that you identified your strongest feeling at the time was anxiety.

LEIGH-ANN: Yes, that's right.

THERAPIST: And when you considered what you were thinking that made you feel this way, you identified the thought that concerned you most was "I can't trust this guy."

LEIGH-ANN: That's right. I felt really uncomfortable.

THERAPIST: Something that I've noticed over the past few weeks of working together is that in several of the situations in which you felt uncomfortable, the underlying thought you identified had to do with the question of trust.

LEIGH-ANN: That's true. I don't know if I can trust anybody.

THERAPIST: Do you think that this concern could be related to some of the traumatic experiences that you have had in your life?

LEIGH-ANN: I think so.

THERAPIST: How? In what way?

LEIGH-ANN: Being molested as a child by my friend's dad has made it hard to trust people. And then later on after the rape—that also makes me feel that way. I can't trust anybody.

THERAPIST: I understand. It sounds as though that belief is a really important one to examine since it's having a major effect on your daily life, including just casual interactions with other people. Shall we examine this belief more carefully today with the 5 Steps?

LEIGH-ANN: OK.

At this stage of the program, the Therapist Tracking Sheet for Client's Trauma-Related Cognitions worksheet plays an important role in commencing a deeper dive into trauma-related beliefs. Starting in Session 1, the therapist, ideally, has been noting the client's articulated trauma-related beliefs as they emerge, either in the context of their responses to the therapist's direct questions or spontaneously as psychoeducation topics are discussed (or via other earlier CR practice). Taking out this worksheet and reviewing it with the client at the beginning of a session can assist greatly in collaboratively finding a trauma-related thought to use for CR work.

Reviewing PTSD Psychoeducation Worksheets and Earlier CR Home Assignments

The therapist should keep nearby the previously completed psychoeducational handouts as well as the client's completed CR home assignment worksheets. One strategy is to return to the psychoeducational How Trauma Affects Thoughts and Feelings handout and to examine distressing thoughts related to traumatic experiences previously identified by the client. From there, the therapist can explore whether a particular thought is still distressing to the client and, if so, initiate a 5 Steps of CR exercise to work on that thought. For example, the therapist returned to this worksheet with Donata:

THERAPIST: Let's return to the handout How Trauma Affects Thoughts and Feelings and look at some of the thoughts you previously described as related to your abuse experiences. I can see that when we completed this back in Session 3, you indicated that you thought that "The world is an unsafe place." When you look back on that thought now, overall, do you still believe it's true?

DONATA: Yes, I think so.

THERAPIST: How do you think some of your traumatic experiences may have contributed to that belief?

DONATA: What my parents did to me—and how my parents hit me or ignored me or both. Or made me do crazy things like fly that plane filled with drugs. And then their so-called friends would be high and hanging around our house—making me do things to them. I never knew when something bad was going to happen. There was no such thing as being safe.

THERAPIST: Yes, Donata, you've had some really difficult experiences of not being able to feel safe, even in your own home growing up. And that makes it hard for you to feel safe anywhere right now?

DONATA: Right.

THERAPIST: How does not feeling safe interfere with your day-to-day life?

DONATA: I'm always nervous that something's going to happen—that the voices are going to get me or someone else is. I have trouble sleeping, and I jump at the slightest sound. It's even hard for me to go out of my apartment sometimes, even to come here.

THERAPIST: Yes, it makes sense, doesn't it? Feeling unsafe and that the world is a dangerous place—is a belief related to your traumatic experiences earlier in your life. And this belief seems to contribute to a lot of the anxiety you experience in your daily life. It sounds as though we should examine this belief more closely together, right?

DONATA: OK.

A related strategy is to review previously completed home assignments, such as the tracking of upsetting situations and thoughts from the Common Styles of

Thinking Worksheet and/or earlier 5 Steps of CR practice. Although the objective of these early CR assignments is for the client to learn the skill of the 5 Steps using more basic (and less trauma-based or affectively laden) scenarios and thoughts, even these more day-to-day situations are often related to the client's trauma history and PTSD symptoms.

Drawing Upon Symptom Assessments

The benefit of readministering the PTSD (and depression) self-assessments at regular intervals throughout the program is that it allows for close tracking of areas of distress that can be readily used to identify upsetting thoughts for thorough examination with the 5 Steps of CR. As the sessions proceed and the time comes to directly focus on trauma-related thoughts with CR, the measures administered in Sessions 7 and 10 (and onward) serve as very useful tools to aid in the identification of trauma-based and core beliefs for in-session CR work.

When a client's Session 7 PCL-5 indicates continued high scores on particular items (i.e., a 3 or 4), these symptoms can be discussed at the beginning of the session in the context of talking about the score changes (since the Session 4 PCL). For example, if Item 7 ("Avoiding external reminders of the stressful experience—for example, people, places, conversations, activities, objects, or situations") was highly endorsed, this can open the door for a brief discussion with the client about why that particular symptom is currently so upsetting to them. The therapist can then ask the client to think of a particular time during the past week when they found themselves having this avoidance symptom. From there, a 5 Steps of CR can be initiated based on that particular situation. The same method can be used with a depression measure as well—such as the Beck Depression Inventory–II (BDI-II), where, for example, the client may endorse Item 3 ("Past Failure") with a score of 2: "As I look back, I see a lot of failures." From this item, a brief examination of a more specific thought can lead to a core belief ("I am a complete failure in all ways") or trauma-based belief ("I should have been able to save my brother"), which can then be evaluated with the 5 Steps. See Exhibit 9.1 for a step-by-step method for using the PCL-5 and BDI-II items in this manner.

Using a Standardized Trauma Beliefs Measure

Another strategy for identifying trauma-related beliefs is to use a standardized instrument to directly measure them, such as the Posttraumatic Cognitions Inventory (PTCI; Foa et al., 1999). The PTCI includes common trauma-related beliefs endorsed by people with PTSD, regardless of type of traumatic event. Given the universality of the beliefs on the PTCI in clients with PTSD, most clients endorse at least several of the items, which provide

EXHIBIT 9.1

Translating PCL-5 and BDI-II Scale Items Into Core and Trauma-Related Beliefs for Examination With the 5 Steps of CR: Procedure and Examples

Step-by-step procedure

1. Identify a specific item on the scale that received a high distress rating.

2. In Step 1 of the 5 Steps, the "Situation" can be either
   - a recent event that triggered this symptom or thought (e.g., "I saw on the news last night a story about a murder–suicide that happened this week") or
   - a memory or symptom that was noticed at a particular moment (e.g., "Thinking about the trauma yesterday," "I had two flashbacks last week").

3. Help the client create a workable thought for Step 3, based on the Step 1 situation and the highly endorsed scale item (e.g., "It was my fault that I let the abuse go on for so long. I'm to blame").

4. Proceed through the 5 Steps from there.

Example from PCL-5

PCL Item 7:	"Avoiding external reminders of the stressful experience (for example, people, places, conversations, activities, objects, or situations."
Step 1 (situation):	"I didn't go to the Department of Motor Vehicles to renew my license in time last week because it's in the same neighborhood as where I think the man who raped me lives."
Step 2 (feelings):	"Anxiety/fear; guilt/shame."
Step 3 (thoughts):	"It was my fault I was raped by him." "I could get raped again by the same man."

Example from BDI-II

BDI-II Item 3:	"Past failure: As I look back, I see a lot of failures."
Step 1 (situation):	"My cousin called me to tell me she was getting married."
Step 2 (feelings):	"Sadness/depression, guilt/shame, anger."
Step 3 (thoughts):	"I've done nothing right in life." "I am a mess and damaged goods." "I will never have a normal life like everyone else (because of what I've experienced)."

Note. PCL-5 = PTSD Checklist–5; BDI-II = Beck Depression Inventory–II; CR = cognitive restructuring; PTSD = posttraumatic stress disorder.

an efficient way to identify specific distressing beliefs that can then be examined with CR. Once a particular distressing thought on the PTCI has been identified, it is relatively straightforward to establish a connection between that belief and the person's traumatic experiences and to then use the 5 Steps of CR to examine the evidence supporting and not supporting that belief.

Since trauma-related thoughts and beliefs can change over the course of treatment, the therapist may choose to track changes over time by repeatedly administering the PTCI (e.g., in conjunction with regular monitoring of PTSD symptoms and depression severity). Table 9.1 includes common trauma-related thoughts and beliefs on the PTCI endorsed by clients with serious mental illness (SMI) and PTSD.

TABLE 9.1. The 10 Most Commonly Endorsed Thoughts or Beliefs on the Post-traumatic Cognitions Inventory (Foa et al., 1999) in 432 Persons With SMI and PTSD

Thought or belief	Belief rating
1. You never know when something terrible will happen.	5.73
2. I have to be especially careful because you never know what can happen next.	5.73
3. You can never know who will harm you.	5.71
4. I have to be on guard all the time.	5.39
5. The world is a dangerous place.	5.20
6. I feel isolated and set apart from others.	5.19
7. People can't be trusted.	5.12
8. People are not what they seem.	5.09
9. My life has been destroyed by the trauma.	4.87
10. I can't rely on other people.	4.80

Note. Belief ratings based on 1 = *totally disagree*, 7 = *totally agree*. SMI = serious mental illness; PTSD = posttraumatic stress disorder. Data are from Lu, Yanos, et al. (2022), Mueser, Gottlieb, et al. (2015), and Mueser et al. (2008).

TECHNIQUES FOR EFFECTIVELY TARGETING TRAUMA-RELATED BELIEFS VIA THE 5 STEPS OF CR

Once the transition into this trauma-based phase of CR work has begun (using the strategies just discussed), the stage has been set to systematically delve into and help the client evaluate specific trauma and core belief-related material. There are some important techniques to attend to so that the use of the 5 Steps of CR has as much impact as possible at this important stage of the intervention, and they are outlined next.

Developing Workable Trauma-Related and Core Beliefs in Step 3

As introduced in Chapter 8 in this volume, a *workable thought* is one that is a very clear conjecture or believed statement that is potentially subject to falsification. In addition, a workable thought is phrased as a full, clear statement about something explicitly related to the client, where the distress it causes is obvious. Using a combination of the general strategies outlined in Chapter 8 in this volume in conjunction with those discussed in the previous section to identify trauma-related and core beliefs will often suffice to articulate a workable thought in Step 3, and the remainder of the 5 Steps can proceed from there. Sometimes, however, additional strategies are required in order to ensure that these trauma-related upsetting thoughts are understandable, well-defined, and therefore workable before proceeding into Step 4. Following are some specific helpful techniques for the therapist to attend to.

Make Sure That the Belief Components Are Clearly Stated and Well-Defined

It is not unusual for clients who have experienced trauma and lived with untreated PTSD (coupled with suffering from symptoms from a co-occurring psychiatric condition like chronic depression, bipolar disorder, or schizophrenia) to describe their current struggles in quite broad and highly distressing terms (e.g., "My life has been destroyed by the trauma," "I'm a bad mother").

While this is understandable given the shifts in cognition that occur as a result of having PTSD, it is crucial that the therapist work with the client to make sure that their thoughts are clearly articulated and well-understood by the therapist before moving on to Step 4. In other words, therapists should not assume they understand what a client means when describing a particular trauma-related (or core) thought unless it is crystal clear, nor should they pretend to understand why a thought is associated with a specific distressing emotion unless it is equally clear. These links need to be directly addressed and made more comprehensible as needed within Step 3. Lack of attention to the clarity of the thought and its associated feeling can impede effective work in Steps 4 and 5 and therefore the ability to successfully refute underlying trauma-related thoughts and beliefs.

When discussing these types of thoughts and before beginning to evaluate evidence, the therapist should ask specific questions to better understand what the client means by general phrases or beliefs and clarify how those are directly connected to their particular emotion(s), as needed. Given that the same phrase or characteristic (e.g., "bad mother") can be defined in myriad ways, the client's personal definition determines in large part how the therapist will (a) help the client link that particular belief to their trauma(s) and (b) guide them through evaluating the evidence for and against that thought in Step 4. Other examples of how commonly held trauma-related and core beliefs may be more specifically articulated for more effective examination with the 5 Steps are provided in Exhibit 9.2.

Zero in on a Specific Trauma-Related Belief

General distressing beliefs are important for the transition into trauma-related CR work, and they can be made more explicit (and therefore, easier to refute) by helping the client more overtly and specifically link the thought to the trauma. This helps to ensure that the trauma-related component is clear and directly related to the client's experience, which will aid in helping the client to challenge it in Step 4.

One way to do this is to ask clients first to add "because" onto the end of their belief statement and then to finish the sentence. For instance, a client's index trauma was surviving an armed robbery in adolescence after an older sister had been shot and killed by burglars. The client often felt depressed and guilty in everyday situations and, after a discussion of their thoughts contributing to those emotions, stated, "I don't deserve anything good anyway." Prompts by the therapist to add a "because" to that thought uncovered something directly trauma-related that could be examined more closely: "I don't

---

EXHIBIT 9.2

Examples of How Commonly Held Trauma and Core Beliefs Can Be Clarified and More Specifically Articulated for Enhanced Effective Examination With the 5 Steps of CR

- "My life has been destroyed by the trauma." → "I'll never have a house of my own or enjoy life."

- "My life has been destroyed by the trauma." → "I will never be able to have a rewarding, trusting relationship with someone."

- "I'm a bad person." → "I think horrible thoughts about others and don't contribute to society by having a regular job."

- "I'm a bad person." → "I don't stick to anything I start, and I'm mean to my partner sometimes."

- "People are not what they seem." → "People will take advantage of you if given the opportunity, so no one can be trusted."

- "People are not what they seem." → "People pretend to care but then act selfish."

- "I'll never have normal feelings again because of the trauma." → "I'll never be able to feel love again."

- "I'll never have normal feelings again because of the trauma." → "I'll never be able to not be painfully anxious around other people."

- "I'm a bad mother." → [Therapist: "How would you define what a good mother is?"] Client: "Someone who spends time with her kids and doesn't lose their temper and helps them with their homework."

- "I'm a bad mother." → [Therapist: "How would you define what a bad mother is?"] Client: "Someone who cries all the time and gets stressed out and doesn't bake cookies for their kids ever."

Note. CR = cognitive restructuring.

deserve anything good in life because my sister died and I didn't, and not having a good life is my punishment for surviving."

A related strategy is to simply ask the question, "Why is this the case?" following a client's identification of a highly distressing belief. For example, in a scenario related to a time that Donata avoided a mental health clinic group picnic invitation due to paranoia and anxiety (Steps 1 and 2), the thought in Step 3 might be "I have to be on guard all the time." In answering the therapist's question ("Why is this the case?"), Donata could reveal the link between this ongoing debilitating belief and past traumatic experiences as follows: "I have to be on guard all the time now because I was physically abused by my parents and their friends and bullied in school." This level of detail allows for a deeper, more meaningful, and more effective examination of the evidence in Step 4, and it likely will lead to a more potent outcome in terms of insight and reduction of trauma and PTSD-related distress.

Additional examples of using "because" to link general distressing thoughts to more specific trauma-related thoughts include the following:

- "I'm shameful because I didn't tell anyone about the sexual abuse, and I didn't stop it, and I felt some sexual feelings, which means I'm bad or not normal."
- "Nobody can ever be trusted because I was physically abused by my parents and boyfriend."
- "I won't ever be able to be self-sufficient because the car accident took away my independence forever."
- "The voices are right when they say I'm a total failure because I didn't do enough to stop my mother from ending her life."

Identify and Explore the Deeper Meaning of the Thought

Sometimes the thought that the client has chosen as the most upsetting one from their generated list in Step 3 may seem somewhat superficial or "close to the surface," even though it clearly caused the client significant distress. When this is the case, the therapist can guide the client to explore further to see if the thought has a deeper meaning. As introduced in Chapter 8 in this volume, this type of below-the-surface thought is commonly known as a *core belief.*

While it is crucial to ensure that overt and specific trauma-related beliefs are addressed during this phase of treatment, the therapist can and should also target core beliefs as needed. Core beliefs often develop early in life and, following a traumatic event, may become even more extreme, entrenched, and debilitating. Thus, they also tend to be strongly related to a client's ongoing general distress and to the perpetuation of their PTSD symptoms. In addition, they often serve as the gateway to the identification of a more specific trauma-related belief to examine down the line. Thus, focusing on an upsetting core belief serves as another useful way to implement trauma-focused work with the 5 Steps of CR. Identifying and examining core beliefs allows for a more comprehensive and sustainable shift in distressing thoughts and their behavioral impact, as well as a potentially larger reduction in PTSD symptoms.

One powerful method of arriving at and extracting a core belief is via the downward-arrow technique (Burns, 1999). Here, the therapist initiates a series of questions about each upsetting thought (and also teaches clients to ask themselves these questions), such as, "If this thought were true, what would it say about me as a person?" Additional questions (e.g., "If this belief were true, what does this mean to me?" "If this happened, what would happen next?" "What would be the worst thing about that?") can get at the deeper meaning and beliefs underlying strong emotional reactions to seemingly minor events (Clark, 1989).

This technique plays an important role in this trauma-focused stage of the intervention. Following is an example of how to move from a more surface thought to a core belief using the downward-arrow technique with Edmundo:

THERAPIST: In Step 1, you noted that this week you went to the pharmacy and became upset while you were there. Then in Step 2, you chose "fear/anxiety" and then "shame" as your most upsetting emotions. In Step 3, we identified a few thoughts related to the situation, and you chose the most distressing one as "The clerk yesterday at the store looked at me like he was going to try something with me after I left." Let's take a closer look at that thought, OK?

EDMUNDO: Yeah, I guess. I thought about this all week. I don't know why it has been bugging me this much.

THERAPIST: It does seem like an important one. First thing, can you help me understand what you mean by "try something with me"? I just want to make sure we are on the same page.

EDMUNDO: Sure, like, maybe he was going to give me a hard time—like, find me and mouth off or, like, want to brawl or something.

THERAPIST: OK, thank you. Now I get it. Let me ask you this, Edmundo. If your thought were true—that there was a good chance the clerk would give you a hard time after you left the store— what would that say about you that this could possibly happen?

EDMUNDO: That he somehow could peg me as someone who can be taken advantage of.

THERAPIST: OK. And if that were the case, what might that say about you?

EDMUNDO: That I'm weak. That I'm known as someone who doesn't take care of his own business and never protected his little brother. Someone who isn't up to the task in life, then or now.

THERAPIST: And if that were actually true about you, Edmundo, what would that mean about you?

EDMUNDO: Well, that people just know.

THERAPIST: That people know what?

EDMUNDO: That, that everyone knows I'm totally worthless.

Once the core belief (which is often directly linked to a past trauma as in Edmundo's case) is identified, there is often an increase in the client's emotion. This is normal and indicates that the therapist has hit on something fundamental to the client's ongoing distress and PTSD symptoms. From there, the therapist can gently guide the client through the remainder of the 5 Steps of CR to help them evaluate the accuracy of this important long-held, core belief ("I am totally worthless"), or the therapist can steer the client toward a more specific thought that explicitly mentions the trauma, such as ("I am totally worthless because I didn't do enough to help my brother and it's my fault he killed himself"). Thus, in some instances, there is high value in helping the client pinpoint and challenge more global core beliefs (e.g., "I am unlovable"), and in other instances, there is value in identifying more specific trauma-related beliefs ("I am unlovable because my parents told me so while they were beating me as a child"). Focusing on either type of belief with the 5 Steps of CR typically leads to reductions in distress.

EVALUATING EVIDENCE FOR AND AGAINST TRAUMA-RELATED BELIEFS

As described in Chapter 8 in this volume, teaching clients how to identify and understand high-quality evidence for and against their thought in Step 4 is crucial to learning the 5 Steps of CR and maximizing their distress reduction. The same Step 4 strategies described in Chapter 8 in this volume are useful in this phase of therapy as well. That said, given that trauma-related and core beliefs tend to be more ingrained and more distressing than other types of upsetting thoughts, some additional tips and techniques may prove useful when helping clients work with these types of beliefs. Throughout these sessions, ongoing use of the Tips for Finding Good Evidence Information Sheet is recommended as a way to help clients systematically identify and examine important evidence bearing on their trauma-related beliefs.

As also illustrated in Chapter 8 in this volume, along with using the Tips for Finding Good Evidence Information Sheet, the therapist's primary role is to act as a guide in helping the client find evidence pertaining to their thought. One useful strategy is for the therapist to employ a Socratic teaching approach in which questions or statements are posed in a guiding, curious, and nonjudgmental style, often framed as potential hypotheses, to move the client along the path toward objectively evaluating the evidence for and against their thoughts. The critical feature of Socratic questioning is that the student (client) is asked questions that eventually lead to specific conclusions but is not told the answers to the questions or the conclusions, so that the student (client) reaches their own conclusions and is more likely to believe them. Using the Socratic questioning style to teach clients how to generate and evaluate evidence pertaining to a belief, with frequent pauses to reflect together on the answers to questions and any conclusions reached by the client, is an effective approach to developing this critical skill and facilitating the client's ability to doing it independently.

The Socratic method of asking questions can be used in a broad range of ways to teach the client strategies for examining evidence pertaining to their trauma-related thoughts. Three primary lines of questioning can be helpful when examining trauma-related beliefs:

- Prompt the client to consider what is similar versus what is different in their current life compared with when their trauma(s) occurred in the past.

- Explore any exceptions to absolutist beliefs that developed in the past, however minor (e.g., one person who could be trusted in their old neighborhood).

- If the traumatic event occurred in childhood, ask questions about their understanding of a typical child's ability to have control over their own environment and decisions.

Following is a snippet of client–therapist dialogue focused on strategies for exploring evidence for and against Edmundo's belief that "I am totally worthless because I didn't do enough to help my brother and it's my fault he killed himself." In addition to the general strategies used for Step 4, also note the specific aforementioned elements useful for working with these sorts of trauma-related beliefs, in particular the therapist's use of the Socratic method:

THERAPIST:	Now that we've identified this very distressing thought in Step 3 and we've noted a few pieces of evidence that you think support your belief that "I am totally worthless because I didn't do enough to help my brother and it's my fault he killed himself," what do we do next, Edmundo?
EDMUNDO:	We turn it around. Like, we say what doesn't make it true. Although to be honest, I'm not sure if there is anything, really.
THERAPIST:	Well, that's why it's so important to dig into this step of the skill—because a thought this upsetting that you have been holding onto for all this time is something that we should look into to see if it may not be totally accurate, right?
EDMUNDO:	Yeah, that's true.
THERAPIST:	OK, let's work together on this. You said you were about 15 when you got involved with the gang in your neighborhood and your younger brother was about 13. Let me ask you this: Would a child of that age, 15—especially one who had a difficult at-home life like you described—be able to make a healthy decision about getting involved in that world?
EDMUNDO:	I thought I was all tough and mature, but I really was just a scared kid. No, I guess not.
THERAPIST:	Right. And so would that maybe also apply to your ability or lack thereof to keep your brother from joining a gang too?
EDMUNDO:	Yeah, I guess so. I was a kid, and I wasn't his parent, even though he was younger than me. That was a job for my dad and mom and even my grandma, but they didn't do what they were supposed to. They were the adults.
THERAPIST:	Yes, I agree. Should that be written down here—under the evidence that doesn't support your thought? It sounds like these might actually be two pieces of evidence for that side? How should we phrase those?

EDMUNDO: Um, I guess, "I was just a kid, so I didn't know enough to make the right decision about not joining a gang and keeping my brother away from it either."

THERAPIST: Good, I've got those two pieces of evidence down here now. What about the part related to your parents?

EDMUNDO: It's not a kid's responsibility to keep themselves out of that kind of danger. It's the role of the parents. They are adults.

THERAPIST: Excellent, Edmundo. I've written that down as well. We now have three pieces of evidence here against your thought. [The therapist reads each aloud and shares the worksheet with the client.] Now let's take a look at the part of your thought related to your belief that you are worthless, which is something you've said you still believe about yourself in general, right?

EDMUNDO: Yeah. I've always felt that way about myself, and it got even more ingrained back when my brother killed himself, and I still feel it to be true.

THERAPIST: Yes, and we've talked about that "feeling" as related to the CST emotional reasoning, which serves as an indicator that your thought may not be totally accurate. It can be helpful to take a look at what might be different now about you and your life compared with back then. What would you say is not the same about you when you were a kid in the gang and around the time your brother died?

EDMUNDO: Well, I am not in that world anymore. I worked hard to remove myself and start a new life.

THERAPIST: Yes, absolutely. And in your new life, are there things that you have done or are doing that don't support your belief that you are worthless?

EDMUNDO: I'm coming to the mental health clinic. I'm taking medicine. I'm doing this therapy with you. I go to PT. I'm trying at least to get healthier.

THERAPIST: Edmundo, exactly. I'm writing all of those down here on our worksheet. What about things related to your efforts with your partner and kids? Is there anything there that we should note that runs counter to your belief that you are worthless?

EDMUNDO: I know I'm not perfect with them, but I am trying to provide more, with the SSDI and the part-time job I got as a start. I pay attention to my kids and show them love as much as I can. So I don't do what my dad did to me.

THERAPIST: I'm going to also note all of those on our sheet here. So would a worthless person do those important things you just mentioned?

EDMUNDO: I guess not.

THERAPIST: Here's another thing that I've heard you mention before that I want to ask more about. Your thought suggests that you didn't put enough effort into helping your brother, but is that 100% true? I've heard you mention briefly before that there were a few times that you tried to help. I think it is important for us to spell out those instances and see if they provide any evidence against your thought here.

EDMUNDO: Well, there were at least three times where I went to his apartment and tried to get him to go with me to the urgent care so he could get his depression and drug use under control. Each time, I brought some information pamphlets with me and sat with him for, like, 2 hours. One time, I even spent the night—trying to get him to go. But he wouldn't, not once.

THERAPIST: And how might those events be considered evidence that doesn't support your thought here, Edmundo?

EDMUNDO: Yeah, those were actual times I made a major effort to help him. I'm not sure what more I could have done in those situations, really (see the Tips for Finding Good Evidence Information Sheet for other, more general types of queries to initiate with clients).

See the Tips for Finding Good Evidence Information Sheet for other, more general types of queries to initiate with clients.

CRAFTING NEW, MORE ACCURATE, AND BELIEVABLE TRAUMA-RELATED THOUGHTS IN STEP 5

The basic strategies for assisting clients in modification of inaccurate beliefs in this step (see Chapter 8, this volume) are similarly fruitful for trauma-related and core beliefs. However, given the long-standing and ingrained beliefs associated with trauma that clients are working on in this program, the process of modifying these typically inaccurate beliefs is often slower and more gradual than with other sorts of thoughts. This is perfectly normal, and time for this "chipping-away" strategy is built into the program.

To carry this out, in Step 5, the therapist should focus on helping the client to gradually debunk core and trauma-related beliefs by starting with a thorough review of Step 4 evidence. Following this review, a straightforward way to help clients consider either fully refuting or at least slightly dialing back their phrasing of this thought is to ask, "Now that we see all the evidence, would you say that your thought is completely, 100% true?" From there, the therapist can help the client make whatever changes they are comfortable with to modify the thought to make it more accurate. Sometimes a friendly negotiation occurs around making more minor adjustments to the phrasing or semantics of the thought rather than major changes that require complete rejection of the old thought.

Focusing on small changes in trauma-related beliefs in Step 5 when clients cling to their old beliefs confers several important benefits to them, including (a) enhanced trust that the therapist's goal is not simply to "completely change all of my thoughts at once," (b) greater initial acceptance of the new thought, and (c) providing time for client to "try on for size" new beliefs between sessions.

For example, in the previous dialogue, Edmundo's original thought was "I am totally worthless because I didn't do enough to help my brother and it's my fault he killed himself." Rather than expecting him to make a large change (e.g., "I am not at all worthless, and my brother's death was in no way my fault"), the therapist could help him see that he could make a more realistic and comfortable initial modification (e.g., "I have made some progress in my life, and I did try to help my brother somewhat, so I am not completely worthless"). It likely would be more productive for the therapist to guide him toward developing that sort of middle-ground new thought in this initial 5 Steps exercise on this specific trauma-based subject. From there, the therapist and Edmundo can work together to help him internalize the new thought and potentially continue to chip away at it more over time in future 5 Steps practice. See Edmundo's completed 5 Steps of CR worksheet in Figure 9.1.

In subsequent sessions or through home practice, there are usually additional opportunities to continue to work on this newer belief and to hone it further while gradually weakening the old one. Using the 5 Steps of CR (Alternate Worksheet With Ratings; described in Chapter 10, this volume) can facilitate this process. This version of the skill worksheet includes a "believability" rating scale as well as a "distress" rating scale, so that even subtle differences in thought conviction and negative emotions before and after the 5 Steps of CR process can be highlighted.

As trauma-based beliefs often change gradually during this phase of the intervention, individuals may continue to feel some distress even after challenging a trauma-related thought and replacing it with a similar but more accurate one. In these situations, developing Action Plans can be an effective way of helping clients cope with any persistent distress while guiding them through the process of gradually modifying and incorporating their new outlook on their trauma into their lives.

FIGURE 9.1. Example of 5 Steps of CR Worksheet Completed by Edmundo, Addressing Trauma-Based Belief

1. Situation

Ask yourself, "What happened that made me upset?" Write down a brief description of the situation, including just the facts.

Situation: "I went to the pharmacy the other day and got really upset while I was there."

2. Feeling

Circle your strongest feeling. If you circle more than one, that's OK. If none of these fit, you can write one in.

(Fear/Anxiety)   Sadness/depression   (Guilt/Shame)   Anger

3. Thought

Ask yourself, "What am I thinking that is leading me to feel this way?" Use your Guide to Thoughts and Feelings handout to identify thoughts related to the feeling(s) circled above. You may have more than one thought related to the feeling(s). Write down your thoughts below, but then choose ONE thought to work on. Choose the thought that is most distressing to you right now, and circle that thought.

Thoughts:

The clerk yesterday at the store looked at me like he was going to try to start with me after I left.

He pegged me as someone who is weak or can be taken advantage of.

I'm someone who doesn't take care of my own business and never protected his little brother—someone who isn't up to the task in life then or now.

I'm totally worthless.

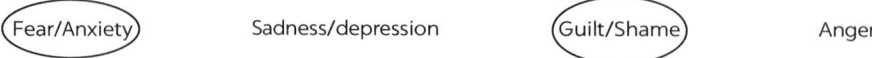

I'll never ever be able to get out of debt now and won't be able to contribute to my family.

Is this thought a Common Style of Thinking? If yes, circle the style:

All-or-nothing   Mind reading   (Over-Generalizing)

Must/should/never   (Catastrophizing)   Emotional reasoning

Overestimation of risk   Self-blame   Mental filter

Write the thought you chose from Step 3 here:

Upsetting thought: "I am totally worthless because I didn't do enough to help my brother and it's my fault he killed himself."

4. Evaluate Your Thought

Now ask yourself: "What evidence do I have for and against this thought?" First, write down all the evidence that DOES support your thought. Then, write down all the evidence that DOES NOT support your thought. You can use your Tips for Finding Good Evidence Information Sheet to help come up with evidence that DOES NOT support your thought.

(continues)

FIGURE 9.1. Example of 5 Steps of CR Worksheet Completed by Edmundo, Addressing Trauma-Based Belief (*Continued*)

Things that DO support my thought:

I am the older brother, and it's my role to protect him.

I am the one who introduced him to the guys in the first place.

I did some bad stuff back then myself, and he probably learned from me, and that contributed to his problems later on.

There were times that I didn't give him enough attention when I knew he was suffering.

I have failed at lots of jobs and have not been as good of a father and partner as I need to be.

Things that DO NOT support my thought:

I had a bad home life and was scared and just a kid myself when I got involved in the gang. I didn't know what I was even doing.

It was my parents' job to protect him (and me) from danger and that life, and they didn't do a good job of it.

Just because I have felt worthless, it doesn't mean that is a fact. It's emotional reasoning.

I worked hard to get myself out of that lifestyle and create a new life.

I do things nowadays that are healthy and good for myself and my family. I come to the mental health clinic, take medicine, doing the CR for PTSD program, going to PT to help my injury.

I am working to provide more for my family financially now.

I show my kids love, unlike the life and family I grew up in.

I tried with my brother—went to apartment several times, tried hard to get him to go with me to the emergency room and rehab, but he wouldn't go.

There didn't seem like more I could do for him because he wouldn't listen. He was far gone.

5. Take Action!

Next, ask yourself, "Do things mostly support my thought or do things mostly NOT support my thought?"

☐ NO, the evidence does not support my thought.

If the evidence does NOT support your thought, come up with a new thought that is supported by the evidence. These thoughts are usually more balanced and accurate (and helpful).Write your new thought in the space below. Remember, when you think of this upsetting situation in the future or when a similar situation happens, replace your unhelpful automatic thought with this new and more accurate thought.

My new thought: "I have made some progress in my life, and I did try to help my brother, so I am not completely worthless."

☐ YES, the evidence does support my thought.

If the evidence DOES support your thought, decide what you need to do next in order to deal with the situation. Ask yourself, "Do I need to get more information about what to do?" "Do I need to get some help?" "Do I need to take steps to make sure I am safe?" Complete the Action Plan Worksheet to help you answer these questions and create a solid plan to deal with the situation.

Note. In some cases, you may decide that the evidence does not support your upsetting thought and change it to a more accurate and helpful one. If so, you may also find it helpful to make an Action Plan to deal with that situation. Thus, in some situations, you may find that doing both things—coming up with a new and more accurate thought AND ALSO creating an Action Plan—can be very helpful. CR = cognitive restructuring; PTSD = posttraumatic stress disorder.

EFFECTIVE USE OF ACTION PLANS FOR TRAUMA- AND PTSD-RELATED SYMPTOMS AND SITUATIONS

As discussed in Chapter 8 in this volume, Action Plans are a valuable way to assist clients in learning how to systematically and effectively approach (rather than avoid) challenging life problems that need attention. This skill maintains its importance as the client begins to work on trauma-related thoughts and core beliefs with the 5 Steps of CR. It is most common for Action Plans to be developed when the client decides in Step 5 that their original upsetting thought is mostly supported by the evidence (i.e., accurate) in Step 4, as well as when there is a lingering problem or distressing (PTSD) symptom that the client needs to develop a healthy and effective plan to address. Once more overt trauma-related work begins in these midtreatment sessions, the Action Plan plays an increasingly useful role. In conjunction with modifying inaccurate beliefs in Step 5, the therapist should look for opportunities to help clients develop practical Action Plans aimed at internalizing more accurate thoughts about their traumatic experiences into their daily lives, enhancing their functioning, and further reducing trauma- and PTSD-related distress.

Often, the most basic and impactful Action Plan in this phase of therapy is one whose goal is to help clients develop effective methods for internalizing their new and more accurate thoughts, as a challenging next step for clients can be how to integrate this new and important perspective into their lives. Creating a detailed Action Plan of strategies to assist the client in how to remember and practice new and more accurate thoughts can make a major difference in sustained reduction of PTSD-related distress. Examples of specific Action Plan elements that can effectively meet this goal include the following:

- Write down the new thought, and put it in several places in your home (e.g., bathroom mirror, refrigerator door, nightstand, etc.) so that it is prominently displayed).
- Keep copies of the new thought on your person (e.g., in a wallet, purse, car, cell phone screensaver or notes page, etc.) for similar impact.
- Review your completed 5 Steps of CR worksheet weekly to remind you of the systematic process and the accuracy of the new thought.
- Tell supportive people about the new thought, and ask them to remind you about it as needed.

There are several additional scenarios, described next, in which assisting clients in developing detailed Action Plans can directly impact their PTSD-related symptoms and distress and improve day-to-day functioning.

Distressing PTSD Symptoms

Action Plans can be developed to help people manage PTSD and other upsetting symptoms that have been determined to not be the result of inaccurate thinking. For example, overarousal (e.g., difficulty sleeping, constantly feeling on edge) and reexperiencing symptoms (e.g., intrusive memories, nightmares) can be distressing, even in the absence of inaccurate or exaggerated thinking (or after correcting inaccurate thinking). Similarly, while cognitive restructuring may help clients overcome avoidance of safe situations that are reminiscent of traumatic events, they may still feel anxious when first confronting these situations.

Distressing symptoms may be identified through the routine monitoring of PTSD and depression (i.e., PCL-5, BDI-II), review of home assignments at the beginning of sessions, and/or discussions or brief check-ins with the client about the past week. Action Plans that address distressing symptoms are generally aimed at bolstering effective coping efforts designed to either reduce symptoms or minimize their effects on functioning. Possible coping strategies for symptoms can be elicited from the client, the therapist, or other trusted written or online resources, and some can come directly from the Wellness Plan Worksheet previously developed in Session 1. Examples of coping strategies are provided in Exhibit 9.3.

EXHIBIT 9.3

Coping Strategies for Common PTSD Symptoms

Symptom: Reexperiencing the trauma (e.g., intrusive memories, flashbacks)

    Breathing Retraining

    Soothing pets

    Positive self-talk (e.g., "I can handle this")

    Thought stopping

    Acceptance (e.g., "just acknowledging memories without giving undue attention to them")

    Grounding (shift awareness to present, such as feeling of body against chair)

    Don't watch news or trauma-related TV shows/movies.

    Stay active during the day.

    Prayer

Symptom: Overarousal (e.g., hypervigilance, increased heart rate and breathing)

    Breathing Retraining

    Physical exercise

    Meditation or prayer

    Recognize triggers, and increase awareness (e.g., negative thoughts, sounds, smells).

    Maintain a sense of humor.

    Find your own space—a room or corner that is safe—and make it soothing.

Symptom: Difficulty sleeping

    Avoid caffeine 5 hours before bedtime.

    Set a bedtime and waking time, and stick to it.

    Don't nap, even if you had a poor night's sleep.

    Do something relaxing before going to bed (e.g., warm bath, reading, watching TV).

    Get regular exercise.

    Don't stay in bed trying to sleep for more than an hour.

    Use Breathing Retraining to fall asleep initially or to fall back asleep.

(continues)

EXHIBIT 9.3

Coping Strategies for Common PTSD Symptoms   (*Continued*)

Symptom: Nightmares

  Remind yourself of the differences between dreams and reality.

  Interact with soothing objects (e.g., blanket, photos) or pets.

  Positive self-talk, reassurance

  Write down or draw picture of the nightmare.

  Get out of bed to interrupt a leftover feeling.

  Create a different end to the nightmare.

  Put feet firmly on ground, look in a mirror, or splash cold water on your face to
    ground yourself.

  Lights on or nightlight

  Use Breathing Retraining to regulate emotions.

Symptom: Problems with concentration

  Remove distractions when trying to concentrate.

  Use underlining and note taking when reading.

  Schedule rest breaks after concentrating for a set number of minutes.

  Play computer games to improve concentration.

Symptom: Avoidance of safe, trauma-related stimuli

  Grounding (for numbing or detached feelings)

  Set gradual goals, and take small steps.

  Get someone to accompany you at first.

  Use Breathing Retraining or self-talk when in a previously avoided situation.

  Use distraction when you are in a previously avoided situation (e.g., looking at magazines in
    store).

Note. PTSD = posttraumatic stress disorder.

PTSD-Related Sequelae Contributing to Current Problem Situations

As the result of trauma history and ongoing PTSD symptoms, clients often experience multiple ongoing challenges in different areas of their lives, such as family and romantic/sexual relationships, parenting, work or school performance, physical health maintenance, and drug and alcohol use. Targeted Action Plans can greatly assist a client in gaining confidence and competence in managing and rising above these common difficulties. Frequently, these particular areas of functioning that need attention are the same ones that the client identified as wanting to improve during goal setting in Session 3. Thus, clients are often highly motivated to work on these personally meaningful areas of their life, and it is easy to engage them in formulating Action Plans to take concrete steps toward addressing them.

For example, as illustrated, Leigh-Ann and her therapist worked on her PTSD-related anxiety and the associated trauma-related belief that was triggered when a man approached her to strike up a conversation at a recent outdoor recovery meeting. While they were able to help Leigh-Ann modify her thought ("I can't trust anybody because of what happened to me") and change it to something more accurate and less distressing via the 5 Steps ("Some men are dangerous, but not every man or every person is"), it was clear that Leigh-Ann still needed specific strategies for dealing with future situations in which a man might approach her to talk, especially since she had just started a new restaurant job where she would frequently need to interact with men. She wanted to be able to better manage PTSD symptoms like hypervigilance, feelings of panic, responding defensively, and "shutting down" in these professional situations, so she and the therapist developed a comprehensive Action Plan of immediate in vivo strategies to enact in situations where Leigh-Ann became triggered in the presence of men while at work. See Leigh-Ann's Action Plan in Exhibit 9.4.

EXHIBIT 9.4

Example of a PTSD-Symptom-Based Action Plan Completed by Leigh-Ann

Instructions: Follow the steps below to develop a helpful Action Plan.

1. Define the goal: What situation requires action?

Think about what change you would like to see in this situation. Be as specific as possible.

To be calmer and handle myself better when men (customers, manager, coworkers, etc.) approach me at the restaurant where I work.

2. Brainstorm possible strategies: What can you do to change the situation?

Use your creative problem-solving skills to think of all the possible things you could do to reduce your distress or address the problem in this situation. When you have made a list of different strategies, think carefully about each one, and place a star (*) next to the best one or ones.

Just quit now. Then I don't have to deal with this. Find a job where I don't have to deal with men as much.

Remember part of my new thought that I've worked on—"Not every man is dangerous"—and say it in my head before responding.**

Remind myself that I am at work and there lots of people around to help me if something was actually dangerous.**

Take one BRT breath before I respond, and say, "Calm"—but in my head, not out loud.

** Make a little fist behind my back to ground myself so I feel less panicky in the moment.**

3. Plan on how to put into practice the strategy (or strategies) you chose: What steps can you take to make this happen?

Consider these questions:

What information do you need to have?

Do you need to get some help?

Who can support you in taking this action?

What obstacles or challenges could interfere with the plan?

How could you prevent or deal with these obstacles or challenges?

Write down the plan below. Be specific about the actions you will take.

Do a practice role-play or two with my therapist of a situation like this so I can get more comfortable with it. Do BRT every day so that it is second nature in the moment I need it at work. After the interaction at work, give myself a second to go into the restroom to do more BRT if I need to and to repeat the other parts of my Action Plan.

(continues)

EXHIBIT 9.4

Example of a PTSD-Symptom-Based Action Plan Completed by Leigh-Ann   *(Continued)*

4. Set a time or a situation to follow up your plan: When and how are you going to take this action?

Ask yourself: When do you want to begin your plan? Is there a specific situation or type of situation where you want to use your plan? When is that situation likely to come up again next?

My therapist and I will do a quick role-play now in our session. Next week, when I am at work, it is likely that a guy will talk to me. I will try out this plan.

Note. PTSD = posttraumatic stress disorder; BRT = Breathing Retraining.

CLOSING TRAUMA-FOCUSED CR SESSIONS

Given the shift into trauma-related content in this phase of the program, there may be an uptick in client distress during these sessions. This is completely normal and should be viewed as a positive indicator that the therapist is helping the client to tap into important and distressing trauma-related beliefs and PTSD symptoms and to be guided to their more adaptive resolution. While some level of resultant vulnerability is to be expected, it is important to help the client return to a more emotionally regulated state prior to the end of each session. In doing so, the therapist increases the client's confidence in their ability to effectively cope with and manage the impact of previously avoided distressing trauma-related material and associated PTSD symptoms, which can enhance good session attendance as well as engagement in trauma-based CR work in subsequent sessions.

To help the client prepare for the session end in order to "send them back out into the world," two skills from the program can be practiced toward the end of the session. Initiating Breathing Retraining practice to close out the session is an excellent way to regulate emotional or physiological arousal that may have accompanied the trauma-based CR work. Assisting clients in developing a quick Action Plan for immediate postsession use can provide them with simple, concrete strategies to cope with residual PTSD symptoms and distress following the sessions and between visits. Elements from the previously completed Wellness Plan Worksheet should ideally be incorporated in the Action Plan. The aforementioned strategies also serve to increase client's ongoing and independent mastery of these important coping skills.

TRAUMA-RELATED CR HOME ASSIGNMENTS

As with the prior CR sessions, the therapist should end each of these more trauma-centered sessions with a collaboratively developed home assignment focused on continuing to use the 5 Steps of CR worksheet to address ongoing distress. Ideally at this stage of the program, the client's outside practice focus should be on using the 5 Steps every day to more fully incorporate the skill into their daily life and further hone their ability to use it quickly and effectively in response to distressing thoughts and beliefs. This includes using the 5 Steps to deal with any stressful situations, including ones in which PTSD symptoms and trauma-related beliefs are triggered, in addition to other upsetting situations.

Whether or not the particular situations and thoughts examined via home assignments are directly trauma-related may be something to be determined on an individual basis. Once clients are in the thick of trauma-related in-session CR, many of them are ready and able to work on similar material on their own between sessions. However, others may have more difficulty working on trauma content outside of sessions for varying reasons. For example, some clients may have difficulty identifying trauma-related beliefs without the therapist's help. Others may find themselves emotionally or physiologically flooded when attempting to address trauma-related thoughts on their own outside of the session. Some of these challenges involving home practice assignments can be addressed by using the following suggestions:

1. Negotiate that the majority of the daily 5 Steps home practice will be based on looking at more general stress or distress in which the client is not expected to delve further into trauma material; however, for one 5 Steps home practice per week, the client will try to use the 5 Steps to work on a currently distressing PTSD symptom (e.g., avoiding a particular activity).

2. Develop together a short list of trauma-related beliefs that the client currently endorses, and make a plan together for the client to work on one (or more) of them on their own.

3. Collaborate on a plan for the client to practice Breathing Retraining before beginning 5 Steps work on a specific trauma-related belief between sessions, as well as during and/or after, as needed.

For other strategies to address more general home assignment challenges, see Table 11.1 in Chapter 11 in this volume.

CONCLUSION

A smooth transition from introducing the basic use of the 5 Steps of CR to addressing trauma-related thoughts (and core beliefs) is crucial, as direct elicitation, evaluation, and modification of these types of beliefs are the cornerstones of the CR for PTSD intervention. In most cases, the initial shift should begin around Session 7, and by Session 9. Clinicians should keep in mind several important variables related to the timing of this transition, including the client's mastery of the CR skill thus far. Clinicians can apply the previously initiated 5 Steps of CR strategies (Chapter 8, this volume) to eliciting clients' trauma-related beliefs and assisting them to evaluate and modify these distressing thoughts. By helping clients to recognize and connect ongoing thinking and behavioral patterns in their day-to-day lives to their past traumatic events, this important material is effectively brought into focus for 5 Steps practice.

As needed, therapists can utilize a variety of additional strategies to elicit trauma-related content for use with the 5 Steps. These techniques include reviewing prior completed psychoeducational handouts and home assignments outlining trauma-related beliefs; utilizing items previously recorded on the Therapist Tracking Sheet for Client's Trauma-Related Cognitions; and examining elevated PTSD symptom items on the PCL-5, depression on the BDI-II, and common trauma-related cognitions on the PTCI.

Specific strategies for addressing trauma-related (and core) beliefs via the 5 Steps can greatly assist in teaching clients how to systematically evaluate the current veracity of these thoughts. Action Plans play an important role in further helping clients approach, rather than avoid, ongoing distressing PTSD symptoms and problematic life situations. They also serve an important role in helping clients plan how to remember and more fully integrate their new, more accurate beliefs into their daily lives. Ongoing encouragement for and strategizing about between-session home practice of CR is crucial in this stage of treatment to increase comfort with the 5 Steps and maintain motivation to address PTSD symptoms. Taken together, these trauma-based CR sessions can substantially reduce client trauma-related distress and PTSD symptoms over time and also move clients toward their personal goals established in Session 4.

10

Solutions to Common Challenges

Therapists may encounter a variety of obstacles when delivering the Cognitive Restructuring (CR) for posttraumatic stress disorder (PTSD) program. These can include complications associated with general sorts of therapy-process challenges, as well as those specifically related to clients' mastery and practice of the CR skills. For example, some clients may seem reluctant to fully engage in the program as a whole, and others may actively avoid delving into trauma-focused content. Some may have difficulty using the 5 Steps of CR in the moment when they are acutely upset or may cling to distressing beliefs despite overwhelming evidence against them. In addition, persistent emotions (like guilt/shame and anger) plus a variety of specific and often stubborn PTSD symptoms (such as nightmares and dissociation) can present special challenges that require unique applications of CR. In this chapter, we describe strategies for addressing and overcoming this full range of common challenges. (Note: For strategies to address challenges specifically related to learning difficulties, cognitive impairment, and symptoms of psychosis, see Chapter 12, this volume. For strategies related to working effectively with persons with borderline personality disorder, see Chapter 13, this volume.)

CLIENT CHALLENGES IMPACTING PRODUCTIVE INTERVENTION PARTICIPATION

Therapists may encounter different problems when working with clients that can interfere with their ability to participate fully and benefit from the CR for PTSD program, including therapy-process-related issues (e.g., irregular attendance

https://doi.org/10.1037/0000423-010
Treatment of Posttraumatic Stress Disorder in Serious Mental Illness: The Cognitive Restructuring Program, by K. T. Mueser and J. D. Gottlieb

and/or home practice efforts, self-defeating beliefs about improvement) and avoidance of trauma-related thoughts and feelings. Utilizing cognitive restructuring to address these challenges allows for the thoughtful and collaborative examination of these types of potential difficulties within the framework of the CR for PTSD model.

Therapy-Process-Based Challenges

As is the case in most psychotherapeutic interventions, there are sometimes engagement challenges—such as poor attendance, lack of disclosure, compromised working relationship, home skills practice nonadherence, and so on—that negatively affect the flow of the intervention and therefore the uptake of the therapy skills. Underlying these types of client behaviors are often anxious or hopeless beliefs about their performance or success in the intervention, their therapist's view of them, and the utility of certain components of the treatment (i.e., home practice assignments).

The therapist may suspect some of their client's thoughts in this realm and should note these sorts of beliefs as potentially responsible for these engagement challenges. Given how common these types of beliefs and behaviors can be, it is useful for therapists to be on the lookout for them and to gently but directly address them with their clients.

Should these challenges be evident in sessions prior to the initial teaching of CR (i.e., before Session 4), the therapist can initiate an empathic, nonjudgmental discussion about what might be getting in the way of the client's engagement. This includes frequent use of normalizing and validation ("It's not uncommon to feel hopeless about positive changes, given what you've experienced. Many people with PTSD find themselves feeling that way"), reminders about empirical data ("Research on this program has found that people who followed through with the sessions got more relief than those who didn't—even people who experienced their traumas many years earlier and had PTSD for a long time"), brief problem solving ("What are three things we can plan together to help you to try the home assignments?"), and cheerleading ("You've been through so much in your life, and you've made it this far—sitting across from me right now and participating in this program. I have faith in you that you can do this!").

As the client moves into the CR phase of the program, the thoughts and beliefs underlying these sorts of obstacles and challenges should be directly evaluated via the 5 Steps of CR. This serves the secondary purpose of providing an opportunity for additional in vivo CR practice. In the following example, the therapist probes to better understand and help address Leigh-Ann's frequent cancelling of sessions:

THERAPIST: Leigh-Ann, I've noticed that you've cancelled a couple of our recent sessions lately. I was hoping we might be able to look into that together if you were willing?

LEIGH-ANN: Yeah, I know. I'm sorry about that. I feel super guilty about it.

THERAPIST:	I want you to know that this is hard work, and I understand that it may feel difficult to keep at it. It is very common for people with PTSD—and other challenges and experiences, like the ones you've had to struggle with—not to make it to all of the appointments. I wonder if we can talk a bit about that right now. It seems important—especially since we are now on Session 8 and so we are about halfway through the program.
LEIGH-ANN:	OK.
THERAPIST:	As you have learned so far in here, it can be helpful to take a closer look at our thoughts underlying some of our actions, especially as they may be related to having PTSD. Taking this past week as an example, what sort of thought was going through your mind when you left me that voice message about cancelling our session?
LEIGH-ANN:	Well, I don't know. I got kind of anxious and then just felt so overwhelmed.
THERAPIST:	So it sounds as though your primary emotions were anxiety and feeling overwhelmed. And what sort of thoughts did you have that were making you feel that way?
LEIGH-ANN:	Ugh, I had a flood of thoughts. To be honest, I've had these kind of often since we started working together. Not that it hasn't been helpful. It's just hard.
THERAPIST:	I completely understand, and I am very glad you are willing to talk about this. Would it be OK if we talked this through using our 5 Steps of CR skill to help us along?
LEIGH-ANN:	Yeah, that would be OK.
THERAPIST:	OK, that's great, Leigh-Ann. I've started a 5 Steps of CR worksheet here for us. Step 1, Situation: "Calling to cancel my CR for PTSD appointment last week." Step 2, Feelings: "Anxiety/fear." And I also wrote in "Overwhelmed." Does this capture your experience? And now, what about Step 3? What are some of your thoughts related to these feelings? Let's get them down on paper.
LEIGH-ANN:	OK. I guess there's kind of a lot of them. First is, like, "Some of these traumas—like the thing with my friend's stepfather—happened so long ago, there's no use in working on it now. It won't ever get better." And then I also have been thinking, "You probably think I'm too screwed up or crazy to help." And then also when I hadn't done my CR home assignment, "I have to do the skills totally right, or it's not worth it." Stuff like that.

THERAPIST: Those thoughts are really quite common, actually. And it makes perfect sense that if you are thinking that way about yourself, this program, or me, you would feel anxious and overwhelmed. These are all really important thoughts. To get us moving forward from here, which one of these thoughts is most distressing to you still—right now as we sit here together?

From there, once the therapy-process thoughts are articulated and written down in Step 3, the therapist and client can proceed as usual—choosing the thought to work on, classifying that particular belief as a Common Style of Thinking (CST), and so on. As demonstrated previously, clients often have multiple thoughts related to this theme, which can be examined individually—either in session as time allows or out of session as a home assignment task. Creating an accepting environment for clients to feel they can admit these doubts can make a significant difference in terms of dropping out of treatment versus sticking with the program, getting "unstuck," and moving forward to get the most out of it and complete it. (For further discussion and an example of using the 5 Steps of CR to uncover and address clients' concerns pertaining to the therapy relationship, see Chapter 13, this volume.)

A brief note on session cancellations: Although avoidance of trauma-related work is a common reason for cancellations in the CR for PTSD program, other factors may play a role as well. For example, some clients experience significant symptom relief from the earlier phase of the program and the initial CR sessions, and as the burden of their PTSD symptoms decreases, they may begin to focus on other areas of their life and therefore cancel sessions. Thus, it is important for therapists to explore and work to understand their clients' underlying thoughts and reasons related to session cancellations and to avoid making assumptions about their cause.

Avoidance of Trauma-Focused CR

Although many clients readily begin addressing trauma-related beliefs with the 5 Steps of CR around Session 7, given that avoidance of trauma-related stimuli is a hallmark PTSD symptom, it is not unusual for some clients to be reluctant to transition into working on these sorts of thoughts and symptoms. There are a variety of ways that this reluctance manifests itself throughout this phase of CR treatment, including but not limited to the following:

• Unwillingness to acknowledge the connection between current distress, general upsetting beliefs, and trauma-related thoughts and beliefs.

• Reluctance to engage in 5 Steps of CR practice related directly to trauma-related beliefs.

• Refusal to work on symptoms (and associated thoughts) identified in recent PTSD Checklist–5 (PCL-5), Posttraumatic Cognitions Inventory, and/or depression inventories.

- Highly anxious responses to suggestions or invitations to work on trauma-related thoughts and beliefs.

When this is the case, clinicians should first ensure they understand the client's specific concerns related to these suggested activities. From there, the clinician should empathize with and normalize the client's concerns and fears, which often will include reminding them of what they have learned in the earlier psychoeducational sessions regarding the understandable nature of avoidance in PTSD. In addition, it is helpful to spend some time discussing ways to help the client feel more comfortable shifting into this phase of the program. This can involve the developing an Action Plan that may include elements from the previously created Wellness Plan augmented use of Breathing Retraining, as well as new strategies to cope with symptom triggers before, during, and after these sessions. Equally important in these sessions is the therapist's reiteration that the client is "driving the bus" with regard to the pacing of work on trauma-related material.

A key strategy for helping clients increase their confidence in addressing trauma-related and core beliefs is to initiate the 5 Steps of CR to address specific concerns about transitioning to this phase of the intervention. Some common anxiety-inducing *metacognitive beliefs* (i.e., thoughts about thoughts) to elicit and evaluate during this phase include the following:

If I start to work directly on my trauma-related thoughts and feelings,

- I'll completely fall apart.
- I won't be able to handle it at all. I'll be a basket-case.
- I'll have to go back to the hospital.
- I'll return to using drugs to numb myself because it will be too much.
- I'll screw up whatever gains I've worked so hard to make in my mental health treatment and my life.

As noted in Chapter 9 in this volume, although addressing these fears with the 5 Steps is suggested above for clients who seem to be avoiding the process, it is recommended that a brief discussion take place with all clients regarding their thoughts about transitioning into trauma-related CR before beginning this phase of therapy.

DIFFICULTY LEARNING AND USING COGNITIVE RESTRUCTURING OR OTHER PROGRAM SKILLS

Clients may experience different challenges learning and using the skills taught in the CR for PTSD program. Useful strategies for addressing these difficulties are provided next.

Cognitive Impairment and Associated Comprehension Challenges

Although the skills in the CR for PTSD program are taught in a linear and straightforward manner, occasionally some clients have difficulty learning the CR skills. These difficulties can occur for a variety of reasons, including the common problem of cognitive impairment in the serious mental illness (SMI) population. However, if therapists are aware of the client's learning challenges (cognitive impairment and otherwise), specific steps can be taken throughout the program to minimize their effects on learning and outcome. (For more information on understanding skill learning and cognitive impairment challenges within the SMI population and for comprehensive alternative teaching strategies to successfully manage these obstacles within the context of the CR for PTSD program, see Chapter 12, this volume. Chapter 12 also includes details regarding cognitive impairment as it pertains specifically to clients with schizophrenia spectrum disorders.)

Challenges Initiating the 5 Steps of CR in Distressing Situations

Clients are often able to use cognitive restructuring on their own to deal with a recent upsetting experience but have difficulty using the skill in the moment when they are feeling distressed. This difficulty can be related to the fact that people with PTSD symptoms are often highly emotionally reactive in situations that might ordinarily be expected to cause much milder levels of distress. They may spontaneously recoil in fright, withdraw into depression, or become angry or hostile without being able to clearly identify their specific feelings in the moment or remember to use the 5 Steps of CR. It can take time for people to be able to use the 5 Steps of CR in vivo when they are upset, even after they have mastered the basic steps. Therefore, the therapist should normalize the challenge of learning how to use CR in the moment and provide encouragement that with continued practice the person will eventually be able to use the skill in these situations.

High levels of anxiety, in particular, can interfere with remembering how to use the 5 Steps of CR. A helpful option is to encourage clients to first use Breathing Retraining (and/or another self-soothing strategy) to reduce their physiological arousal or emotion flooding, and then to recognize that this distress reaction is related to a particular thought they are having. From there, they can begin to initiate the 5 Steps, following either all five of the steps or just an abbreviated version. For example, it can be helpful to explore whether the client is able to first identify a CST in these types of situations. If they can recognize when a thought reflects a CST, the formal evaluation of evidence can be skipped for the moment, and they can instead focus on the fact that because their thought falls into a CST category, that automatically means that it is likely not 100% accurate. This recognition can serve to reduce at least some distress in the moment. The client can then delve into the remaining steps at a later time if need be (or with the therapist in a subsequent session).

WHEN USING THE 5 STEPS OF CR DOES NOT SUFFICIENTLY REDUCE DISTRESS

As discussed in Chapter 9 in this volume, sometimes using the 5 Steps of CR leads to new, more accurate, and more believable thoughts that are associated with only modest reductions in distress, particularly when working with strong and long-held trauma-related beliefs. In these situations, especially when it is the first time that the client is addressing a particular trauma-related thought, it is important to reinforce the client's use of cognitive restructuring by pointing out that as they become more familiar with their new view and incorporate it into their life, their conviction in it may further increase while the distress related to their old perspective continues to decrease. However, additional work may be required when the client finds the old thought continuously reasserting itself in multiple situations, causing ongoing distress.

Dealing With Recurrent, Stubborn, and Highly Distressing Traumatic Thoughts

Trauma-related thoughts and the negative feelings associated with them are sometimes repeatedly triggered (as automatic thoughts, for example), despite some previous success via CR at disputing those beliefs. Clients may find this discouraging since their "old thinking" keeps reasserting itself again and again in their lives, and they may feel they are making no progress.

There are several strategies for helping clients overcome these sorts of recurrent trauma-related beliefs. First, the therapist should continue to normalize the client's experience of an old thinking pattern returning, while at the same time providing encouragement that with ongoing 5 Steps skill work, over time their beliefs and ways of thinking will in fact change ("I want you to know that it is absolutely normal to have your old thinking about your experience come back here and there. You've thought that way for a long time, even with the recent CR work we've done. It can take some time to fully feel like the new thought is part of you. But I can assure you that the more we work on it and the more you practice, the more that your new way of thinking will start to be more present and feel more comfortable to you"). One useful analogy for conveying this is to describe thought patterns as similar to the path worn by a river, and that with many years of thinking a particular way, it is only natural for the water (thoughts) to flow down a particular path (way of thinking). However, with practice, the client can learn to form new paths or ways of thinking that are more accurate and eventually feel more natural.

Second, for some clients, helping them simply recognize that an old trauma-related thought is a Common Style of Thinking and therefore is not accurate can bring relief without necessarily emphasizing the importance of replacing that thought with a more accurate one. For example, one client learned to say to himself when he recognized an inaccurate trauma-related thought, "There goes my stinking thinking!" This approach emphasizes that what is most critical is for people to recognize that their thoughts are not necessarily accurate and that while they cannot necessarily rid themselves of those thoughts, they need not pay them heed either. This is a central message reflected in mindfulness approaches to depression (Segal et al., 2002) and therapies such as acceptance and commitment therapy (Hayes et al., 2012), dialectical behavior therapy (Linehan, 1993), and metacognitive therapy (Wells, 2009). This strategy is also useful in assisting clients who have cognitive impairment (see Chapter 12, this volume).

Third, to highlight an important strategy discussed in Chapter 9 in this volume, Action Plans can play a significant role here in enhancing the client's coping with persistent trauma-related intrusions as well as in continuing to work on internalizing new and more accurate thoughts. Specifically, Action Plans can be created to address a number of different relevant goals, such as (a) how to manage recurring old and inaccurate trauma-related beliefs and associated feelings, (b) how to remember new and more accurate thoughts when old thoughts are triggered, (c) how to cope with PTSD symptoms triggered by specific situations that may compromise conviction in newly developed thoughts, and (d) how to reduce the impact of trauma-related distress on interactions with others. For an example, see Donata's Action Plan (Exhibit 10.1) for dealing with her distress when her recurrent old thoughts of worthlessness are triggered by her auditory hallucinations.

Teaching Clients to Rate Their Beliefs and Distress

In general, it is important to reinforce the client's use of CR even when only modest reductions in distress occur in order to encourage them to continue to hone their CR skills with the expectation of reaping greater benefits over time. This includes situations in which the client's use of CR is associated with only a very small improvement in negative feelings. A useful strategy for drawing attention to these small changes in beliefs and associated distress is to teach clients how to numerically rate their conviction in old and new thoughts as well as the degree of distress associated with them. These ratings can provide more fine-grained evidence of concrete changes in thoughts and beliefs and related distress following CR, which allows the therapist to highlight that even small improvements in distress are associated with the uptake of new and more accurate thoughts, thereby reinforcing their use of the CR skill.

To highlight the subtle improvements that occur following CR, the therapist can use the 5 Steps of CR (Alternate Worksheet With Ratings) to teach the client how to rate their conviction in their thoughts and the levels of associated distress. In this approach, the first three steps of the 5 Steps of CR are the same as usual. However, at the end of Step 3, after clients have identified the most upsetting thought associated with the situation, they are taught how to rate their level of conviction in this thought's accuracy on a Belief Scale ranging between 0 (*completely untrue*) and 100 (*completely true*). They are also taught to rate how upsetting this thought is on a Distress Scale ranging between 0 (*not upsetting*) and 100 (*extremely upsetting*). From there, the evaluation of the evidence for and against the upsetting thought in Step 4 occurs in the same way as in the usual 5-Step approach.

EXHIBIT 10.1

Example of an Action Plan Completed by Donata

Instructions: Follow the steps below to develop a helpful Action Plan.

1. Define the goal: Think about what change you would like to see in this situation. Be as specific as possible.

To not get really upset and start to dissociate when my voices tell me my old thought all the time—"you are worthless"—that I now know is not true.

2. Brainstorm possible strategies: What can you do to change the situation?

Use your creative problem-solving skills to think of all the possible things you could do to reduce your distress or address the problem in this situation. When you have made a list of different strategies, think carefully about each one, and place a star (*) next to the best one or ones.

Do BRT and a grounding thing right when they yell it at me.*

Write down my new thought that we worked on in a few places like my phone and on my fridge.*

Keep my written 5 Steps so I remember all of the good evidence I came up with to review when the voices yell at me and I doubt my new thought.*

Make a recording of my new thought and play it back.

Ask the counselor at the senior center to help me remember my new thought and this plan.*

3. Plan how to put into practice the strategy (or strategies) you chose: What steps can you take to make this happen?

Consider these questions:

What information do you need to have?

Do you need to get some help?

Who can support you in taking this action?

What obstacles or challenges could interfere with the plan?

How could you prevent or deal with these obstacles or challenges?

Write down the plan below. Be specific about the actions you will take.

I will make a few copies of the new thought in session today, and I will type it into my phone this week. I may forget or get distracted, so I will ask the counselor to remind me to put up the signs around my apartment. I will get a folder to keep my completed 5 Steps worksheet so it is private and will keep it in my kitchen. If and when the voices start to tell me again I am worthless, I will review the worksheets and write out a new one too. I will keep using BRT every day so I am good at it when I need it for this plan.

4. Set a time or a situation to follow up your plan: When and how are you going to take this action?

Ask yourself: When do you want to begin your plan? Is there a specific situation or type of situation where you want to use your plan? When is that situation likely to come up again next?

Today I will type the new thought into my phone. Tomorrow I will call the counselor to ask her to remind me later this week. I will put up the new thoughts in my apartment tomorrow a.m. and set up my 5 Steps folder. The voices may come at me at any time, so I will make sure I will get this all set up by Thurs.

However, at the start of Step 5, the client does not make a decision about whether the evidence overall does or does not support the accuracy of their upsetting thought. On the 5 Steps of CR (Alternate Worksheet With Ratings), the client is instead prompted to first provide a second conviction-level rating of their initial thought (on the Belief Scale) now that they have carefully examined the evidence. That second Belief Scale rating is then compared with their first rating to determine whether generating and evaluating evidence for the thought reduced their conviction in its accuracy (as reflected by a potential reduction in their Belief Scale rating).

Any reduction in the client's Belief Scale rating means that they do not believe their original thought is as accurate now as they initially believed, which serves as a prompt to come up with a new, more accurate thought to replace the old one. This new thought should be rated higher on the Belief Scale than the second rating of the old thought (if it is not, more work is needed to develop a more believable thought). After a new thought has been developed that the client rates more believable than the old thought, they provide a new rating on the Distress Scale for how upsetting they find the new thought. When this method is used, the new thought is almost always associated with at least some reduction in distress compared with the old thought.

The 5 Steps CR (Alternate Worksheet With Ratings) is helpful in guiding clients to more closely evaluate gradations in changes in their beliefs and emotions, which makes smaller and more modest improvements in the accuracy of thoughts and reductions of negative feelings more salient. For Edmundo, this granulated rating-scale version of the 5 Steps of CR made a big difference in helping him feel less stuck in his persistent self-blame for his brother's suicide:

THERAPIST: Edmundo, I think we've both noticed over the past few sessions that upsetting thoughts related to your brother's suicide have impacted you greatly. And although we've worked on a few different 5 Steps of CR practices around this, it hasn't really felt to you like you've been able to get much relief from your guilt and shame and sadness. This is common for people with PTSD, and we have talked about this previously in terms of the Common Style of Thinking of excessive self-blame. I'd like to use a different version of our 5 Steps of CR worksheet together to see if we can find some additional ways to help you get some relief.

The therapist and Edmundo proceeded through Steps 1–3 together using this worksheet, where they settled on a very upsetting thought about which he had high conviction (rated at 80 on the Belief Scale and 90 on the Distress Scale) to examine more closely: "I'm totally to blame for my younger brother's suicide because I let him join into the gang life and he would definitely still be alive today if I had been a better person and family member."

When working on Step 4, Edmundo, with the therapist providing some good Socratic questioning, was able to come up with evidence that did not support his upsetting thought, and they then proceeded to the rating section of Step 5 as follows:

THERAPIST: OK, you did a great job just now of coming up with some very solid evidence that does not support your thought that you are totally to blame for your brother's suicide. Let's review some of this evidence: "I tried multiple times to get him out of the gang life after I left, but he wouldn't listen," "He was addicted to drugs for a long time," "He was someone, even as a kid, who was really depressed," and "He had his own demons and trauma that had nothing to do with me." Now that you've worked on all this evidence, let's look back at the original thought. On a scale of 0–100, now how accurate do you think your original thought is?

EDMUNDO: Um, I guess I can see this a little more clearly now somehow after all this time. I never got to spell it out like this and understand how he made his own choices. I don't believe it as much now. It still hurts, though. Maybe like 50.

THERAPIST: OK. Well, that's actually a pretty decent-sized difference between your first rating, which was 80, right?

EDMUNDO: Yeah, I guess it really is.

THERAPIST: Let's move on to the rest of Step 5 together so we can help you come up with and solidify a new way of thinking about this, based on your evidence.

DIFFICULTY LETTING GO OF UPSETTING TRAUMA-RELATED AND CORE BELIEFS

Although clients readily admit high levels of distress and impairment in their lives as a result of PTSD symptoms and their associated trauma-related beliefs, they sometimes have difficulty or appear reluctant to modify those thoughts or let them go. This can occur despite systematically accumulated and clear evidence gathered from use of the 5 Steps of CR indicating their trauma-related thought is inaccurate. One reason for this discrepancy is that when traumatic events occurred many years ago, such as in childhood, the associated core beliefs (about oneself, other people, and the world) coalesced early in life, therefore making it difficult for the client to be able to see things another way. To help clients move forward from this seeming intractability, two strategies are recommended, as discussed next.

Increasing Believability of New Thoughts

In addition to utilizing the 5 Steps of CR (Alternate Worksheet With Ratings; as described previously), another strategy to maximize the believability of the new thought (discussed in Chapters 8 and 9, this volume, and worth reviewing here) is to formally incorporate some of the evidence that was identified as supporting the old thought into the new one. Coupling some evidence that the client perceived as supporting the old thought into the new one can help make the new thought more balanced and therefore more acceptable to clients. This strategy was illustrated in client–therapist dialogues within previous chapters (such as with Leigh-Ann in Chapter 8, this volume) and is particularly useful in situations where the client is continuing to struggle to believe their new thought over time.

If the client still does not believe the new thought and therefore remains upset going forward, it becomes even more important for the therapist to continue to help the client reformulate the new thought so that it does increase in believability. As described in Chapters 8 and 9 in this volume, that typically takes the form of "backing off" of the initial new thought if it is not believable to the client and helping the client rewrite it in a more tentative manner that feels more acceptable and adoptable. Although the change may be merely the modification of a word or two, this "semantic hedging" can make a tremendous difference in the client's willingness to accept the new thought in the moment.

Using this strategy in conjunction with the rating system from the 5 Steps of CR (Alternate Worksheet With Ratings) provides an effective combination. For example, following the previous dialogue, Edmundo came up with a new, more accurate thought in Step 5. However, after some therapist prompting, he admitted that his believability in the new thought was not very high (40) and that his distress level had reduced a bit with this new thought but not much (from 90 to 60). From there, the therapist helped him reformulate and modify the thought further into something more believable for Edmundo that then reduced the associated distress more significantly.

Initial new Step 5 thought (low believability and therefore little distress reduction):

> I'm not at all to blame for my younger brother's suicide because he made his own choices.

Reformulated Step 5 thought (higher believability and therefore substantially reduced distress):

> Even though I wish I had the opportunity to do more for my brother and I may have been somewhat to blame for his struggles at first by bringing him into the street life, he made it very hard to help him later on and had his own demons. We both had a hard life that was not our fault, and so there are tragedies that happen as a result: because of this, his suicide is not really my fault.

Using the Payoff Matrix to Explore Reasons for Clinging to Trauma-Related and Other Upsetting Beliefs

Sometimes clients may cling to a long-held trauma-related belief, even after concluding that the evidence does not support it and identifying a new thought they think is more believable. This often occurs without the appearance of being obstinate and even after the completion of several 5 Steps of CR worksheets over time on different variations of the same theme or belief. Clients may also continue to hold onto old beliefs despite understanding that just because a belief feels true, it does not mean it is true (i.e., the emotional reasoning CST). For example, the client may say, "I know the thought isn't true, but I keep coming back to it again and again" or "I know the evidence doesn't support this thought, but I still think it's true."

In the case of Leigh-Ann, who held tightly to the belief that she was to blame for the history of sexual assaults perpetrated against her, it became clear after she completed a few similarly themed 5 Steps of CR exercises that she was reluctant to let go of this thought, despite a good amount of solid evidence to the contrary. For many with PTSD, some of these ingrained beliefs may have become part of the person's guiding principles in life (for better or for worse), and although they may find them somewhat distressing (e.g., "You can never let your guard down"), they are also personally meaningful and continue to serve some function in their lives (e.g., providing a perceived sense of safety). Empathic but direct exploration by the therapist of these patterns can help the client become unstuck in their trauma-based beliefs and begin to look at their experiences and life with a fresh perspective not dominated by trauma.

More specifically, the therapist can explore with the client the perceived value and costs of holding onto the belief versus letting it go in favor of a more accurate one. A recommended strategy for facilitating this comparison is to construct a Payoff Matrix with the client aimed at understanding what they have to gain by continuing to hold onto the belief and what the costs are of giving it up. Collaboratively developing a Payoff Matrix (which can be understood as a combination of a functional analysis and a decisional balance exercise) assumes that adhering to a belief that is not supported by available evidence is not irrational but serves an important purpose for the person. Once the perceived costs and benefits of holding onto an inaccurate belief have been identified, those perceptions can be the focus of further attention.

The Payoff Matrix is a 2 × 2 table with four quadrants. The horizontal axis is split into two halves for the belief in question and the alternative belief, and the vertical axis is split into two halves for the advantages and disadvantages of each belief (see the Payoff Matrix worksheet). The therapist works with the client to identify the advantages of holding onto the belief in question (upper left quadrant), the disadvantages of holding onto that belief (lower left quadrant), the advantages of accepting the alternative belief (upper right quadrant), and the disadvantages of giving up the old belief and adopting the new one (bottom right quadrant). Like generating evidence for and against a thought when teaching the 5 Steps of CR, the therapist first helps the client write down all of the perceived advantages and disadvantages of the old belief, regardless of how accurate they appear to be. Sometimes just becoming more aware of the high cost that the individual is paying to hold onto an old belief can help to shift the balance to a greater readiness to endorse the new belief. Often, however, it is also useful to more closely examine some of these perceptions, such as why the client sees holding onto the belief as beneficial or what the perceived costs are of giving up the belief in favor of a more accurate one. The bird's-eye view that the Payoff Matrix provides can create a needed shift in the client's perception and increase willingness to let go of long-held and unhelpful core and trauma-related beliefs.

Leigh-Ann and her therapist completed a Payoff Matrix to understand how continuing to hold on to a distressing belief ("I'm to blame for the fact that I have been sexually assaulted as a teen and then again as an adult") may have both perceived benefits as well as important consequences. As they worked on this exercise in session, it was uncovered that part of Leigh-Ann's reluctance to let go of this belief was related largely to her ambivalence about what it said about the safety in the world and her own safety if she actually did not cause these assaults. When clients have a recapitulation of the same belief themes over the course of the CR sessions, this exercise can help them gain a new perspective on the utility of continuing to ruminate about these types of thoughts. See Table 10.1 for Leigh-Ann's completed Payoff Matrix worksheet.

Similarly, if despite multiple 5 Steps of CR exercises, Edmundo continued to cling to his beliefs (from Chapter 9, this volume; "I'm totally to blame for

TABLE 10.1. Example of a Completed Payoff Matrix for Leigh-Ann

Instructions

The thought or belief I am having trouble letting go of is this: "I'm to blame for the fact that I have been sexually assaulted as a teen and then again as an adult."

List the advantages and disadvantages of keeping this thought or belief versus changing it to a more accurate one. Be as specific as possible.

Advantages of keeping this thought or belief	Advantages of changing this thought or belief
In what ways does holding onto your thought or belief make your life seem more manageable, safer, or easier to handle? Does the thought or belief provide you with a sense of control, security, or predictability of the future?	How could changing your thought or belief improve your life? Consider whether changing your thought or belief would reduce distressing feelings and free you up from concerns about past events.
• If I was responsible for my own abuse, then the world seems safer since I can prevent such things from happening again. • It makes me feel like I have more control of my life.	• I would feel better about myself if I accepted that the abuse was not my fault. • I might be able to enjoy sex more in the future if it didn't make me feel ashamed about what happened with my friend's father and my neighbor.

Disadvantages of keeping this thought or belief	Disadvantages of changing this thought or belief
In what ways does holding onto your thought or belief make your life more difficult? Consider the role that the thought or belief plays in causing upsetting feelings for you and preventing you from doing things you would like to do.	What are the possible disadvantages of changing your thought or belief? Would changing the thought or belief lead you to feel less control, security, or ability to predict what is going to happen?
• I feel bad about myself and ashamed when I have memories of these incidents. • It's hard for me to try to move on and trust anyone, and I am lonely because of that. • I am not able to enjoy sex and feel like I won't be able to in the future as a result of this belief.	• If I accept that the abuse wasn't my fault, then the world seems scary and unpredictable. If an adult can abuse an innocent child, then anything could happen.

my younger brother's suicide because I let him join into the gang life, and he would definitely still be alive today if I had been a better person and family member" and "I am totally worthless because I didn't do enough to help my brother and it's my fault he killed himself"), the Payoff Matrix would be a potentially useful exercise to initiate with him as well. Thus, the Payoff Matrix serves as an important tool for the therapist to understand the impact of these long-held beliefs on clients' worldview and self-view so that the therapist can help clients to recognize and untangle these perspectives and therefore gain some newfound relief from the ongoing distress caused by maintaining these highly upsetting beliefs.

UNRESOLVED DISTRESSING FEELINGS ABOUT PAST SITUATIONS

Even with extensive and successful 5 Steps of CR work around highly distressing PTSD-related beliefs, some clients continue to experience upset and interference related to thoughts or memories about past traumatic events. Strong feelings of shame, guilt, anger, or rage about events that occurred many years ago may persist even after examining and modifying the thoughts underlying them. These emotions often surface when recent events trigger relevant memories, when a trauma anniversary is upcoming, or when clients are preoccupied or ruminate about their traumatic experiences. Strategies for addressing these often complex emotions within the treatment model are discussed next.

Guilt and Shame

As mentioned in previous chapters in this volume, clients who have a trauma history of childhood sexual abuse often have unresolved, complicated feelings of shame and guilt, which often manifest in chronic self-blame types of beliefs. Following 5 Steps of CR work and the Payoff Matrix exercise, clients who continue to struggle with these emotions may benefit from Action Plans that incorporate compassion or forgiveness for oneself, as in compassionate mind approaches (Gilbert & Irons, 2005; Neff, 2011). Training in the compassionate mind assumes that the ability to feel compassion for oneself is an attribute that can be learned through practice addressing self-attacking cognitive styles with strategies such as practicing empathic (self)-understanding, considering alternative perspectives, and using positive imagery (Gilbert & Choden, 2014; Lee, 2005).

Persistent Anger

Anger is generally viewed as a negative emotion, but there are some important distinctions between anger and other distressing feelings. Anxiety, depression, and guilt are invariably unpleasant feelings, and most people want them to go away for those reasons alone. Anger, on the other hand, is associated with thoughts of having been wronged. This externalization of blame can be energizing and contribute to feelings of righteousness and having some control over an unjust situation. Thus, while people are readily motivated to use cognitive restructuring to reduce distress associated with other emotions, they are often less motivated to use it to reduce their anger. However, strong angry feelings can be disruptive and interfere with functioning, including relationships, school or work performance, and feelings of well-being.

Several strategies can be helpful when teaching CR to clients who struggle with anger. When clients describe angry feelings, the therapist should not automatically assume that they find these feelings unpleasant or unwelcome. Care must be taken to first explore the situation with the client, including the associated thoughts and feelings, to determine whether anger or some other emotion should be the focus of cognitive restructuring. It is normal for people to feel either angry, anxious, or both when they perceive a threat (i.e., the fight-or-flight response). Strong fear can be paralyzing, leaving the person feeling vulnerable and defenseless and contributing to avoidance and hypervigilance. Similarly, feelings of depression or shame can be immobilizing due to beliefs of helplessness and low self-worth. Anger can serve as a defense against these vulnerable feelings, replacing them with a sense of empowerment and activation. Clients sometimes reject the use of cognitive restructuring to address their angry feelings, as they may see the skill as an attempt to invalidate or make their anger go away, when in truth they feel that their anger is justified.

As detailed in Chapter 8 in this volume, a useful strategy for addressing situations involving anger is to help the client understand and identify additional negative emotions underlying or accompanying their anger and to make these feelings (e.g., anxiety, shame) the focus of cognitive restructuring. Recognizing the link between anger and other upsetting emotions involves exposing one's vulnerability, and thus it requires a good therapeutic relationship between the client and therapist. However, if clients are able to use CR to address these other more vulnerable emotions, their angry feelings often dissipate.

Another effective 5 Steps technique is to apply the metacognitive strategy described in the earlier section related to exploring fears and thoughts related to engaging in specific CR for PTSD therapy exercises. In this case, the therapist would help the client to acknowledge and challenge unhelpful beliefs they may have about willingness to work on anger within the context of this program (e.g., "If I try to let go of my anger, that will mean that my abuser will have won" or "If I stay angry and alert about this, then I won't be vulnerable to another assault").

Similarly, clients may benefit from completing a Payoff Matrix to evaluate what they are gaining from holding onto anger and what it is costing them. When a client perceives that holding onto anger protects them from future victimization, the therapist can systematically guide the client through the Payoff Matrix by asking questions such as these: "How effective is the anger at protecting you? Is it possible to protect oneself without remaining angry? Has the anger ever caused bad things to happen that would otherwise not have occurred? What has been given up in order for you to maintain the high level of alertness? Is it worth it?" This examination of the benefits and costs of maintaining the anger can challenge the perceived costs of giving up the anger and provide clarity to clients about the price they are paying by holding on to this emotion.

Helping clients recognize that feelings of vulnerability often underlie anger takes time, and there is sometimes a need for other strategies to address anger. After a review of all the available evidence, if the client firmly believes that the evidence supports the thought, the therapist should accept this and move on to developing an Action Plan to address the situation. Even if the therapist believes the evidence does not support the thought, it is always the case that it is the client's perception that drives the decision making in CR.

Developing an effective Action Plan depends on what the nature of the situation is and how the client has handled it up to that point. Different Action Plans are required to address anger related to three types of upsetting situations. Some common anger-based Action Plan themes include (a) a recent situation that the client is angry about, (b) events that occurred long ago that the client is still angry about, and (c) a pattern of maladaptive angry responses to a variety of situations.

A potentially useful strategy for crafting helpful Action Plans for some clients with strong, angry feelings about prior abusive experiences is to collaboratively develop plans that explore the value of forgiveness of others (Freedman & Enright, 1996; Reed & Enright, 2006; Weinberg et al., 2017). There are many different ways to forgive, and useful guidance is available to clinicians and clients for exploring the potential benefits of forgiveness (Enright, 2001).

Aside from attempting to reduce distress related to unresolved feelings associated with the past, Action Plans can focus on minimizing the negative effects of those feelings on present functioning or current personal goals. For example, clients who experience persistent feelings of rage related to a past abuser with whom they have no contact could develop an Action Plan designed to minimize the impact of those feelings on their current relationships.

Like all Action Plans, each of these requires establishing a specific agreed-upon goal to drive the problem-solving nature of the skill and help the client develop a reasonable and acceptable plan to initiate. Some typical goals of these sorts of Action Plans are as follows:

- To develop consistent, healthy coping strategies to use in the moment to deal with irritability and anger related to current stressors.
- To reduce maladaptive or dangerous behavioral patterns resulting from anger (i.e., verbal outbursts, aggression, etc.).
- To learn assertiveness skills for expressing angry feelings appropriately while preserving important relationships (work, family, romantic partner, etc.).

- To learn more effective social skills for managing upsetting feelings in day-to-day interactions (Mueser et al., 2024).
- To reduce persistent anger related to past traumatic events.
- To minimize disruptive effects of anger on functioning, life goals, and well-being.
- To explore strategies related to forgiveness of others.

USING CR TO ADDRESS PERSISTENT PTSD AND OTHER STUBBORN ASSOCIATED SYMPTOMS

As described in previous chapters in this volume, using the PCL-5 (and Beck Depression Inventory–II) to identify and target ongoing interfering symptoms is an effective first step toward assisting clients in addressing these with the 5 Steps of CR. There are some PTSD symptoms, however, that may be persistent and pose special challenges. These include nightmares, dissociation, and hypervigilance/overestimation of danger. Strategies to address these are discussed next.

Nightmares

Nightmares in people with PTSD typically involve dreams that are thematically related to the individual's traumatic experiences but are not a simple repetition of those events. Sometimes there is no apparent relationship between the content of the nightmare and the person's trauma history. Regardless of the nature of the nightmares, they are often a major source of distress and interfere with sleep both by abruptly waking up the person and by creating perpetual anxiety about going to sleep. A consequence of this anxiety is that people often postpone going to sleep until long after they are exhausted, and/or they are prone to using alcohol and drugs to cope with their sleep problems (Nishith et al., 2001), thus increasing their vulnerability to substance use problems.

Cognitive restructuring can be used to help clients cope more effectively with nightmares and often to overcome them. To implement this approach, the therapist should explain to the client that nightmares can be due to unresolved concerns or problematic beliefs related their traumatic experiences and that the first step to addressing them is to begin keeping a short journal of the nightmares they experience. The journal can be kept by the person's bed, and when they are awakened by a nightmare (or the next morning), they can briefly write down what happened in the nightmare. The therapist should ask the client to bring the journal to each session. As part of the session agenda, the therapist and client can review the nightmare content in the journal entry. Sometimes there is an obvious relationship between a particular nightmare and the client's traumatic events. At other times, a common theme that appears to be related to the person's traumatic experience may emerge across several nightmares or even after several weeks of journal review. After a particular issue or theme related to trauma has been identified, the therapist can help the client identify the feelings and beliefs related to it and then use the 5 Steps of CR to examine those beliefs more closely (e.g., "I'm helpless and have no control over my life because of the abuse I suffered as a child"). Addressing and resolving trauma-related issues that underlie nightmares can reduce both the frequency of the nightmares and the distress associated with them.

The 5 Steps can also be used to help clients deal with anxiety or other negative feelings they have about trying to get back to sleep after a nightmare. Under these circumstances, CR can help clients to address Common Styles of Thinking that may interfere with coping with the nightmares—such as catastrophizing ("I can't stand it if I have another nightmare tonight. I won't be able to go through the day tomorrow if I don't get at least 6 hours of sleep"), all-or-nothing thinking ("I'm a basket case because I keep having nightmares"), or jumping to conclusions ("I'm always going to have nightmares")—and develop more adaptive self-statements for coping with these experiences.

In addition, Action Plans are useful for dealing with nightmares and can involve journaling the content of nightmares (as previously described), developing additional strategies to cope with nightmare distress instead of using alcohol and drugs, and taking steps to improve overall sleep hygiene. While improved sleep hygiene may not have a direct impact on nightmares per se, it may improve the quality of sleep when the person is able to sleep and decrease some of the disruptive effects of the nightmares on sleep overall.

Dissociation

Dissociative symptoms are a common posttraumatic reaction in which individuals experience a break in the usual connections between thoughts, feelings, and behaviors (e.g., flashbacks, numbing, depersonalization, derealization). These symptoms are frequently distressing because they can interfere with the person's ability to relate to others and to integrate experiences into their sense of self. CR can be used to reduce distress associated with these symptoms as well as the symptoms themselves.

Flashbacks involve the momentary reexperiencing of an event in which people lose their connection with the present and feel as though the event is actually happening again. Flashbacks tend to be brief but can be extremely upsetting. CR can be used to address flashbacks in two ways. First, since flashbacks involve the reexperiencing of upsetting events, the 5 Steps of CR can be used to examine distressing thoughts the client has about those events (e.g., "I'm tarnished because of what happened"), as well as concerns about the flashbacks themselves (e.g., "I'm never going to be able to live a normal life if I continue to have flashbacks").

Second, flashbacks are often triggered by specific stimuli, including intense emotions. Teaching clients how to recognize distressing feelings that precede flashbacks can facilitate their ability to use CR to cope right away, thus preventing flashbacks from occurring. Clients can be taught to keep a log of their flashbacks, including the time when the flashback occurred, the situation, possible trauma-related stimuli, and any thoughts or feelings that preceded it. The therapist can review this log with the client to identify possible precipitants of flashbacks (e.g., thoughts of being trapped, feelings of anxiety and panic, a trauma-related stimulus, etc.) and then engage the client in practicing how to recognize those thoughts, feelings, or stimuli and to initiate CR as soon as they are detected.

Numbing, depersonalization, and derealization symptoms are disturbing because they interfere with individuals' connection with others and the world around them. CR can be used to cope with these symptoms based on the assumption that historically they served a protective function in shielding the person from extremely distressing thoughts and feelings. As clients develop new skills for dealing directly with negative feelings (i.e., Breathing Retraining, CR, freestanding Action Plans), they no longer have a need for these symptoms to protect themselves from that intense distress. The therapist should provide this rationale to clients to increase their motivation and willingness to approach this distressing symptom and associated upsetting emotions.

Since numbing and related symptoms are a learned response to distress that has been reinforced over many years, skills practice is needed to preempt this response. The therapist can facilitate clients' use of the 5 Steps to address the upsetting feelings that precede numbing and related symptoms by assisting them in increasing their own awareness of those situations and associated emotions. This recognition can be accomplished by teaching clients to maintain a log of when these experiences occur, as previously described in this section when addressing flashbacks.

Hypervigilance or Overestimation of Danger

People with PTSD often have exaggerated perceptions of danger that interfere with their lives, prevent them from achieving their goals, and result in chronic anxiety, hypervigilance, and sometimes paranoia. Repeated use of the 5 Steps of CR is often effective at reducing these appraisals of risk and vulnerability as well as the upset and functional interference associated with them. However, some clients experience only minimal reductions in distress after reviewing the evidence and concluding that their initial perceptions of risk were exaggerated. They therefore continue to report high levels of anxiety associated with any risk, no matter how small.

For clients who are preoccupied by excessive concerns over relatively low-risk situations, the Action Plan proves very useful. Note that this sort of Action Plan can be implemented following the end of a 5 Steps practice when clients decide that the evidence does support their belief regarding a high-risk situation and they therefore remain distressed, or when clients do modify their thought somewhat in Step 5 but still find themselves anxious or worried. In addition, when overestimation of risk is a more chronic experience, the therapist can help the client initiate a freestanding Action Plan (i.e., not tied to a particular 5 Steps example to address this frequent interference).

The specific goal of the Action Plan is determined by the client's acceptance level regarding the general and specific risks they face in their life. For those who accept the degree of risk inherent in their current lives, the goal is to reduce the distress associated with those risks (e.g., using Breathing Retraining, reminding oneself that such risks are low, thinking of positive outcomes associated with the acceptable risks). For clients who do not accept the risks associated with their current lives, the goal instead is to help them explore how to make changes in their lives that could further reduce their risk to a perceived acceptable level. Such changes could involve modifying one's habits (e.g., halting substance use to reduce chances of victimization) or living situation (e.g., making long-term plans to move to a safer neighborhood).

CONCLUSION

A wide range of strategies can be used to overcome common obstacles encountered throughout the CR for PTSD program, such as therapy-process challenges, reluctance to deal with trauma-related material, difficulty using the skills in times of acute distress, persistent upsetting beliefs despite clear evidence against them, and only minor reduction in distress when replacing inaccurate thoughts with new, more accurate ones. CR and associated techniques (including stand-alone Action Plans and the Payoff Matrix) can and should be used creatively to deal with these common challenges. These same strategies are also highly effective in helping clients to manage a variety of stubborn emotions (like guilt/shame and anger) as well as problematic posttraumatic symptoms (including nightmares, dissociation, and hypervigilance) that can greatly interfere with functioning and personal goals.

11

Skill Generalization and Termination

The effectiveness of the skills taught in the Cognitive Restructuring (CR) for posttraumatic stress disorder (PTSD) program depends on the extent to which clients are able to use and transfer them from the therapy sessions to their daily lives. Trauma survivors with co-occurring serious mental illness may face particular obstacles in learning how to use the skills in their personal lives due to problems such as severe symptoms (e.g., psychosis), cognitive impairment, interpersonal conflict, or multiple stresses. This chapter describes strategies to enhance skill generalization as a cornerstone to a successful ending to the CR for PTSD program and provides guidelines for a fruitful termination process.

SKILL GENERALIZATION

There are two broad approaches to maximizing the generalization of skills taught in therapy to clients' daily lives: increasing the client's competence in the skills and increasing environmental supports for using them. *Competence* resides within an individual and is the ability to use a skill effectively in appropriate situations. *Environmental supports* reside outside the person and are facilitators of the individual's use of a skill in day-to-day situations. Attention to both approaches is critical for clients to gain the maximal benefit from the CR for PTSD program.

Increasing Competence Within Sessions

The greater competence clients develop at cognitive restructuring over the course of treatment, the more likely it is that they will continue to be able to use the skill after the program ends. The ability of clients to use cognitive

https://doi.org/10.1037/0000423-011
Treatment of Posttraumatic Stress Disorder in Serious Mental Illness: The Cognitive Restructuring Program, by K. T. Mueser and J. D. Gottlieb

restructuring independently can be improved by strengthening their skills within treatment sessions and promoting their use of the skills in natural settings.

Cognitive restructuring is a relatively complex skill that is taught by focusing on the specific components of the skill and gradually building the client's competence through repeated practice and successive reinforcement of approximations to the skill (i.e., shaping). To shape clients' competence at using cognitive restructuring, the therapist needs to actively engage them in repeatedly practicing the skill during treatment sessions and provide feedback and guidance to hone the skill over multiple efforts. This requires more than just talking about the 5 Steps of CR or leading the client through the steps of the skill; the client must be actively involved in trying to use cognitive restructuring in the session. Shaping the specific components of the cognitive restructuring skill involves explaining and demonstrating the steps (with the therapist initially taking the lead), prompting the client to use the steps of the skill (with the client taking the lead), reinforcing the client for steps that were performed well, providing additional prompts or instructions to teach other steps, and then gradually fading the instructions and prompts during sessions as the client becomes more able to perform the skill independently. Once clients are able to use the overall skill on their own, their competence is reinforced by the natural impact of cognitive restructuring on reducing negative feelings (i.e., negative reinforcement), and they no longer need to depend on the therapist for reinforcement in learning or using the skill.

Home Assignments: Increasing Competence by Promoting the Use of Skills in Natural Settings

Progress in the CR for PTSD program depends on the ability and willingness of clients to practice cognitive restructuring on their own. Home assignments designed to facilitate this are a cornerstone of this program. Independent use of skills is naturally reinforced, increasing the chances that clients will use the skills again in the future. Difficulties using skills independently provide valuable information to the therapist, who can focus on teaching those aspects of the skill the client has not mastered. We have found that clients who completed more home assignments during the CR for PTSD program improved significantly more in PTSD and other outcomes than those who completed fewer home assignments (Mueser et al., 2008). Thus, as previously mentioned, it is crucial that the therapist explain the value of home assignments at the outset of the program and remind clients of its importance throughout the 16 sessions.

Once clients begin trying to use skills on their own, the therapist modifies home assignments to shape the skills in order to make them as effective as possible and more likely to be maintained after completing treatment. Tailoring the skills to the individual client and maximizing the effectiveness of home assignments have been addressed in previous chapters in this volume. Some of these options include modifying Breathing Retraining (BRT) and developing home assignments that focus first on having clients practice the skill in comfortable, nonstressful situations and then later on encouraging clients to try the skill in more challenging ones (Chapter 5, this volume). Similarly, as discussed in Chapters 7–9 in this volume, the Common Styles of Thinking (CST) skill is introduced and practiced as an initial CR skill. Then, the 5 Steps of CR skill is taught, focusing initially on more basic annoyances, stressors, and upset feelings to help the client learn the skill. Once the client has demonstrated basic understanding and some independent use of the skill, the emphasis shifts more overtly to trauma-related and core beliefs work.

Addressing Obstacles to Adherence to Home Assignments

Despite the importance of outside practice, clients do not always follow through on home assignments, especially early in treatment. While this is not uncommon in most cognitive behavioral therapy interventions, targeting and helping the client overcome obstacles to follow-through is critical to success in the CR for PTSD program. It is important for the therapist to not give up on developing home practice tasks with a client and to follow through on their progress during these sessions. In all cases, any home assignment should be collaboratively agreed upon between client and therapist to ensure that the client understands both the rationale, utility, and logistics of the task and is willing to try to complete it.

Generally, it is helpful to conceptualize the completion of a home assignment as *any* attempt by the client to use skills taught in session on their own, regardless of whether a written assignment was completed. Thus, if a client reports successfully recognizing and challenging CSTs related to negative feelings on several occasions over the past week but did not use the worksheet, the therapist should first reinforce the client for following through and using the skill. Then, the therapist can explore strategies for helping the client use the worksheet for the following week's home assignment to further embed and generalize CR use.

If no written home assignment was completed and the client did not try to use the skills, the therapist should problem-solve with the client about obstacles to completing the next home assignment before the following session. Common problems include (a) forgetting or getting distracted; (b) misplacing the worksheet; (c) not understanding the assignment or being unsure how to use the skill; (d) becoming triggered by PTSD symptoms while attempting to do the assignment; (e) being worried about perceived therapist negative judgment of their experiences, distress, and/or their ability to carry out the home practice task sufficiently; and/or (f) feeling preoccupied or overwhelmed with other life problems or crises. When addressing lack of follow-through on a home assignment, the therapist always should first explore the reason for not doing the assignment, as the differing reasons mentioned earlier naturally lead to very different interventions to increase outside practice attempts and success.

Once a discussion about the particular obstacles has occurred, the therapist should again reiterate the importance of outside practice on PTSD symptom improvement and goal attainment and then develop a plan to overcome these specific obstacles (consider a written freestanding Action Plan to facilitate the process). For example, with a client who reports getting easily distracted and overwhelmed when trying to complete home assignments during the week, specific strategies can be reviewed and agreed upon. These include prompting clients to set aside a time of day and a quiet, private place where they can practice the skill; planning to use BRT before attempting the task; and enlisting social support for encouragement and reinforcement. With clients who attempt outside practice between meetings but report struggling with a particular piece of the skill while on their own (i.e., expressing confusion about how to initiate a short inhale in BRT or getting stuck in Step 4 of the 5 Steps), it can be useful in the beginning of the subsequent session to discuss the area of difficulty and then help the client complete that particular exercise before moving on with the rest of the session content. These and other strategies for overcoming home assignment obstacles are summarized in the bottom of Exhibit 11.1.

EXHIBIT 11.1

Strategies for Enhancing Adherence to Home Assignments

Routinely:

- Develop assignments collaboratively with the client to ensure buy-in and feasibility.
- Conceptualize home practice broadly as including any efforts to practice or use targeted skills outside of session, not just completion of written materials.
- Individualize assignments for the client (e.g., be specific, plan when and where the assignment will be done, anticipate and problem-solve possible obstacles).
- Follow up on home assignments at the beginning of each session to demonstrate their importance.
- Reinforce amply any and all efforts to practice or use skills outside of the session.
- Elicit whether the client's use of a skill was associated with any reduction in distress.
- Develop a plan (Action Plan as needed) for the home assignment at the end of each session, addressing any obstacles the client previously encountered to completing assignments.
- Help the client anticipate upcoming stressful or trauma-related situations for which they could anticipate using these skills during the week.

If problems occur with follow-through on home assignments:

- Review the rationale for home assignments, and remind the client of CR for PTSD program study findings that clients who routinely did home assignments had better outcomes in PTSD symptoms and other areas than those who did not.
- Do not apologize for home assignments! Review (or elicit) the rationale that practicing skills taught in session in daily life is a cornerstone of how this program works.
- Have the client practice completing part of the home assignment at the end of the session (or at the beginning of the following session) to troubleshoot challenges and ensure understanding.
- Shape adherence by simplifying assignments, reinforcing efforts and small steps to follow through, and gradually modifying and increasing difficulty as the client succeeds with easier assignments.
- Engage supportive other(s) in helping the client follow through on assignments.
- Address with the 5 Steps of CR any inaccurate or unhelpful thoughts related to the perceived utility of home assignments or the client's ability to complete them (i.e., "I have to do this assignment perfectly, or it's not worth trying").

Note. CR = cognitive restructuring; PTSD = posttraumatic stress disorder.

The following dialogue illustrates how Edmundo's therapist addressed his difficulty in following through on home assignments:

THERAPIST: Edmundo, I've noticed that it seems like it has been a bit of a challenge the past few sessions in terms of working on our 5 Steps of CR skill between sessions. What do you think about that?

EDMUNDO: Yeah, I know. I'm really sorry.

THERAPIST: I want you to know that having some trouble following through on home assignments is not uncommon in this program. You are not alone in that. Also, though, we know from the studies done with this intervention that practicing the skills taught in this program at home is important—it really helps people get even more relief from their PTSD symptoms. And I definitely want that for you! I'm hoping we can talk this through together for a few minutes. Would that be OK?

EDMUNDO: I know. Me too. OK.

THERAPIST: Can you help me understand what might be getting in the way for you? For some people, it's related to forgetting, to being worried about having enough privacy at home to practice, or to not feeling sure the skills will help—that sort of thing. For others, it is about confidence in one's abilities or being afraid of making a mistake. But tell me a little more, Edmundo, about what you think—so we can figure it out together.

EDMUNDO: I don't know exactly. It's on my radar, so it's not that. And I have a ton of stuff that I am stressed and upset about, so I know there are things to work on. And I've seen in our meetings when we've done the skill together, it helps. But every time I go to sit down and write out one during the week, I get super anxious and sad.

THERAPIST: I'm so glad you are sharing this with me. Is there a specific thought that goes through your head that is making you anxious and sad when you start to try the assignment?

EDMUNDO: Yeah, it's something like, "I gotta get this right. If I don't do it well, then there's no point. I did badly in school, and that's how I felt a lot back then. Same thing now, I guess."

THERAPIST: I see. Actually, this thought you are describing is pretty common for a lot of people. Why don't we go ahead and do a 5 Steps together about this situation and your thought that is causing this distress. We can work on it right now.

> I think it could be useful to help get things unstuck. What do you say?

EDMUNDO: That's a good idea. Thanks.

Reducing Reliance on Written Worksheets

In the later sessions (e.g., Sessions 12–16), when attention starts to shift to the generalization and maintenance of skills learned, consideration must be given to how the client can continue to use cognitive restructuring after the program has ended. A few useful strategies can be used to facilitate this goal.

First, if the client has difficulty mastering the 5 Steps of CR, the skill can be simplified to make it easier. For example, as discussed in Chapter 10 in this volume, the client might find it easier to rely on recognizing and challenging the CST to deal with distress and to complete home assignments in the generalization phase of the program that focus on practicing this CST skill rather than the 5 Steps of CR.

Another method for facilitating the maintenance of cognitive restructuring is to reduce or eliminate the client's reliance on written worksheets and handouts. While these materials serve as a crucial aid to teaching cognitive restructuring, reliance on them for the day-to-day handling of upsetting feelings may be impractical. Teaching clients how to use cognitive restructuring without depending on the worksheet can foster skill generalization and maintenance. Competence in using the 5 Steps of CR without a worksheet can be shaped through a combination of in-session work and home assignments:

THERAPIST: Leigh-Ann, over the past several sessions you've done a really good job of learning how to use the 5 Steps of CR to deal with upsetting feelings—both in general and related to the sexual molestation and rape you experienced. Up until now, you've used a worksheet to go through the steps. However, to use the 5 Steps at any time and in any situation, it might be helpful to be able to use the skill without the worksheets. How about if we try working on this problem today without the worksheet?

LEIGH-ANN: OK. I'm willing to try, I guess.

THERAPIST: Good! So what do we do in Step 1 of the 5 Steps of CR?

After the client and therapist review together in session the 5 Steps of CR without the worksheet, a home assignment can be developed for the client to practice in that way on their own. In collaboration with clients, therapists can develop home assignments that are graded in difficulty in order to shape the ability to use the skill without the worksheet. For example, the client might begin practicing the 5 Steps of CR without the worksheet for 2 or 3 days of the following week while continuing to use the worksheet on the remaining days.

Success at using the skill without the worksheet can be followed up with assignments to decrease or altogether eliminate the worksheets. Alternatively, an assignment can be developed that asks clients to try to do the first two or three steps of CR without the worksheet and then use the worksheet for the remaining steps (e.g., Steps 4 and 5), as they tend to be the most involved. In subsequent assignments, the client can practice doing more steps of the skill without the worksheet.

Utilizing mobile phone technology is an excellent way to promote skill generalization, and it also serves as an alternative for clients who have struggled to complete written home assignments and/or who have difficulty keeping track of the traditional worksheets in their daily life. For example, clients can create phone notes to track their use of BRT or to type out abbreviated 5 Steps entries related to an impromptu stressful event. The phone audio recorder feature can be used when clients find themselves in a situation that merits CR by talking through the 5 Steps in the moment.

While initiating the aforementioned strategies with the client, the therapist should introduce the 5 Steps of CR Notecard (2-sided). This is a summarized version of the 5 Steps skill that is made into a small card-sized document. One side shows a condensed list of the 5 Steps, and the other side lists a pared-down set of questions from the Tips for Finding Good Evidence Information Sheet to facilitate client's working through Step 4. These cards are designed to be printed, pasted together, then cut, and, ideally, laminated. Clients should be given multiple copies of the 5 Steps of CR Notecard (2-sided) and should be encouraged to keep these in prominent places where the Notecards can remind them to use the 5 Steps when distressed and can serve a quick walk-through of the skill. Most clients have about three to five cards distributed in various locations (e.g., in a bag, purse, wallet, or car; on a refrigerator or nightstand).

Some clients lack confidence that they will be able to use the 5 Steps of CR without the full, written worksheet. The therapist can acknowledge the client's concern while suggesting that they try it and noting that if it does not work, they can certainly resume using the worksheet. Some clients may find that the optimal approach is to use worksheets for the most upsetting (and/or trauma-related) problems but not for less distressing situations. Therapists should ensure that clients have an ample supply of CR worksheets and the 5 Steps of CR Notecard (2-sided) to take with them once the program has ended.

Increasing and Capitalizing on Environmental Supports for Ongoing Skill Use

Environmental supports can play an important role in assisting clients to learn, use, and maintain skills taught in the CR for PTSD program. Environmental supports include people with regular contact with the client who can prompt or assist them in using the targeted skills (e.g., professionals and other supportive persons). Involving a support person in helping the client practice CR and BRT outside of therapy sessions is the most powerful strategy for developing competence and sustained use of these skills, since teaching the skill is not limited to the restricted time and place of the therapy hour, thus fostering generalization.

Supportive persons can help clients learn and generalize skills by facilitating their completion of home assignments. For clients who have a basic understanding of the skill but who forget to practice it at home, the support person can prompt them. For clients who do not yet have a basic grasp of the skill from their work in the session with the therapist, a support person can help them follow through on their home assignment by providing supplementary prompting and coaching. The greater the role played by the support person in helping the client practice the skills and follow through on home assignments, the more closely treatment needs to be coordinated between the therapist and that support person, whether the person is another mental health professional, a significant other, a family member, or a friend.

Similarly, the maintenance of clients' cognitive restructuring skills after the CR for PTSD program has ended depends on the level of competence achieved by the client at the end of the program. Clients who have basic skill competence but forget to use it during times of stress may benefit from being prompted by support persons to use it at appropriate times. However, some clients with significant cognitive impairment never achieve independent competence at CR by the end of the program, although they benefit from assistance in using the skill provided by the therapist and support person. With these clients, the support person can play a more integral role in helping the client continue to use these skills after the program has ended.

Professional Supports

While clients will have a time-limited relationship with their CR for PTSD therapist, many will have a long-standing relationship with another mental health professional. For example, many individuals may have a longer term therapist. People with a more severe co-occurring condition like psychosis or bipolar disorder may have a case manager or staff at their supported housing. Individuals with an addiction may have a substance use counselor. And people with chronic medical conditions or with a need for oversight in the administration of their psychiatric medications may have an in-home or visiting nurse. Any of these professionals can be a valuable resource for supporting clients' use of cognitive restructuring in their daily lives.

As described in the previous section, and in earlier chapters in this volume, it is helpful for the therapist providing the CR program to have regular contact and coordination with supportive professionals. This coordination can be arranged by having a brief in-person or virtual online meeting (or phone call) at the outset of the intervention that includes the CR therapist and the client and/or other meetings at various points throughout the course of the 16 sessions, as needed. Brief updates every several weeks can inform the professional about clients' progress and any stresses or challenges they are experiencing. These contacts also allow the CR for PTSD therapist to get input from other professionals about how they think the client is doing.

Toward the end of the program, the therapist should explain to the client that they will work together to develop a plan with the professional aimed at helping the client continue to use their skills after the intervention ends. This plan will include a joint session together with the professional (see the Termination section, later in this chapter).

Personal Supports

Personal supports (aka, significant others) like family members, spouses, and friends can also play an important role in helping clients maintain their skills. The decision to involve significant others in treatment is based on three considerations: (a) Is the involvement of this person crucial to the consistent delivery of the CR for PTSD program to the client? (b) Is there strong conflict between the client and their personal support that could undermine the client's ability to make effective use of the program skills? (c) Is there is a clearly supportive person available whose involvement would enhance the client's participation motivation and learning and/or increase the person's understanding of the client's PTSD struggles and needs to enhance recovery?

Some clients depend on a significant other for coordination of mental health services and transportation. A variety of stresses (e.g., poverty, health problems), multiple demands on the significant other (e.g., constraints due to work), and family chaos can all jeopardize the ability of the client to get to the scheduled treatment sessions. In situations in which the client depends on another person for attendance, it is crucial for the therapist to solicit that person's understanding and support for the client's participation in the program and to problem-solve barriers as needed.

Facilitating the support of a significant other should be done in close collaboration with the client and in a manner respectful of their preferences (e.g., not talking about details of their trauma history). One approach is to arrange to have the significant other attend part of a session with the client on a regular basis to inform them about the intervention and progress. For example, the significant other can be invited to join the last 15 minutes of the first session and then to join again every third or fourth session. During these group meetings, the therapist can encourage the client to take the lead in explaining the program, describing skills they have learned and the nature of home assignments, summarizing progress made, and discussing anticipated stressors in the coming week to work on with CR. Depending on the relationship between the client and significant other and the client's need for support, these discussions can also address ways that the significant other can facilitate the client's practice and use skills on their own.

In addition, it is recommended that psychoeducational materials and handouts be reviewed and shared with supportive others, as this information is often new to them and therefore highly valued as a way to help them better understand their loved one's behavior.

ADDRESSING PERSISTENT PTSD SYMPTOMS

Although clients usually experience a significant reduction in their PTSD symptoms over the course of treatment and many no longer meet diagnostic criteria for PTSD at the end, some continue to have symptoms despite having learned cognitive restructuring and generalized its use to their everyday lives. Two approaches can be used when working with clients who have persistent PTSD symptoms later in the program. For most clients, a combination of both strategies is optimal.

Encourage Continued Practice of Cognitive Restructuring

Results from our research trials of the CR for PTSD program have shown that many clients continued to improve in PTSD and other areas following the end of the intervention when they are reevaluated at 6 and 12 months posttreatment (Mueser et al., 2008; Mueser, Gottlieb, et al., 2015). Clients are often relieved to learn that it is common for some PTSD symptoms to persist over time but gradually improve even after the end of treatment with continued skill practice. The therapist should normalize the slowness at which some symptoms improve and point out that when clients have been thinking a certain way for many years, they will need time to learn new ways of thinking. This can help clients understand that overcoming the effects of trauma and PTSD is a long-term process, and it encourages them to stick with the 5 Steps as a crucial tool in aiding their recovery. Any improvements in symptoms over the course of the program can be used as evidence to support its value and the importance of continuing to use it after the program has ended.

Shift Focus to Personal Goals

Clients with PTSD often assume that reducing or eliminating their PTSD symptoms is a prerequisite to pursuing and achieving personally important goals such as finding a meaningful relationship, returning to school or work, or fulfilling other significant pieces of their overall recovery process. These individuals may erroneously conclude that the persistence of their PTSD symptoms is a barrier to living a "normal" and rewarding life. The notion that one can live a fulfilling life while still having PTSD may be surprising to clients (even if this was likely already referred to in the early, engagement-based phase of treatment), but it is generally received as good news.

These particular personal goals will have previously been established in Session 3. While the tracking of these goals over time is an already embedded part of the CR for PTSD intervention (see Chapter 6, this volume), when significant PTSD symptoms persist into the later stages of the program, the therapist can shift attention somewhat away from tackling PTSD symptoms and more toward these goals (usually after Session 12).

The therapist and client should be very familiar with the client's goals at this point in the program, and the client will already be working toward them.

However, if concrete progress has not yet been made, the therapist should explore the steps that the client can begin taking to move forward in these areas. With encouragement, some clients begin working toward their goals more fervently at this point. Others may be still skeptical that they can make important life changes as long as they have PTSD symptoms.

To address this skepticism, the therapist can normalize the client's persistent symptoms by explaining that sometimes PTSD symptoms do not completely go away with treatment and that it is possible to live a happy and rewarding life despite having symptoms. Second, the therapist can note that PTSD symptoms sometimes improve as a result of pursuing specific personal goals. For example, people with PTSD are often more prone to reexperiencing symptoms during unstructured rather than structured time, and so pursuing meaningful activities (e.g., work, school, more involved parenting) can decrease that unstructured time and hence their reexperiencing of symptoms. This specific focus on goals would be useful for a client like Donata, who had frequently found herself overwhelmed by PTSD and voices when she was home alone in her apartment without an out-of-the-house routine.

A helpful adjunctive strategy is to prompt the client to use CR to address perceived or real barriers to achieving their goals and to examine hopeless beliefs that they cannot make progress toward their goals as long as they continue to have PTSD symptoms. Here, the 5 Steps of CR is used to evaluate the validity of the concerns, which result either in altering the client's perception (e.g., "I can take the needed step to being more involved in my kid's school even if I have intrusive trauma memories. I just need to start") and/or in developing an Action Plan to deal with the identified obstacles.

TERMINATION

The CR for PTSD program is a time-limited intervention, and clients are prepared for the ending of therapy from the beginning of the program. Such communication is critical to shaping clients' expectations for the intervention, motivating them to take an active role in learning during the therapy sessions and adhering to outside practice, and preparing them for moving on after the program has ended. Planning for termination, reviewing progress, and identifying needs the client has or may develop in the future can maximize the long-term benefits of participation.

General Termination Approach and Planning

The end date for the program should be jointly determined by the therapist and client based on the client's progress during the program, with 12–16 sessions recommended as the usual program duration. Between Sessions 8 and 10, the therapist should initiate a discussion of the client's progress in the program and additional treatment needs in order to estimate the number of sessions until completion. Additional input from another professional involved in the client's treatment (such as a case manager, a psychiatrist, or an addiction counselor) may also inform this decision. In most cases, completion of the full 16 sessions is most beneficial to ensure that adequate time can be spent working on trauma-related and core beliefs via the 5 Steps of CR and also to enhance skill generalization in the later sessions.

Around Session 10, the therapist should remind the client again of the time-limited nature of the program and clarify the number of sessions remaining. The therapist should also discuss the option of starting to meet every 2 weeks (instead of weekly) to give clients more practice using the skills on their own and to become used to reduced contact with their CR for PTSD therapist. This tapering works well for some clients but may not for others—particularly those who may struggle with attendance, skills practice consistency, and momentum. During this period, the therapist should get input from the client about their possible concerns about termination and their preferences for topics to focus on in the remaining sessions, particularly as related to specific lingering PTSD symptoms as well as movement on their previously outlined personal goals. The client's recent scores from the PTSD Checklist (PCL) and the Depression Assessment Tracking Sheet (i.e., from Sessions 10 and 13) serve an important purpose in these latter sessions, and specific items that continue to be elevated should become the focus of CR in these remaining sessions.

Agenda and Content for the Penultimate Session

The organization of the final two termination sessions depends on whether the client has a long-standing relationship with another professional (e.g., case manager or therapist) who will continue to provide help and support to the client after the program has ended. When a family member or other significant person has been an active supporter of the client's treatment, this person's continued support after the program ends may be critical because they may play a role like that of a professional with a long-term relationship with the client. Guidelines for involving a professional or personal support person in the penultimate session (i.e., Session 15) are provided next. If there is no obvious support person in the client's life, modifications for Session 15 content are outlined as well.

Involvement of a Professional or Personal Support

During the last third of the intervention (i.e., approximately Session 11 or 12), the therapist should discuss inviting the identified mental health professional (or personal support) to part of the scheduled penultimate session, explain the rationale for their inclusion, and outline what can be accomplished in that session, as follows:

1. Review the progress the client has made in the program, including skill mastery, PTSD symptom reduction, and personal goal progress; identify any

specific associated needs the client has or anticipates having in the future; and discuss plans for getting those needs met.

2. Have the client teach the attendee about the 5 Steps of CR and lead them through a brief, basic example of a stressful situation to demonstrate how the skill works and what the client has learned (see the following dialogue).

3. Discuss how the supportive person can continue to support the client in ongoing skill use, management of persistent PTSD symptoms, and continued work toward achieving goals.

As needed, prior to this session, the therapist can help allay any anxieties or concerns that the client may have in leading the support person through the 5 Steps of CR skill. Some clients express insecurities about taking on this role, in which case the therapist can encourage and assure the client that this is just for practice and that the therapist will be right there to jump in and support the process as necessary. By and large, however, clients are eager to demonstrate their CR mastery and look forward to the opportunity to share what they have learned with their supportive person. It is recommended to schedule the support person's attendance at the future session around this time to ensure that they are available on the appropriate date. Typically, attendance for part of the session—about 20 to 25 minutes of the 50- to 60-minute session—is adequate. As needed, their participation can occur via phone or video if in-person attendance is not feasible.

As preparation for that session, the therapist should discuss the terms of the meeting with the professional or support person, with an emphasis on disclosure and privacy issues that have been agreed upon with the client. For example, some clients prefer not to discuss any details about their traumatic experiences in this setting, and this desire should be respected. The general purpose, structure, and plan (agenda) of the meeting should also be described. In addition, the therapist should request that the support person come prepared with a (minor) stressful situation that they feel comfortable sharing in the session so that the client can lead them through the 5 Steps of CR.

In this penultimate session, prior to the arrival of the support person, the therapist and client set their agenda as usual, reviewing the CR home assignment and discussing any final questions or concerns the client may have about leading the 5 Steps. Upon arrival of the support person, if the client has agreed to play the role of the teaching expert in the 5 Steps, the therapist can help initiate the skills practice, as shown with Donata and her case manager, Vern, in the following:

THERAPIST: We're so glad you could join us, Vern. As you know, the CR for PTSD program that Donata has been participating in involves learning and practicing skills for dealing with upsetting feelings, with a focus on those that are related to traumatic experiences. One of the most important skills Donata has been learning is cognitive restructuring. Since she has worked hard and has developed some real expertise in this skill, we thought it might be helpful for her to teach you in a role-play how it works. When we've finished that, we can talk together about how Donata has benefited from the program and how you can continue to support her and the skills she has learned after this program has ended in order to help her with her ongoing overall recovery. Donata, do you want to go ahead and start on the practice with Vern? And remember, just do the best you can, and I'll be right here to jump in and coach you if you need me.

DONATA: Yeah, OK. I'm ready to try. Vern, this is the worksheet we use that tells you what to do. We can start at the top. Do you have a situation that happened that made you upset?

VERN: Well, actually, I do. I was driving to work the other day, and there was this big construction blockade on the road that the GPS in my car didn't account for, and I ended up having to sit in stopped traffic for almost half an hour. I was pretty annoyed and a little anxious during that!

DONATA: That's a good one. We talk about how you felt in the next step here: strongest feelings. I'll write down the situation in Step 1. And do you want to pick anxiety for the feeling on the sheet for Step 2? I can also write in "annoyed" here.

VERN: Yes, both of those, thanks.

DONATA: OK. Now we think about what we are thinking when we feel bad. So, do you know what you were thinking then in the car?

VERN: Well, I knew I'd be late for work for sure. So I started to think, "This is going to ruin my whole day."

DONATA: That's a thought we write down here in Step 3. I'll write that. Our thoughts get exaggerated sometimes, like we catastrophize and think it's the worst. It's called a Common Style of Thinking. Do you think your thought was one of these on the list here?

From there, the client and support person proceed through the remainder of the 5 Steps, with the therapist jumping in as needed when the client requires assistance. When the role play is over, the therapist prompts the client to describe ways they have found CR helpful in coping with negative feelings and stressful situations, including trauma-related beliefs, and ways that this person can support them in using the skill in the future. It is helpful to create a written list or an Action Plan during this discussion, with specific elements delineated, such as "Vern can remind me to write out a 5 Steps once a week" and "If Vern sees me starting to get real upset or yell at the voices, he can help me do Breathing Retraining."

If some time remains following the support person's departure, the therapist and client can spend a few minutes debriefing about the client's experience guiding the support person through the skill, with the therapist providing ample reinforcement for the client's efforts. From there, a final home assignment should be discussed, and the therapist should remind the client that the next session will be the last. The therapist should also provide a basic agenda of this upcoming final session, so that the client can know what to expect. Any concerns about ending can also be briefly discussed at this time. In some cases, it may be helpful for this last CR home assignment to be related to any anxious or upsetting beliefs that client may have about termination. The client can initiate a 5 Steps around their concerns (e.g., "I'll never be able to get any better than this without these treatment sessions each week" or other similar distressing termination-related thoughts).

No Involvement of a Professional or Personal Support

If a client has been referred through a prescriber or primary care doctor or if the CR for PTSD program is delivered in the context of a private practice rather than via a mental health clinic, the client may not have another professional to join the meeting. Similarly, there may not be a ready choice of a personal support in the client's life. When having a support person join is not an option, it is nevertheless recommended that the client have the opportunity to demonstrate their expertise in the 5 Steps skill with the therapist playing the role of the learner. In this case, the therapist should be ready with a benign and not overly personal annoying or stressful situation for the client to assist them with. The role-play practice can proceed as described in the previous section.

The Final Session

In the final session (usually Session 16), the typical agenda is as follows:

1. Review the 5 Steps of CR home assignment (possibly related to a distressing thought about termination).

2. Administer and review the final PCL-5 (and Depression Assessment Tracking Sheet and Posttraumatic Cognitions Inventory, as applicable), and discuss the trajectory of PCL scores over the course of treatment.

3. Discuss progress made toward personal goals from the earlier Goal-Setting Worksheet for the CR for PTSD Program.

4. Complete the Challenging My Most Distressing PTSD Symptoms and Thoughts worksheet.

5. Complete the Summing Up Worksheet.

6. Distribute extra copies of program worksheets and materials.

7. Determine the next steps, share final appreciations, and say good-byes.

PTSD Symptom and Goals Progress

Once the final PCL-5 is administered and scored, the findings should be briefly reviewed by the therapist and client, this time with a broader focus on overall changes in particular assessment items as well as the client's total score. It is helpful for the therapist to have all the previous PCL-5 scores from the outset of treatment at the ready, and it is recommended that they be tracked and presented via the PTSD Assessment Tracking Sheet (a similar strategy can be used to review depression symptoms with the Depression Assessment Tracking Sheet).

During this review, the therapist should point out which particular symptoms have decreased over time as well as which have not changed as much. This information will be useful in the next part of the session when the therapist helps the client note their most distressing PTSD-related thoughts and specifically the ways they have learned to challenge them over the course of the program. In addition, a brief discussion should be initiated here about what the client attributes the symptom reductions to, and their attributions should be reinforced and expounded upon by the therapist. In many cases, the client's final PCL-5 score will fall below 33, which is the threshold for a designation of "probable PTSD" (see Chapter 3, this volume). When this occurs, the therapist should inform the client that they "no longer have a diagnosis of PTSD," as this can create a meaningful, emotional, and proud moment for clients.

Following the assessment review, the therapist should proceed with a brief discussion about the client's progress toward the personal goals that were established at the outset of treatment. This serves as a very useful part of the final session because it allows the client to focus on the ways in which learning to understand and manage their PTSD better may have allowed them to become less stuck in their lives and move toward the specific, meaningful things that they have wanted for themselves. It also serves to promote their own more general recovery goals. This final focus on goal attainment also allows for an understanding that even when people have lingering PTSD symptoms, they can still make progress toward their goals and use the skills they learned in the program to help them. Specific plans for ongoing goals work can be delineated further in the subsequent part of this session by working collaboratively on the Summing Up Worksheet (details follow).

Reviewing Changes in PTSD-Related Thoughts

Following the symptom assessment and goal review, the therapist should guide clients through developing a summary list of their most distressing trauma-related and core beliefs (typically about three–five thoughts) that have been worked on during the therapy. This discussion can help clients gain further insights into how they have been able to modify their previous distressing and inaccurate beliefs into new, more balanced and accurate beliefs that are also less upsetting. Having a written sheet documenting these changes also serves as a salient reminder for clients when they find themselves struggling with the old thoughts at any point after treatment ends. To help organize this information, it is recommended that the therapist guide the client through the Challenging My Most Distressing PTSD Symptoms and Thoughts worksheet. This worksheet focuses specifically on PTSD symptoms and associated beliefs and is designed to highlight trauma-related thoughts that the client modified through CR and/or effective Action Plans. For some clients, these symptoms may no longer be present, and the worksheet summarizes what worked; whereas for others, some of the symptoms may persist, and the worksheet serves to remind them how to cope with them most effectively.

Clinical material for this exercise can come from a few different sources that have been tracked over time: (a) the Therapist Tracking Sheet for Client's Trauma-Related Cognitions, (b) completed 5 Steps of CR worksheets, and (c) the therapist and client's collaborative review of the most prominent trauma-related beliefs addressed via CR. An example of this exercise follows, as discussed by Leigh-Ann and her therapist:

THERAPIST: Leigh-Ann, I'd like us to use this worksheet to review (a) some of the distressing PTSD-related beliefs that we worked on during the course of our time together and (b) the ways in which you have been able to use cognitive restructuring to start to see things a bit differently and cope better with those symptoms and distress. I have some of your very well-done past 5 Steps of CR worksheets here if we need a memory jogger of some of the most important thoughts we worked on.

LEIGH-ANN: OK, yeah. This is a good idea. I know we've talked about a lot, and it would be good for me to get to have this list because I'm a little worried I will go back to my old way of thinking after this, and I really don't want to.

THERAPIST: That's a very common concern, and while it may be true that sometimes our old thoughts creep back in during moments of stress, you now have the tools to pull yourself back to a more realistic and healthy way of thinking about your experiences. This document will help guide you over time as needed.

LEIGH-ANN: OK, that helps to think of it this way.

THERAPIST: So let's talk about a couple of different thoughts that were addressed in this program. Do you have one in mind that you'd like us to start with?

LEIGH-ANN: Well, I know one of the big ones for me was blaming myself for being molested by my friend's dad. I've carried that around for years, and it has made me so ashamed. "It's my fault that he singled me out. I did something to invite this."

THERAPIST: Yes, that is a really important one that we spent a good amount of time on. Let's put that down first, with the feeling of shame. Over time, you've been able to identify it as a Common Style of

	Thinking, and after working on it with the 5 Steps of CR, you've started to see that it isn't entirely accurate. What should we write down in these other columns to reflect that?
LEIGH-ANN:	Yeah, I have. It's been a relief, for sure. We've talked about it like excessive self-blame, and that's what it is. The new way you helped me look at it after we used the skill is more like, "A child can't be held responsible for that kind of thing. It is always the adult's fault, and this guy was really a messed-up person." We can write all that down so I remember.
THERAPIST:	Yes, very good, Leigh-Ann. Another theme that we worked on quite a bit was related to some of your beliefs about being able to ever trust people again. Should we include that one and also indicate how you are seeing that now? ...

See Table 11.1 for Leigh-Ann's completed Challenging My Most Distressing PTSD Symptoms and Thoughts worksheet.

Summarizing Achievements and Next Steps

The final exercise in this termination session involves a review of the CR for PTSD program components, the client's major takeaways, and a plan for how the client can go forward to continue to make progress from here.

The Summing Up Worksheet pulls together the client's experiences in the program by summarizing what has improved, what still needs to be worked on (such as continued work on client goals or symptom management), which particular skills will be most helpful to achieve those continued improvements, and how the client can remember to use those skills. If the client had support persons (either professional or personal) who participated in the prior session, the previously discussed role of these people in helping the client continue to use the skills should be included in the list. If specific stresses are known to trigger or worsen PTSD symptoms in the past (e.g., anniversary dates of losses, family gatherings), these can be discussed and planned for along with the skills the client can use to cope with them.

THERAPIST:	We have spent the last few months working together to help you learn about, understand, and manage upsetting emotions related to your past traumatic experiences. You've worked really hard and have done well. I'd like us to summarize the progress you've made, the specific skills you've learned, and ways you can continue to use them after we end today.
LEIGH-ANN:	Thank you. It was hard, but that means a lot.
THERAPIST:	You did such a beautiful job, Leigh-Ann, even though there were some very difficult times. I'm very proud of you. Let's get some of this down on paper on our worksheet here so you can have a copy of it. First, we spent some time talking about the

TABLE 11.1. Example of the Challenging My Most Distressing PTSD Symptoms and Thoughts Worksheet, Completed by Leigh-Ann

Upsetting trauma-related situation or reaction	Related distressing feeling(s)	Upsetting thought and Common Style of Thinking	New, more accurate thought and/or Action Plan
Blaming myself for being molested by my friend's dad	Shame	"It's my fault that he singled me out. I did something to invite this." (self-blame) "I'm damaged goods because of what happened to me, and I'm not worth loving." (self-blame)	"A child can't be held responsible for that kind of thing. It is always the adult's fault, and this guy was really a messed-up person."
Wondering/thinking if I am able to ever trust people again	Anxiety Sadness	"I can't trust anybody because of what happened to me." (catastrophizing, overgeneralization)	"Some men are dangerous, but not every man or every person is."
Getting triggered around men in recovery meetings and mostly at work at the restaurant	Anxiety/fear Anger	"It feels like every guy definitely sees that I am vulnerable, knows there is something wrong with me, and is going to hurt me in some way. I am not safe." (mind-reading, emotional reasoning, overgeneralization)	"Not every man is dangerous." "People I work with don't know about my past unless I tell them." "I am safer now because I don't drink, and at work, there are people there to help if there is any real danger." Action Plan: Remind myself of new thoughts. Do BRT quietly in triggering moments. Use other grounding strategies from my written plan.

Note. PTSD = posttraumatic stress disorder; BRT = Breathing Retraining.

common effects of trauma, such as symptoms of PTSD, feelings of depression and guilt, and interpersonal difficulties like having trouble trusting men or anyone. As we have talked about these problems, you have learned that your reactions to your traumatic experiences are normal and are like those of others with similar experiences. In what ways did you find learning about the symptoms of PTSD helpful?

LEIGH-ANN: It was good to know that I wasn't crazy or anything like that. I never realized that other people have these same symptoms—like the memories, the feelings, and everything that goes with it. I had always kept it all to myself because I felt like an alien compared to other people my age.

THERAPIST: That's absolutely right. It's good to know you aren't alone in how these experiences affected you. Second, early in treatment you learned an important skill for dealing with tension and anxiety and other PTSD symptoms—Breathing Retraining. Over the course of the program, I've been so pleased to hear about how you have practiced this skill and learned how to use it in a variety of situations where you have felt anxious. How has the Breathing Retraining been helpful? In what situations have you found it useful?

LEIGH-ANN: Lots of times. Sometimes I feel really tense when I'm out in public. And when I have to deal with the kitchen guys at work, they can be triggering to me. The BRT helps calm me down and keeps me even-keeled. Also, it helps when I'm trying to sleep after a stressful day.

THERAPIST: Any other situations?

LEIGH-ANN: I still sometimes, although now less often, have those memories of the rape. I use the BRT then, and it helps me calm down.

THERAPIST: Yes, that's made a major difference for you, which is so important. The third thing that you learned in the program is the skill of cognitive restructuring, and you have done such great work with the 5 Steps of CR! There were many occasions where you were able to look more closely to realize that your thoughts and long-held beliefs about the traumas you experienced were not accurate, and you were able to change those thoughts to more accurate and less upsetting ones. You've also seen that sometimes the thoughts associated with upsetting feelings are, in fact, accurate, and when that happens, you know how to take action to address the problem rather than avoiding it or pretending it doesn't exist. As we've worked together, I've been really impressed with the progress you've made in learning and using the 5 Steps of CR. What stands out for you as having been the most helpful part of cognitive restructuring?

LEIGH-ANN: I used to just isolate my true self or be really irritable with everyone in my life—coworkers, neighbors, potential friends—because I thought I was totally damaged goods due to what had happened in my life. I still get down sometimes, but the 5 Steps of CR helps me figure out when I'm overreacting to a situation or when there really is a problem.

THERAPIST: And have you found that your overreactions are sometimes related to your traumatic experiences?

LEIGH-ANN: Yes. I used to react like I was still a child and couldn't protect myself. Now I know that things are different now. I'm not vulnerable the way I was as a child or even as much as I was a few years ago. And I am starting to blame myself less for the traumas, feel less guilty about that—and just a little less guilty overall about other things that come in life.

THERAPIST: That's so good to hear you say that. I'm making sure we get all of this down on the worksheet so you can take it with you and look at it regularly to remind yourself how far you have come. You've done a great job of applying these cognitive restructuring and Action Plan skills. And just like any other skill, you'll get better and better with more practice over time. I have found that many clients continue to improve after they have finished this program. For this reason, it's important for you to keep using the skills that you've learned here so that you can maintain all that you have gained and move even closer to what you want for yourself in life.

Ending the Final Session

In the final part of the last session, the therapist should make sure that the client has a complete collection of the handouts and worksheets done in this session as well as past sessions, including completed 5 Steps of CR worksheets and Action Plans. In addition, clients should be given a packet of blank worksheets so that they have clean copies to use going forward. If another mental health professional is involved, it is recommended that the therapist provide some clean copies to that person as well to facilitate the client's ongoing skill use.

The agenda and exercises outlined in this chapter provide a setting for a warm, comprehensive, and collaborative termination session. The therapist should allow the client the opportunity to share any final thoughts about their experience. From there, the clinician should conclude this final session by providing genuine and personalized positive feedback and encouragement to the client. The therapist should let the client know how proud they are of the client and how much they have enjoyed working together with the client. Typically, this particular structure, combined with the clinician's own personal style of ending a final therapy session with clients, serves to create a valuable and satisfying experience for both clinician and client.

CONCLUSION

From the outset of the CR for PTSD program, the therapist aims to help clients generalize the skills taught in session—especially cognitive restructuring, which is the core of the program—to their daily lives. Generalization is fostered by strengthening the client's competence at skills within the session, tailoring skills as needed to the individual client, collaboratively developing home assignments for the client to practice skills outside of sessions, and facilitating environmental supports for using the skills in the client's day-to-day living. Attention to the generalization of skills taught in sessions over the course of the program also facilitates the maintenance of skills over time after the program has ended.

Despite mastering the skills taught in the program, some clients may find that PTSD symptoms persist. When faced with such symptoms toward the end of treatment, the therapist has the combined tasks of encouraging the client to continue using the skills with the expectation of long-term benefits in symptom reduction and shifting the emphasis of treatment somewhat more toward helping the client achieve personal goals. As clients approach this late stage of treatment, regardless of whether they still experience PTSD symptoms, the therapist helps them conceptualize Breathing Retraining, cognitive restructuring, and Action Plans as personal life skills applicable to dealing with any unpleasant feelings and as useful tools for addressing obstacles to personal goals. This shift in emphasis—toward desired life changes and skills that promote coping and self-reliance—empowers trauma survivors by helping them see themselves not as helpless victims of circumstances beyond their control but as the masters of their own destiny.

Termination plays a vital role in the CR for PTSD program as it is crucial to empowering clients to take control over their lives and avoid dependency on the therapist. Clients are prepared for termination from the outset of the program, with specific plans based on the client's needs drawn up as they near the end. Central to these plans is addressing the issue of how clients can continue to use and hone their skills as they pursue their personal life goals and what role available professional and personal supports can play in these efforts. By reinforcing the client's skills and responsibility for change throughout their work together and collaboratively planning for life after the program has ended, the therapist ensures that graduation from the program is not experienced as a loss by the client but instead as another step forward in their life and toward their overall recovery.

SPECIAL CLINICAL CHALLENGES AND POPULATIONS

12

Working With People With Psychosis

As reviewed in Chapter 1 in this volume, there is a strong association among trauma, posttraumatic stress disorder (PTSD), and psychotic disorders (e.g., schizophrenia spectrum disorders). Trauma in early life increases the vulnerability of individuals to developing a psychotic disorder, which subsequently increases their chances of interpersonal victimization in adulthood. As a result of the high exposure to trauma over their lifespan, people with a psychotic disorder have much higher rates of PTSD than those in the general population, which interacts with and worsens the course of their psychosis. Effective treatment of PTSD in people with a psychotic disorder is critical to reducing the burden of these symptoms on them and enabling them to regain control over their lives.

There are some unique challenges that clinicians may encounter when providing the Cognitive Restructuring (CR) for PTSD program to people with psychosis. This chapter addresses these common challenges and provides strategies for overcoming them. The primary focus of this chapter is on the psychotic symptoms themselves and the resultant increased sensitivity to stress, regardless of the client's primary diagnosis (e.g., schizophrenia spectrum disorder, bipolar disorder, depression with psychotic features, borderline personality disorder). However, we also consider several other issues more common in schizophrenia and related disorders (but nevertheless present in other disorders as well), including working with individuals with significant negative symptoms or cognitive impairment and responding to questions raised by clients about the accuracy of their primary diagnosis in light of the discovery of untreated PTSD.

https://doi.org/10.1037/0000423-012

Treatment of Posttraumatic Stress Disorder in Serious Mental Illness: The Cognitive Restructuring Program, by K. T. Mueser and J. D. Gottlieb

HIGH SENSITIVITY TO STRESS

Clients with psychotic symptoms are often highly sensitive to the effects of stress, which can create challenges when dealing with trauma-related thoughts and feelings, both in session and out of session. Individuals' reactions to stress vary from one client to the next, with common responses including intense feelings of anxiety, cognitive disorganization, and increases in psychotic symptoms (e.g., worsening of auditory hallucinations).

The therapist should be aware of the client's signs of stress, be attentive to when they occur in sessions, and take immediate steps to contain and reduce them as needed. Therapists should not end a treatment session early (and reschedule a new one) when a client experiences significant distress, as this can inadvertently reinforce avoidance of trauma-related memories and increase the fear associated with them, which can increase the client's anxiety about continue participation in the CR for PTSD program. Actively working with clients to manage and reduce their distress in the moment provides the best opportunity for helping them process their traumatic experiences and changing the underlying beliefs leading to their PTSD.

The most effective tool for dealing with acute distress in the session is to use Breathing Retraining. When significant distress is detected, the therapist can pause to lead the client in practicing this skill. If necessary, this can be done multiple times in the same session, such as when the client is working on examining a challenging negative belief related to a traumatic event. With clients who are prone to experiencing severe distress in sessions, the therapist may find it helpful to begin and/or end each session by practicing Breathing Retraining together.

Clients may report experiencing similar effects of stress related to the completion of home assignments, especially those involving the practice of CR. Several strategies can be used to address this problem. First, home assignments should always be collaboratively created so they are not overly demanding and only gradually become more challenging. For example, early on, a plan might be made for the person to practice the 5 Steps 1 or 2 days per week rather than every day. Second, clients should be reminded not to work on trauma-related thoughts and beliefs early during the program but rather to stick with more minor everyday negative feelings until their skills have developed further. Third, a plan can be made for the client to practice Breathing Retraining before doing any CR home assignments.

PERSISTENT HALLUCINATIONS

One of the hallmark symptoms of psychosis is hallucinations. Clients with a schizophrenia spectrum diagnosis are more prone to having persistent hallucinations, even when receiving and adhering to optimal pharmacological treatment. While the broad range of hallucinations can include auditory, visual, tactile, olfactory, and gustatory hallucinations, auditory hallucinations are most common, occurring in about 70% of clients (Mueser et al., 1990). Auditory hallucinations most frequently involve hearing one or more voices either talking directly to the person or talking about the person. Although a small percentage of individuals have auditory hallucinations that are positive in nature, for most people the voices are negative, saying antagonistic and highly critical things to them or about them and sometimes telling them what to do (i.e., command hallucinations). People with auditory hallucinations usually find them very distracting and intrusive, and they are a frequent source of distress, especially when the person perceives the voices as having some power or control over them (Chadwick & Birchwood, 1994).

The content of auditory hallucinations is often influenced by adverse life events they have experienced, including traumatic ones (Bentall et al., 2012; Kingdon & Turkington, 2004), further contributing to the high levels of distress they can cause. For individuals with PTSD, auditory hallucinations can also be a type of reexperiencing symptom (e.g., a combat veteran who hears the voices of fallen comrades calling to them, a young adult who hears the voice of a high school bully). The hallucinations can also occur in the form of a running commentary about the person, their traumatic experiences, and what those traumatic experiences say about their worth, morality, and responsibility (e.g., a childhood sexual abuse survivor whose voices call them derogatory names and tell them that they wanted and enjoyed the abuse).

In the CR for PTSD program, these voices may become more pronounced and distressing during sessions in which trauma-related thoughts and beliefs become the focus of cognitive restructuring, potentially interfering with important work if not dealt with empathically and effectively by the therapist. There are several options available for addressing distressing hallucinations that clients may experience in and between therapy sessions.

As described in the High Sensitivity to Stress section, it can be useful for the therapist to lead the client in practicing Breathing Retraining when their voices get worse in a session (e.g., growing louder and more vociferous, saying more critical or hurtful things) and to then resume working on the same material after the client feels calmer. This can be done multiple times within a session if needed. Also as previously described, clients with persistent troubling auditory hallucinations may benefit from beginning each session with the therapist leading them in practicing the Breathing Retraining exercise together.

In addition to frequent use of Breathing Retraining in session, when sessions shift to teaching cognitive restructuring, use of the 5 Steps of CR to delve into the content of the distressing voices can help the therapist and the client to identify, examine, and challenge trauma-related beliefs that are reflected in what the voices say about or tell the person. This can be especially effective because the content of auditory hallucinations often reflects what clients think and feel about themselves, but they do not recognize these thoughts as their own (Garety & Hemsley, 1994). For example, Donata experiences frequent intrusions from highly critical voices. In the following example, the therapist works to understand what the voices have recently said to Donata and the upsetting feelings the voices have caused, to make a connection between the voices' antagonistic statements and Donata's own thoughts about herself, and to then examine those distressing thoughts via the 5 Steps of CR:

THERAPIST: You mentioned when you came in a few minutes ago that the voices were really yelling at you as you sat in the waiting room for our appointment earlier. I know that has been an ongoing upsetting problem for you, and so I thought it might be helpful for us to work on this together using the 5 Steps of CR.

DONATA: Um, OK. But how would we do that, though?

THERAPIST: Well, as you've learned, the 5 Steps of CR can be helpful for any kind of distress you are having at all. So we can take a closer look at your experience with the voices earlier today and see how that is affecting you. Then we can go through the 5 Steps skill to help figure out if there is another way to look at or deal with the situation. How does that sound to you?

DONATA: Now I get it. That's probably a good idea.

THERAPIST: OK, let's start with Step 1. How would you describe this upsetting situation, Donata?

DONATA: Sitting in the waiting area and the voices hissing at me: "You are disgusting, and everyone hates you, and you should just leave because no one wants to help you here."

THERAPIST: That does sound very upsetting. I understand. Good job describing that so well, Donata. I've written that down. And then we go to Step 2. What do we do here?

DONATA: We say how it made us feel—scared, angry, ashamed. All of that. Still feeling it. They don't stop.

THERAPIST: Excellent job with being clear on how this situation has made you feel. Let's go to Step 3. What are your thoughts about the situation when the voices yell those mean things at you?

DONATA: That they are right—that I am disgusting and that everyone does hate me and no one wants to help me here. I did almost leave.

THERAPIST: I'm so sorry, Donata. I know you've put up with this a lot. I am very glad you didn't leave, though, so that we can work on this right now together! So it sounds like your thought is this: "The voices are right. I am disgusting, and everyone hates me, and no one wants to help me here." Do I have that correct?

DONATA: Yeah, you do. I can't get it out of my mind.

THERAPIST: That's completely understandable given how you've described how persistent the voices can be. And it makes sense that you would feel all those emotions from Step 2—scared, angry, and ashamed—if you are allowing yourself to believe what your voices are telling you, right? Let's take a closer look at this thought of yours, though, to see if it is totally accurate—if the voices are right or not.

DONATA: OK, I'll try.

THERAPIST: Do you think that your thought that "The voices are right. I am disgusting, and everyone hates me, and no one wants to help me here" might be a Common Style of Thinking? And if so, which one? Let's take a look.

The 5 Steps can also be used to address thoughts that the client has about their experience with their hallucinations, even when they are not necessarily trauma-related. For instance, many clients have beliefs—such as "My voices control me and everything around me" or "I can't have a life if the voices are always around and criticizing me"—the accuracy of which can be examined via this skill. This strategy of evaluating beliefs about voices with CR is frequently used in broader cognitive behavioral therapy for psychosis interventions (Beck et al., 2009; Chadwick et al., 1996; Fowler et al., 1995; Kingdon & Turkington, 2004; Morrison et al., 2004) and can be an effective way to help clients find some relief from hallucination-related distress, especially early in this intervention when the focus is on learning CR and applying it to everyday distress before moving into more trauma-focused work.

While the 5 Steps of CR can be helpful in identifying and changing trauma-related beliefs that are reflected in or underlie distressing voices, Action Plans can also play an important role in dealing with these hallucinations. Clients with persistent hallucinations may experience these distressing symptoms at any time in their daily lives, so it can be useful to help them develop Action Plans for coping more effectively with these voices when they occur outside of sessions. In addition to using Breathing Retraining as a relaxation skill that can calm the person and reduce the severity of hallucinations, there are a broad range of other strategies for coping with distressing voices—such as distracting oneself by engaging in another task, listening to music or watching a video, engaging in positive self-talk, mindfully "just noticing" the voices without giving them undue attention, exercising, taking a walk, or engaging in a conversation with someone (Fowler et al., 1995; Gingerich & Mueser, 2011; Kingdon & Turkington, 1994; Morrison et al., 2008). In the context of developing Action Plans, the therapist can explore different coping strategies with the client for dealing with the problematic voices, help them select and practice specific strategies (preferably some of which are new to the client), and then plan with the client to try the strategies on their own between sessions. See Exhibit 12.1 for Donata's Action Plan for how to cope better when the voices are yelling at her and saying critical things.

EXHIBIT 12.1

Donata's Action Plan for Coping With Distressing Voices

Instructions: Follow the steps below to develop a helpful Action Plan.

1. Define the goal. What situation requires action?

   Think about what change you would like to see in this situation. Be as specific as possible.

   "To handle it better when the voices are yelling at me, distracting me, telling me what to do, and saying critical things."

2. Brainstorm possible strategies. What can you do to change the situation?

   Use your creative problem-solving skills to think of all the possible things you could do to reduce your distress or address the problem in this situation. When you have made a list of different strategies, think carefully about each one, and place a star (*) next to the best one or ones.

   Try to outshout them. That worked one time before, but I was embarrassed about doing it.

   Just give in and do what they say to do so they will maybe shut up.

   Sit down somewhere, close my eyes, and do 15 breaths of Breathing Retraining. **

   Remind myself that when we did the CR, I figured out that the voices aren't always right about me. The bad things they say about me aren't true. **

   Say alphabet backwards in my head to try to focus my brain and thoughts on something else. **

   Put on my headphones and listen to jazz. **

3. Plan on how to put into practice the strategy (or strategies) you chose.

   What steps can you take to make this happen?

   Consider these questions:

   What information do you need to have?

   Do you need to get some help?

   Who can support you in taking this action?

   What obstacles or challenges could interfere with the plan?

   How could you prevent or deal with these obstacles or challenges?

Write down the plan below. Be specific about the actions you will take.

Keep practicing BRT in session and on my own so I keep getting better at it and it comes really naturally when I get upset from the voices. Write down my new thoughts from CR about the voices, and keep one in my purse. Keep my headphones in my purse at all times so I know where they are and I have them with me when I am out of the voices start up. Tell my case manager, Vern, about this plan so he can remind me.

4. Set a time or a situation to follow up your plan.

   When and how are you going to take this action?

Ask yourself: When do you want to begin your plan? Is there a specific situation or type of situation where you want to use your plan? When is that situation likely to come up again next?

I will call Vern, my case manager, after today's CR for PTSD session to tell him about the plan. I will find my headphones in my room tonight and put them in my purse. Then I will be ready to try out the plan the next time the voices bother me, which will probably be this week.

Note. BRT = Breathing Retraining; CR = cognitive restructuring; PTSD = posttraumatic stress disorder.

Action Plans can also be used to solidify gains made in the 5 Steps of CR when thoughts or beliefs related to the distressing voices have been successfully challenged and replaced in session with new and more accurate thoughts or beliefs. These new, more accurate, and more believable thoughts often directly contradict what the voices are saying or implying about the person, and they require time and practice to replace the old ways of thinking. Sometimes, the voices can temporarily get worse or more vociferous as the person tries to resist or correct them. Developing an Action Plan to help the client remember the new and more accurate thought when they hear their voices can increase the chances that this thought will bring some relief in the moment to the person and that in the long run it will replace the inaccurate thought echoed by the voices. Action Plans aimed at helping clients recall more accurate thoughts when they are having distressing hallucinations out of session can employ a variety of different options. These include practicing in role plays with the therapist to remind the client of the new thought, rehearsing how to remember the new thought out of the session when not hearing voices, posting the new thought in prominent places (e.g., on a refrigerator or cell phone), using a relaxation exercise to calm down when hearing the voices before reminding oneself of the new thought, and involving a significant other to remind the person of the new thought and situations where they may need help remembering it.

DELUSIONAL ELABORATION OF TRAUMATIC EVENTS

Similar to how adverse and traumatic life events are often reflected in the content of auditory hallucinations people experience, they can also influence the formation and elaboration of acute paranoid and/or delusional beliefs (Bentall et al., 2012; Kingdon & Turkington, 2004). People with PTSD and a psychotic disorder have sometimes experienced traumatic events that they can accurately and plausibly describe but that also form the basis for a delusional elaboration that goes far beyond the event itself.

For example, as a child and adolescent, Donata experienced severe childhood physical and sexual abuse and neglect, and following the onset of her initial psychotic episode, her understanding and description of these traumatic experiences became tangled with some distressing delusional details. She developed an ongoing set of beliefs and associated memories that she was forced to engage in dangerous illegal drug-related cartel-like activities as a teenager, including "being forced to scuba dive underneath transport boats to hide bags of cocaine." In fact, Donata's description of her most distressing traumatic event on her screening PTSD Checklist–5 (PCL-5; "index trauma") was this: "My parents and their friends beating me up when I was growing up and making me run drugs for them by forcing me to fly a helicopter on a cocaine drop." In all cases, we recommend allowing the description and wording of the index trauma to come from the clients themselves. This same guideline holds true when working with someone with psychosis who describes their verified traumatic events (in Donata's case, childhood physical and sexual abuse) within a framework of delusional elaboration.

Not all paranoid or delusional beliefs can be readily traced to traumatic events, and thus it is important for the clinician to try to distinguish between trauma-related delusions and delusions unrelated to trauma. The importance of the distinction is that the clinician needs to develop an understanding of the nature of the symptoms and thoughts behind trauma-related delusions to identify broader trauma-focused beliefs that can eventually become the focus of cognitive restructuring. In Donata's case, it was clear that her delusional beliefs were very tied to her traumatic experiences, and the key to helping her with her debilitating PTSD (and associated distress from psychotic symptoms) was to guide her toward identifying nonpsychotic core and trauma-related beliefs at the root of the delusional elaborations in order to begin to work with them via CR. Addressing these sorts of beliefs via the 5 Steps, in turn, can have ameliorative ripple effects by reducing many or all of the cognitive distortions and associated delusional details based on these underlying beliefs.

Working with clients with trauma-related delusional beliefs can present several unique challenges to the therapist. The delusional elaboration of the traumatic events or the client's current delusional beliefs may be more immediately distressing to the client than memories of the traumatic events themselves. Thus, the client may be drawn more to these particular beliefs and want to focus the discussion or much of the session on the details of these concerns.

Clients with delusions have also usually encountered numerous people who have been skeptical about their assertions or have outright called them false or delusional (e.g., family members, friends, mental health professionals), and therefore, they are often eager for validation of their beliefs, especially from a clinician. The therapist needs to work collaboratively with the client about their delusional beliefs to grasp their essential concerns and their relationship to the trauma, while avoiding colluding with the client and reinforcing their conviction in the delusional belief itself.

When working with clients with delusional elaboration about traumatic events, it is important to focus primarily on the distress the client experiences (related to their beliefs), via empathy and validation, without attempting to determine the veracity of their belief or nor attempting to help the client see what is and is not true about the delusional belief. To avoid colluding while still maintaining a strong therapeutic alliance and working relationship with the client, the therapist must strike a delicate balance between being sure to not overtly state their opinion about the truth or falsity of the belief itself. Instead, it is preferable to seek a common ground with the client, such as by focusing primarily on using the 5 Steps of CR to address the distress the client experiences or (if necessary) by "agreeing to disagree" about the likelihood that certain events happened without dwelling on them.

When using cognitive restructuring to address distress related to a delusional belief, the therapist's primary goal is to identify the core (nondelusional) thought underlying it and then use the 5 Steps of CR to explore that trauma-related belief.

This process typically necessitates gentle redirection by the therapist and skilled Socratic questioning to help steer the client away from rumination about the delusional details and toward the true heart of the distress—the trauma-related belief. This process is illustrated next, where the therapist uses the structure of the 5 Steps collaboratively with Donata to understand important aspects of her delusional beliefs as they pertain to deeper, nonpsychotic, highly distressing trauma-related thoughts:

THERAPIST: I'm so glad you just brought up what was so upsetting to you last night. This is exactly the kind of thing we want to talk through in here. We've identified the upsetting situation in Step 1—"Thinking about and getting upset how when I was growing up, my parents making me do that thing." And in Step 2, you had said a few minutes ago that remembering that situation has made you feel three emotions—"anxiety," "sadness," and "shame."

DONATA: Yeah, always. It's horrible what I did. Flying that helicopter and more than once! So they could do their drug drops. They knew I'd do it. I couldn't say no. And then the boat diving. I barely knew how to swim, but I had to scuba dive. No one has believed it.

THERAPIST: Donata, I appreciate you reminding me of some of these details again, and I want to reiterate that I strongly believe that your past experiences have certainly been beyond what any person should have to go through. I have so much empathy for you and your courage to get to where you are today. And these upsetting beliefs have very understandably continued to be on your mind after all of this time. I can tell how upset these memories of yours are making you. And it makes perfect sense for you to have these kinds of emotional reactions, given that you have experienced your past this way. Let's try to get to some more specific thoughts that are upsetting so we can work through this together. In Step 3 here, we want to figure out what some of your distressing thoughts are that are causing the anxiety, sadness, and shame. What is going through your mind as you think about this situation?

DONATA: I had to do all these different crazy things, like the helicopters and the boats, just so my parents could have their friends and their life. Also, put down that my older brother didn't have to do them. Only I did.

THERAPIST: OK, yes. Let's write those two thoughts down here under Step 3. Let me ask you this. Donata, what does it say about you that

	you believe you were in the position to have to do these dangerous and extraordinary things on behalf of your parents and that your brother didn't?

DONATA: That there was or is something wrong with me. That I was a burden to them.

THERAPIST: I see. Let's put that down as well. And if it was true that there was or is something wrong with you, that you were a burden to your parents, why would that be the case?

DONATA: Because ... because something I've always thought deep down is that it was all my fault that my family did all these terrible things—the drugs, hurting me, keeping those friends around, all of it.

THERAPIST: And when you think that thought—"It was all my fault that my family did all these terrible things"—how do you feel?

DONATA (TEARFUL): Ashamed.

THERAPIST: I know this is very hard, but I'm so glad you are sharing this with me. You are doing a great job, Donata. Let's go forward from here together with the skill now that we've identified your most distressing thought: "It's all my fault that my family did all these terrible things." How does that sound to you?

Once Donata and the therapist are able to delve beneath the delusional details to get at the heart of the trauma-related belief, the therapist can guide her through the remaining steps of the skill—Step 3(b), identifying the Common Style of Thinking (CST; Donata chose self-blame), and into Step 4, providing evidence that supports the belief followed by evidence that does not support the belief (a snippet of which is illustrated next). Note the therapist's style of focusing on the facts related to Donata's childhood and on the distress caused by the delusional elaboration—while not getting into a discussion about the truth of the delusional details themselves:

THERAPIST: OK, you've done a really nice job so far with Step 4. Let's talk a little more about some other things that don't support your thought that it was all your fault that your parents did all these terrible things. You've mentioned to me in earlier sessions that you think your parents likely had some mental illness symptoms themselves and had their own drug addictions that they weren't willing to get treatment for. What kind of role do you think that might have played in their parenting and your childhood experiences?

DONATA: Yeah, they couldn't be normal parents. They were high all the time. I thought it back then, but I realize now. They couldn't be loving. Or even make sure I had nutritious food or a clean place to sleep a lot of the time. They let their so-called friends have their way with me. And used me to do their dirty work, like with the boats and planes.

THERAPIST: These are all very good observations. So actually, it was their behavior that resulted in the terrible things they did rather than yours. Is that right?

DONATA: Yes, I guess so.

THERAPIST: Should we put that down in the worksheet here?

DONATA: OK, that's right.

THERAPIST: So you've identified those pieces of evidence—those specific things that your parents did and did not do. Now we can ask a question: How much did their ability to look after your safety and mental and physical health line up with the way a parent should look out for their child's safety and well-being? What do you think?

DONATA: It doesn't line up at all, I guess. I've heard from other people I've known in my life that their parents didn't do the kinds of things that mine did.

THERAPIST: Sounds like that's another piece of evidence we should note here on the worksheet?

DONATA: Yeah, for sure.

Once the client is able to make a decision about the accuracy of their thought (based on the evidence developed in Step 4) in situations where they decide that the evidence does not in fact support their initial belief, the therapist can help them create a new, more accurate belief reflecting a truer perspective on their traumatic experience. The shift in the client's perception of the core, trauma-related belief should be reflected in the new thought. As such, the delusional detail is likely viewed as unnecessary to include in the new thought.

For instance, Donata was able to move from one thought ("I had to do all these different crazy things, like the helicopters and the boats, just so my parents could have their friends and their life") to a nonpsychotic and more core, trauma-related (and therefore workable) thought ("It was all my fault that my family did all these terrible things") and then, at the conclusion of the 5 Steps, to a more accurate and substantially less shame-inducing and distressing thought that was supported by the Step 4 evidence ("I was put in a position that no child should be put in. That was not my fault"). Figure 12.1 provides the full details of Donata's 5 Steps, delineated in her worksheet.

FIGURE 12.1. Example of a 5 Steps of CR Worksheet Completed by Donata Addressing Trauma-Related Belief (via Examination of Delusional Belief)

1. Situation

Ask yourself, "What happened that made me upset?" Write down a brief description of the situation, including just the facts.

Situation: Thinking about and getting upset how when I was growing up my parents making me do that thing.

2. Feeling

Circle your strongest feeling. If you have more than one, that's OK (If none of these fit, you can write one in.):

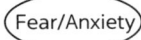 Fear/Anxiety   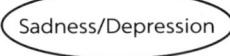 Sadness/Depression   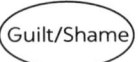 Guilt/Shame   Anger

3. Thought

Ask yourself, "What am I thinking that is leading me to feel this way?" Use your Guide to Thoughts and Feelings Information Sheet to identify thoughts related to the feeling circled above. You may have more than one thought related to the feeling(s). Write down your thoughts below, but then choose ONE thought to work on. Choose the thought that is most distressing to you right now, and circle that thought.

Thoughts: I had to do all these different crazy things, like the helicopters and the boats, just so my parents could have their friends and their life.

My older brother didn't have to do these things, only I did.

There was or is something wrong with me.

I was a burden to them.

(It was all my fault that my family did all of these terrible things)

Is this thought a Common Style of Thinking? If yes, circle the style:

All-or-nothing	Mind reading	Overgeneralization
Must/should/never	Catastrophizing	Emotional reasoning
Overestimation of risk	(Self-Blame)	Mental filter

Write the thought you chose from Step 3 here:

Upsetting thought: It was all my fault that my family did all of these terrible things.

4. Evaluate your thought.

Now ask yourself: "What evidence do I have for and against this thought?" First, write down all the evidence that DOES support your thought. Then, write down all the evidence that DOES NOT support your thought. You can use your Tips for Finding Good Evidence Information Sheet to help come up with evidence that DOES NOT support your thought.

Things that DO support my thought

My parents were always yelling at me and telling me I was dumb and in the way.

They didn't act that way as much to my brother.

The kids at school knew that my family was messed up, and they would bully me and say that I was a freak and made my parents crazy.

(continues)

FIGURE 12.1. Example of a 5 Steps of CR Worksheet Completed by Donata Addressing Trauma-Related Belief (via Examination of Delusional Belief) *(Continued)*

Other parents didn't do these horrible things, and maybe that's because their kids were smarter or easier to be with—it's hard to know that for sure, but I really think so.

Things that DO NOT support my thought

My parents were addicted to drugs, and so were their friends.

They also had some mental illness. I think I can see that now.

They never got any treatment or tried to get better from the drugs or mental illness.

Because of the drugs and mental illness, they weren't able to be normal parents and do normal parent things—be loving to me, make sure I was clean and fed, keep me safe from their dangerous friends.

Because they were sick and addicts, they used me for their dirty work, like with the boats and planes.

It was their own behavior and actions that caused the terrible things they did to me and their own lives, it was not my behavior as a kid.

Most parents don't do the kinds of awful things my parents did—but that's not because their kids are better or worse than I was—it's because parents should look out for their child's safety no matter what.

5. Take action!

Next, ask yourself, "Do things mostly support my thought, or do things mostly NOT support my thought?"

☐ NO, the evidence does not support my thought.

If the evidence does NOT support your thought, come up with a new thought that is supported by the evidence. These thoughts are usually more balanced and helpful. Write your new thought in the space below. Remember, when you think of this upsetting situation in the future or when a similar situation happens, replace your unhelpful automatic thought with this new and more accurate thought.

My new thought

I was put in a position that no child should be put in: that was not my fault.

☐ YES, the evidence does support my thought.

If the evidence DOES support your thought, decide what you need to do next in order to deal with the situation. Ask yourself, "Do I need to get more information about what to do?" "Do I need to get some help?" "Do I need to take steps to make sure I am safe?" Complete the Action Plan Worksheet to help you answer these questions and create a solid plan to deal with the situation.

Note. In some cases, you may decide that the evidence does not support your upsetting thought and change it to a more accurate and helpful one. If so, you may also find it helpful to make an Action Plan to deal with that situation. Thus, in some situations, you may find that doing both things—coming up with a new and more accurate thought AND ALSO creating an Action Plan—can be very helpful.

NEGATIVE SYMPTOMS IN SCHIZOPHRENIA SPECTRUM DISORDERS

Although psychotic symptoms are required for the diagnosis of schizophrenia, negative symptoms play a prominent role in the disorder. *Negative symptoms* refer to reduced or absent behavioral, mood, motivational, and cognitive processes that are ordinarily present in people but are diminished or absent in people with schizophrenia. These negative symptoms of schizophrenia can be categorized into two types, including expressive deficits and experiential deficits (Kring et al., 2013). *Expressive deficits* refer to reduced behavioral displays of emotions in facial expressions (e.g., blunted affect), vocal characteristics (e.g., monotonous voice tone), and use of gestures and bodily movement (e.g., paucity of gestures). *Experiential deficits* refer to reduced feelings and motivation, such as decreased feelings of pleasure (anhedonia); reduced motivation and effort for social relationships, work or school, or self-care; difficulty initiating and following through on plans (avolition); and general lack of engagement in the world around the person (apathy). Although both expressive and experiential deficits are types of negative symptoms, they are not strongly correlated with each other, and thus a client may have one type of these symptoms without having the other.

Expressive Deficit Symptoms

Negative symptoms such as blunted affect and monotonous voice tone require a few key adaptations when providing the CR for PTSD program. The most important starting point when working with a client with prominent expressive deficits is for the therapist to avoid assuming that they know how the client is feeling during a session based on their nonverbal behavior. For example, clients may be talking about a traumatic event and not appear visibly upset or distressed, but this does not mean that they do not feel distressed. People with blunted affect experience the same depth and range of emotions as people without blunted affect, but they do not communicate their feelings as clearly as others do in their facial expressions and voice tone (Berenbaum & Oltmanns, 1992; Blanchard et al., 1994), which can lead to the inaccurate impression they are experiencing few or no emotions when, in fact, they are. For example, the clinician may mistake the client's lack of emotional expressiveness to mean that they are not fully engaged with the material, are emotionally numb, or are dissociating when in fact they are feeling full and potentially very intense feelings in that moment. Therefore, when working with clients with diminished expressiveness, it is critical to frequently check in verbally with them to find out how they are feeling and to avoid assuming their lack of expressiveness reflects a lack of emotion or engagement.

Just as the therapist may mistake a client's blunted affect as conveying lack of engagement or disinterest, significant others in the client's life may make the same mistake (e.g., someone appears bored when listening to their loved one talk about their day). This can contribute to misunderstandings and conflict in close relationships. Since many clients with blunted affect are not aware of their reduced expressiveness (Mueser, Valentiner, & Agresta 1997), they can benefit from some brief psychoeducation about this symptom and encouragement and practice in using verbal feeling statements when interacting with others. This is especially useful when the client's goals established in Session 4 involve improving interpersonal relationships or reducing social isolation or loneliness.

Experiential Deficit Symptoms

These types of negative symptoms can create additional challenges for clients and therapists in the CR for PTSD program. Motivation to participate in sessions may wax and wane over time, leading to inconsistent attendance and lack of follow-through on home assignments. Clients may struggle with uncertainty as to whether the effort to participate in the program is worth it.

There are several effective strategies that are helpful for addressing these challenges. First, the therapist should always be on the alert for any efforts of the client to follow through on the use of the skills and any gains made either in the therapy session or outside of session and provide abundant reinforcement as indicated. This can be extended to reinforcing regular participation in treatment sessions, such as good attendance and active engagement with the material. Clients with motivational deficits are extremely sensitive to the effort required to make changes or achieve something, and therefore being attentive to and reinforcing any efforts can stimulate further effort.

Second, the therapist should be on the lookout for opportunities to use CR to address thoughts and beliefs that may underlie some of the client's deficits in motivation. There is strong evidence that people with experiential deficits engage in a broad range of negative and self-defeating thinking styles that may serve to maintain their low level of motivation (Granholm et al., 2009; Grant & Beck, 2009; Rector et al., 2005). Furthermore, cognitive restructuring has been shown to be effective at changing the thoughts and beliefs underlying negative symptoms in schizophrenia and thereby reducing the severity of those symptoms (Granholm et al., 2014, 2018; Grant et al., 2012). Thus, directly targeting defeatist attitudes with cognitive restructuring in the program may reduce their impact and enhance motivation and investment in change. Common examples of self-defeating thoughts related to negative symptoms and pertinent to engagement in the CR for PTSD program are listed next. Of note, these sorts of beliefs are relevant to explore even in clients who do not have negative symptoms, as clients with depressive symptoms or feelings of hopelessness often have similar types of thoughts that benefit from CR work:

- "I don't have enough energy or stamina to get through this program."
- "It's too hard to try to complete all the work and practice required in this treatment."
- "I've tried other things for my symptoms in the past, and they never help, so what's the point?"
- "I don't even know how to explain what my upsetting thoughts and feelings are, so why bother trying?"

A third strategy for maintaining and enhancing motivation to continue to participate in the CR for PTSD program is for the therapist to periodically stop and review changes and accomplishments the client has made thus far in the program. Clients are sometimes so preoccupied with the current challenges in their lives that they lose sight of genuine and important gains they have made during therapy. Drawing attention to these small but meaningful steps forward can instill hope for further change in the future.

DIFFICULTIES LEARNING CR FOR PTSD SKILLS

As mentioned in Chapter 10 in this volume, given the complex interplay among cognitive functioning (i.e., attention, memory, planning, abstract reasoning) and PTSD and despite the systematic approach to teaching skills in the CR for PTSD program, it is not uncommon for some clients to have difficulty learning and retaining the CR techniques. For those with psychosis or schizophrenia spectrum disorders (and even those without), these challenges may be in part related to general acquisition difficulties or as a result of cognitive impairment.

Cognitive Impairment in Psychotic Disorders

Reduced cognitive abilities in areas such as attention and concentration, memory psychomotor speed, and executive functions (e.g., abstract thinking, planning, problem solving) are a cardinal feature of schizophrenia (Kahn & Keefe, 2013; Kaulkstein et al., 2010). Decreases in cognitive functioning typically begin prior to the onset of psychotic symptoms (Mollon et al., 2018) and are stable over the course of the illness (Sheffield et al., 2018). Cognitive abilities may be further compromised by the cognitive effects of PTSD in areas such as attention and memory (Johnsen & Asbjørnsen, 2008). Although a reduction in cognitive abilities occurs in most people who develop schizophrenia, this does not mean that all people with the disorder have cognitive impairment, as some individuals have above-average intellectual functioning or even superior intelligence (e.g., the mathematician John Nash) before (and after) developing the illness.

There are several implications for treating clients with impaired cognitive functioning (or other learning difficulties) in the CR for PTSD program. Cognitive challenges can result in slower learning of information and skills, less generalization of skills taught in therapy sessions to daily life, and greater difficulty learning more complex skills. Fortunately, when the therapist is aware of specific impairments the client has, adaptations can be made in the teaching methods to compensate for their effects. Research on the CR program shows that clients with more impaired cognitive functioning improve as much in PTSD and other outcomes as those with intact cognitive abilities (Mueser et al., 2018).

GENERAL STRATEGIES FOR FACILITATING SKILL ACQUISITION

Individuals with general learning difficulties or cognitive impairment require more practice to acquire the information and skills taught in the CR for PTSD program. The most important strategies for teaching skills to these clients include providing new information in small amounts (or "chunks"), breaking skills down into small steps, frequent practice and repetition, and abundant reinforcement for all efforts.

When working with clients who have these learning difficulties, the therapist needs to give greatest priority to teaching the two skills most critical to reducing PTSD symptoms: Breathing Retraining and Cognitive Restructuring. Since more time may be needed to teach these skills and information overload should be avoided, the therapist can consider simplifying the content of psychoeducation in the earlier sessions. As emphasized in Chapter 6 in this volume, it is important for the therapist to not delay beginning teaching cognitive restructuring beyond Session 4. To accomplish this, the therapist may need to focus on only the most important information and concepts about trauma and PTSD in the handouts, such as the specific symptoms the client has and the fact that PTSD is a treatable disorder.

The other parts of the intervention that involve providing information to the client—program orientation and Breathing Retraining—should also be kept as simple as possible. New information should be delivered in small "chunks" to avoiding overwhelming the client, frequent pauses should be taken to review what has been discussed, and regular breaks should be taken to ask the client to describe their understanding of the material ("to make sure we are on the same page"). The introduction and rationale for Breathing Retraining should be provided as briefly as possible to reserve the most time for directly teaching and practicing the skill. The therapist may need to model Breathing Retraining several times in Session 1, and each time the client should practice the skill before they master it. Repeated in-session practice may be necessary to consolidate learning and uptake. In these cases, it can be beneficial to encourage the client to use the abbreviation "BRT" in place of Breathing Retraining for ease of communication.

In general, home assignments should be as easy and specific as possible early in the program to maximize follow-through. A new home assignment should be demonstrated by the therapist and practiced by the client at the end of the session to ensure that the client understands how to do it. After an assignment has been agreed upon, asking the client to summarize it is a useful check. Making plans with the client to arrange for reminders to do their home assignment can also facilitate follow-through (e.g., posting a sign on the refrigerator, putting a worksheet by the bedside table, setting a phone alarm). Significant others and other mental health professionals who work with the client can be important environmental supports for facilitating follow-through on home assignments as well. These and other strategies enhancing follow through on home assignments are further described in Chapter 11 in this volume.

Similar to teaching Breathing Retraining, the introduction and rationale for cognitive restructuring (Thought–Feeling model, CBT Triangle, Common Styles of Thinking) should be kept to a minimum to reserve time for in-session practice. When providing examples of these concepts, the therapist should stick to the simplest possible example (e.g., is a scratching sound outside of one's window at night a burglar or the cat?) and move on once the client has understood the point. If the client clearly understands just one or two of the Common Styles, and can recognize examples of them in their life, the therapist should focus on those specific styles and not try to teach the other ones.

As is the case with most clients participating in this program, learning the 5 Steps of CR is most effective when therapists and clients are actively working through specific examples with the worksheet and spending a minimum of time abstractly talking about the skill. This is especially true for clients with cognitive impairment. Following a brief general reminder (as needed) of how the 5 Steps works and before beginning each step, the name of the step should be clearly stated or elicited (e.g., "The third step is identifying the thoughts that led to the distressing feeling"). The therapist should avoid spending too much time on any one step to get through all the steps and help the client understand the skill as a single, cohesive exercise. In addition, the therapist should frequently pause to review what was accomplished in the previous steps or elicit the review from the client (e.g., when beginning Step 3, briefly review what was done in Steps 1 and 2, and when beginning Step 4, briefly review Steps 1–3).

Specific Strategies for Teaching Cognitive Restructuring

Although the 5 Steps of CR was designed to be as simple and straightforward as possible, for some clients it may not be critical that they master this specific cognitive restructuring skill. If, despite using the aforementioned strategies to teach the 5 Steps, the client continues to have difficulty learning the skill, an alternative cognitive restructuring skill can be taught, such as one of the strategies described in the next sections (and summarized in Exhibit 12.2).

EXHIBIT 12.2

Alternative Cognitive Restructuring Skills to the 5 Steps of CR for Persons With Learning Difficulties

Recognizing the Common Styles of Thinking

- "What thought is upsetting me?"
- "Is this thought a Common Style of Thinking?"
- "What would be a more accurate or helpful way of looking at the situation?"

The 3Cs: Catch it, Check it, Change it (Granholm et al., 2016)

- Catch it: "What am I thinking that is upsetting me?"
- Check it: "Is this thought accurate? Does the evidence support my thought?"
- Change it: "What new thought would be more accurate or helpful?"

Brainstorming multiple perspectives/alternative explanations for upsetting situations

- "What am I thinking that is upsetting me?"
- "What is another way I could think of this situation?" (Generate at least two or three alternative thoughts.)
- "Which way of thinking about this situation is most helpful to me?"

Mindful distancing of upsetting thoughts

- "What am I thinking that is upsetting me?"
- "There goes my stinking thinking!"

Focus on Recognizing and Examining Thoughts That Underlie Negative Feelings

In all cases, it is crucial to establish with the client that the single most critical step in cognitive restructuring is to recognize that when they are upset about something, there is a thought underlying that emotion and that the thought may not be entirely accurate. Two particular alternative CR methods are similar in that they focus on the important steps of identifying thoughts that underlie upsetting feelings and examining those thoughts. First, clients who are able to notice when they are engaging in a CST but are not able to master the full 5 Steps of CR may benefit from just sticking with the CST skill as their main approach to cognitive restructuring. Second, some clients may find the CST too abstract and benefit from learning the even simpler three-step skill of identifying and changing negative thoughts: "Catch it, Check it, Change it" (or the "3Cs"; Granholm et al., 2016).

Focus on Generating Alternative Thoughts or Explanations

For some people, the ability to think of several different perspectives or interpretations of a situation in which they are feeling upset can be more crucial to alleviating distress than trying to determine the absolute correctness or accuracy of any one interpretation (reflected in the "Brainstorming multiple perspectives/ alternative explanations for upsetting situations" strategy in Exhibit 12.2). Because negative emotions are often the result of being stuck viewing a situation from a single perspective, enhancing cognitive flexibility by teaching people how to generate multiple different perspectives on an upsetting situation can in and of itself reduce distress (Suarez et al., 1987). Some clients benefit from just the process of generating alternative interpretations for an upsetting situation, while others benefit more from also choosing which perspective is most helpful to them.

"Distancing" (or Mindfulness) Strategies

While the strategy for generating alternative thoughts or explanations described above generally weakens the individual's conviction in an upsetting thought (and associated distress) by helping them realize that other thoughts (and interpretations) are possible in a particular situation, distancing (or mindfulness) approaches focus instead on lessening the importance the person attaches to the upsetting thought (and hence its negative psychological impact). This can be accomplished by first explaining to the client that they cannot control all of the thoughts in their head (while they can control their behaviors and achieve their goals) and that not all thoughts are accurate, useful, or helpful. This then sets the stage for the client learning how to recognize (or "just notice") upsetting thoughts, while not "buying into" such thoughts or giving them undue excess attention (Hayes et al., 2012).

This approach is especially helpful with clients who find it difficult or impossible to completely replace old, inaccurate, and upsetting thinking styles that have been reinforced over many years with new, more accurate, and less distressing thoughts. Instead of repeatedly disputing the familiar and upsetting thoughts, the client learns how to acknowledge thoughts while at the same time recognizing that the thoughts reflect the client's old thinking style and are not necessarily true. For example, one client learned to respond minimally to his upsetting thoughts by jokingly saying, "Thank you, brain, for that wonderful insight!" This method is frequently used in acceptance and commitment therapy (Hayes et al., 2012) and other mindfulness-based approaches to coping with distress (Linehan, 1993; Segal et al., 2002; Wells, 2009).

CLIENT QUESTIONS ABOUT THEIR PRIMARY PSYCHIATRIC DIAGNOSIS

While the previous sections of this chapter addressed common clinical challenges experienced by clinicians when providing the CR for PTSD program to clients with psychotic symptoms and those with a schizophrenia spectrum disorder, a somewhat different issue sometimes occurs in the CR program when the client raises questions about their primary psychiatric diagnosis. This happens most often during the psychoeducational sessions early in the program as clients are learning about PTSD and associated problems and are trying to relate the information to their own experiences. This issue can also come up earlier, especially soon after clients learn about their PTSD diagnosis, such as during the orientation to the CR program.

Clients are sometimes surprised to learn about their PTSD diagnosis, especially when they received another primary diagnosis may years before (e.g., schizophrenia, bipolar disorder, borderline personality disorder) and are only now being told that they also have PTSD. Understandably, clients often wonder why they were not told about their PTSD diagnosis at an earlier time. Some clients may also question whether their primary diagnosis is accurate or whether the PTSD diagnosis might better explain the symptoms and life challenges they have experienced. While this questioning can occur for people with any serious mental illness (SMI) diagnosis, in our experience it is more common in people with a schizophrenia spectrum disorder (Pratt et al., 2005).

Understanding why clients may question their SMI diagnosis after learning that they have PTSD is key to responding to their concerns. First, clients often personally relate to the broad range of symptoms and major life intrusions associated with PTSD that are described in the educational handouts, such as difficulties with social relationships, problems with work and school, and struggles with anxiety and depression. The PTSD diagnosis may seem to explain more about their life challenges than the primary diagnosis they were previously given and thus be more intuitively appealing. Second, considering that the individual's PTSD may have been only recently diagnosed, they may rightly wonder whether the primary diagnosis could be an error that was made because PTSD was not considered. This is a reasonable question considering that the failure to detect one disorder can certainly lead to the misdiagnosis of a different disorder. (For a broader discussion and guidelines for proper differential diagnosis of PTSD and other SMI symptoms and disorders, see Chapter 3, this volume.)

Third, the PTSD diagnosis may be preferred by clients because it is less stigmatizing than a diagnosis such as schizophrenia. The fact that PTSD is more common and that it is a consequence of (external) traumatic events that are also common may have the effect of "normalizing" the disorder for people. This is in contrast to a psychotic disorder diagnosis, which people may find more alienating and believe sets them apart from others in society.

The most effective approach to addressing these questions is to first explain that it is possible to have both disorders. It can be further explained that since it is known that traumatic events increase the chances of someone developing an SMI, PTSD is also a much more common disorder among individuals with an SMI than in the general population. Some clients may continue to believe that their only diagnosis should be PTSD. Rather than debating about the diagnosis, the therapist can empathically acknowledge the client's concerns and perspective and try to channel their interest and investment in PTSD into diligent work together in the program.

When clients have received a diagnosis of PTSD many years after receiving their primary diagnosis and inquire about the delay in being diagnosed with PTSD, the best way of responding is for the therapist to explain that until recently, the importance of trauma and PTSD in the lives of people with other psychiatric disorders was not sufficiently recognized. This honest response can sometime produce mixed reactions, including feelings of resentment or loss that the client was not diagnosed earlier or was not offered treatment earlier. The therapist should validate and empathize with the client's feelings, while also encouraging them that it is never too late to deal with and overcome the aftermath of their traumatic experiences.

In general, when these types of concerns are raised by clients, they are not a significant obstacle to effectively delivering the CR for PTSD program. The therapist's role in these situations is to validate the client's experience and any associated distress, provide accurate information, and answer their questions as directly and forthrightly as possible. In fact, sometimes these types of candid and sincere discussions can serve to greatly increase the working alliance and therefore the client's engagement in treatment and motivation to overcome their posttraumatic reactions.

CONCLUSION

There are some unique challenges related to working with people with psychosis, including clients' high sensitivity to stress, distressing auditory hallucinations (which can be a direct PTSD reexperiencing symptom and thematically related to the person's traumatic experiences), and delusional elaboration of actual experienced traumatic events. Strategies to address these symptoms in the CR for PTSD program—such as initiating Breathing Retraining to reduce in-session stress, using the 5 Steps of CR to address upsetting voices content (and associated beliefs), and extracting the trauma-related belief underlying delusional content—can provide relief for clients while helping them to cope with and address distressing psychotic and PTSD symptoms.

Two other common clinical features of people with a psychotic disorder (such as schizophrenia)—negative symptoms and cognitive impairment—are important for clinicians to better understand so that they can adopt strategies to assist clients in this program. CR is recommended to address inaccurate beliefs that may underlie reduced motivation associated with negative symptoms (e.g., "It's no use trying"). Effective approaches for working with people with impaired cognitive functioning include teaching simpler alternatives to cognitive restructuring as well as "distancing" (mindfulness) approaches.

Clients with psychosis diagnoses such as schizophrenia (as well as other diagnoses, like bipolar disorder or borderline personality disorder) sometimes raise questions or express doubts about their primary diagnosis after learning that they have PTSD. This is especially common when clients were given their SMI diagnosis many years ago and were only recently diagnosed with PTSD. In these cases, it is important for the therapist to empathize with the client's concerns, provide accurate information, and harness the client's motivation to work on their PTSD symptoms in the CR for PTSD program.

13

Working With People With Borderline Personality Disorder

Borderline personality disorder (BPD) is disorder characterized by unstable interpersonal relationships, difficulties managing emotions, disturbances in self-image, and impulsivity (American Psychiatric Association, 2013). Of particular clinical concern are self-harming behaviors such as cutting or burning oneself and recurrent suicidal threats or behaviors, often resulting in psychiatric hospitalizations. BPD is a common co-occurring disorder in people with major mood disorders (e.g., major depression, bipolar disorder) and occurs somewhat less often in people with schizophrenia or schizoaffective disorder (Mueser, Gottlieb, et al., 2015). As a result of substantial psychosocial dysfunction associated with BPD, it frequently results in long-term disability and is thus included within the broad category of serious mental illness (SMI).

There is a high comorbidity between BPD and other psychiatric disorders such as major depression, substance use disorders, and posttraumatic stress disorder (PTSD; Bolton et al., 2006; Mueser et al., 1998; Zanarini et al., 1998, 2021; Zimmerman & Mattia, 1999). For example, one large epidemiological study in the United States found that 30% of individuals with BPD also had a diagnosis of PTSD (Pagura et al., 2010). People with BPD and PTSD tend to have more severe symptoms, more impaired functioning, and more frequent psychiatric hospitalizations than those with either disorder alone (Bolton et al., 2006; Cackowski et al., 2016; Zlotnick et al., 2003). The high prevalence of PTSD in people with BPD and the associated increased level of impairment in those with both disorders underscore the importance of effectively treating PTSD in these individuals.

https://doi.org/10.1037/0000423-013
Treatment of Posttraumatic Stress Disorder in Serious Mental Illness: The Cognitive Restructuring Program, by K. T. Mueser and J. D. Gottlieb

294 Special Clinical Challenges and Populations

Although there is widespread agreement on the importance of treating PTSD in people with BPD, the question of how treatment should look has generated considerable debate. Much of this debate has been centered around the constellation of symptoms involving affective instability, poor emotion self-regulation skills, self-injury, and suicidal gestures (sometimes referred to as "parasuicidal" behavior) that often contribute to hospitalizations. Some proponents of BPD treatment have suggested that trauma-focused therapy (such as cognitive restructuring or prolonged exposure) may be too stressful for people with BPD (or complex PTSD) and have advocated for a phased treatment approach initially aimed at enhancing emotion regulation and other skills in order to prepare them for later trauma-related work (Bohus et al., 2013; Cloitre et al., 2002; Harned et al., 2014). Others have argued that delaying trauma-related therapy for PTSD in individuals with BPD could deprive them of the most efficacious treatment possible for their symptoms, potentially contributing to worse long-term outcomes (de Jongh et al., 2016).

There is now compelling evidence that PTSD can be effectively and safely treated in people with BPD using trauma-focused therapy, including the Cognitive Restructuring (CR) for PTSD program, without a prolonged stabilization period (Zeifman et al., 2021). Indeed, we included individuals with BPD and PTSD in the two large controlled trials we conducted of the CR program in persons with SMI (Mueser et al., 2008; Mueser, Gottlieb, et al., 2015) and provided the program following the same principles and methods as with the other study participants with SMI and PTSD but not BPD. Approximately 25% of each study sample included participants with BPD ($Ns = 27$ and 55, respectively). The CR program was found to be feasible and well tolerated by the participants with BPD with no adverse events reported. Furthermore, although the participants with BPD had more severe PTSD symptoms at the beginning of the trial than the other participants, they improved at similar rates in PTSD and related outcomes (Kredlow et al., 2017). Thus, the CR program is a viable option for treating PTSD in people with BPD.

In this chapter, we discuss common clinical challenges and recommend solutions for treating people with BPD in the CR for PTSD program.

ENGAGEMENT AND RETENTION IN THERAPY

Individuals with BPD have often had tumultuous relationships with family members, friends, and others during their formative years when growing up, and having intense and unstable interpersonal relationships is one of the defining characteristics of the disorder. Difficulties tolerating distress and poor skills for regulating their own emotions are important factors contributing to these relationship problems. These challenges to good social relationships in BPD can be further worsened when the person also has PTSD, which can lead to being distrustful of others (due to prior victimization) and difficulties being emotionally and physically close to others (due to avoidance of trauma-related stimuli).

As a result of these problems establishing and maintaining interpersonal relationships, individuals with BPD may be more difficult to engage in the CR for PTSD program. It may be harder to establish a strong working alliance between the client and therapist, and clients may be more prone to dropping out of treatment early. These therapeutic challenges are more broadly reflected in the treatment history of most people with BPD, who have typically had multiple therapists in the past (Lieb et al., 2004). Because clients with BPD have often been in treatment with a wide range of different clinicians, an additional challenge is that they may be skeptical that the CR program will be helpful, which can compromise their investment in the program as well as in effort to learn the skills and apply them to their own experiences.

Effective Strategies

To minimize interpersonal struggles during therapy, it is important for the therapist to emphasize during the orientation that the CR for PTSD program is focused on teaching skills to help clients process and deal with their traumatic experiences and that a collaborative approach is taken with all aspects of the program, with the therapist serving as a "consultant" to the client. For example, clients can choose not to talk about a particular topic if they prefer, they can identify topics they would like to discuss in a session during the agenda setting at the beginning of each session, and they can choose to make modifications in the skills taught to suit their needs (e.g., keeping eyes open during Breathing Retraining). The emphasis on the role of teaching skills in the program and the collaborative approach to working together can assuage concerns participants may have about control, manipulation, and the replaying of interpersonal dynamics from past relationships, including therapeutic ones.

When describing the CR for PTSD program, the therapist should do so in a confident and knowledgeable fashion. Rather than asking the client to take their word regarding the effectiveness of the program, the therapist can describe research that has been conducted showing its beneficial effects on PTSD and other symptoms. While clients may remain skeptical, the therapist should encourage them to keep an open mind, to collect their own evidence based on their own experience in the program, and to determine for themselves whether the program is effective. Therapists do not have to convince clients that the program is effective; they only have to encourage them that it is worth giving the program a try.

For clients who have had many negative life experiences, including treatment-related ones, and who continue to vacillate about participating in the program, the therapist can review with them how their current life is going and encourage them to try something different in the spirit of "nothing ventured, nothing gained." With clients who remain on the fence about participating in the program after trying all of the above suggestions, the therapist can suggest that they agree to work together with the therapist for a set number of sessions (e.g., three sessions) and that, after completing those sessions, discuss whether they found the sessions to be beneficial and whether they would like to continue their participation in the program. If the client is interested in continuing to participate in the program, the therapist can discuss with the client whether they want to agree to work for a limited number of sessions (e.g., another four sessions) and then to discuss impressions again or whether they prefer to proceed with the rest of the program as designed.

The most prominent motivation for most people with PTSD engaging in treatment is to get relief from distressing PTSD and other symptoms, which can be especially acute in people with BPD. However, PTSD symptoms often gradually decrease during the program, reducing the intense distress associated with them, which can lead some clients to drop out before completing the program. To avoid this, it is important for the therapist to explore, identify, and track specific personal goals that the client has that are related to their PTSD, such as improving interpersonal relationships, returning to work or getting a promotion, completing their schooling, taking better care of their health, or engaging in more leisure and recreational activities. Over the course of therapy, the clinician works with the client to use the skills taught in the program to help them make progress toward their goals, in addition to working on their trauma-related thoughts and beliefs. Active work toward goals increases the client's investment in participating in the full course of the program and reduces the chances of premature termination.

Despite the therapist's effort to work on both the client's PTSD and personal goals, some clients may want to terminate early or may engage in "therapy-interfering" behaviors such as missing or cancelling appointments or reducing or stopping following through on home assignments. These behaviors may be the result of a variety of different beliefs the client has about therapy, and these have the potential to undermine the long-term effectiveness of the program if not addressed. Gentle exploration with the client about their thoughts—about themselves and their future, the CR for PTSD program, the therapist, and their traumatic experiences—can identify beliefs, which can then be examined more closely using the 5 Steps of CR. When beliefs are related to high levels of distress the client has experienced during the therapy, the therapist can initiate developing an Action Plan to help the client deal more effectively with their distress while continuing in the program. Examples of beliefs that can underlie therapy-interfering behaviors and can be addressed with the 5 Steps include the following:

- Nothing has worked for me. I'm too complicated and have had too much trauma. There's no point to keep trying.
- I've tried this program for X weeks, and it's just not working. It's never going to work.
- This therapy brings up so much bad stuff for me, I can't stand it. It's just not worth the pain.
- I no longer have any hope for myself and my future. It's not worth the effort of trying to change.
- I've made some improvements in the program, and I'm ready to move on right away. I have more important things to do.

Intense Distress, Emotion Dysregulation, and Difficulty Tolerating Emotions

People with BPD tend to experience emotions very intensively and can become overwhelmed by even relatively minor negative feelings. These difficulties tolerating and coping with negative emotions can lead to variety of challenges in daily life, such as overwhelming feelings of anxiety, extreme dependency or demands on others, impulsive behaviors (e.g., self-injury, substance use), with resulting effects on social relationships, ability to work or attend school, and health and self-care. In the CR for PTSD program, intense feelings of distress in sessions can make it more difficult for the therapist to shift the focus from a rehashing by the client of the upsetting or traumatic event to a collaborative conversation focused on learning cognitive restructuring skills. Relatedly, the intensity of distressing feelings that clients experience in their daily lives and the difficulty they have tolerating those feelings can present a challenge to practicing cognitive restructuring for their home assignments. The client may report that they felt too overwhelmed in the situation to remember to try to use the skill.

Effective Strategies

Increased Utilization of Breathing Retraining

Breathing Retraining is a useful skill for helping to manage intense and overwhelming emotions, both when they occur in sessions as well as outside of session. To reduce emotional overarousal when the client experiences intense feelings within a session, the therapist can initiate a short break to lead the client in practicing Breathing Retraining. For clients who frequently are overwhelmed by their intense emotions, the therapist can minimize the level of distress at the outset by beginning each session with a joint practice of Breathing Retraining. Gradually, as the client becomes more adept at using Breathing Retraining, the therapist can hand over to the client the responsibility for using Breathing Retraining to self-regulate emotions at any point during the session where it might be needed or beneficial.

Additional strategies may be useful to facilitate the learning and adoption of Breathing Retraining. Along with frequently practicing the skill in session with the therapist guiding the client through the skill, some clients may benefit from practicing the skill on their own by listening to an audio file of the therapist providing the verbal guidance. Other individualized modifications to the skill can be made in the service of accentuating the effects of the slower, more relaxed breathing, such as mindfully focusing on a relaxing image during the exercise. Some examples of suggested imagery content are provided in Exhibit 13.1.

Breathing Retraining can also be used to facilitate completion of home assignments that may otherwise be derailed by intense emotions. When clients have developed sufficient competency in the skill, the therapist can help them plan to practice the exercise before attempting to complete cognitive restructuring home assignments, including those unrelated to their traumatic experiences. Breathing Retraining can be built into the routine use of cognitive restructuring for clients who are often overwhelmed by their emotions, eventually fostering their ability to use the skill in the moment in the long run.

EXHIBIT 13.1

Examples of Pleasant Imagery to Accentuate the Relaxing Effects of Breathing Retraining

- Imagining oneself laying on a beach or field of grass.
- Feeling the crinkling of fall leaves underfoot while walking through the woods.
- Petting a beloved dog or cat.
- Imagining flying above trees looking down like a bird.
- Picturing a stream with leaves floating down it.
- Hearing the sound and waves of the ocean.
- Envisioning a sunset.
- Conjuring a favorite vacation spot.

Practicing Cognitive Restructuring in the Moment

It is important to emphasize that it takes time and practice to learn the cognitive restructuring skills and that early in the learning process the client may be able to use the skills only after the event has passed or in situations in which resulting stress is not overwhelming. As clients become more practiced and adept, the therapist can encourage them to use their cognitive restructuring skills closer to the timing of the distressing event with events that are increasingly more upsetting and ultimately in the moment as the event is unfolding.

Low tolerance for distressing feelings is often accompanied by negative, self-defeating thoughts about how terrible the feelings are (e.g., "I can't stand these emotions") and beliefs about how the person will never be able to manage those feelings more effectively in the future (e.g., "I can't change. This is the way it's always going to be"). The therapist can look for opportunities to help the client examine, challenge, and modify these thoughts and beliefs using the Common Styles of Thinking skill and the 5 Steps of CR skill. This can be achieved most effectively immediately after the client has experienced a brief period of intense emotion during a session and some regulation has been restored through the use of Breathing Retraining. While the emotions are still fresh, the therapist can help the client use CR to examine their thoughts and beliefs about the feelings they just experienced and to change extreme, inaccurate thoughts to more accurate and realistic ones. Once this has been accomplished, the therapist and client can work out an Action Plan to help the client remember the new and more accurate thought in situations where their feelings become overwhelming. Additionally, the therapist can prompt the client to remember the new thought as appropriate during subsequent sessions.

Expanded Use of Action Plans

Action Plans can be used more broadly to help clients consider the full range of possible options for managing situations in which they become overwhelmed by their emotions. This can be especially useful early in the process of learning cognitive restructuring before the person has learned how to examine their thoughts in situations where they experience intense distress. For example, in addition to the use of Breathing Retraining, an Action Plan can contain other self-soothing and calming strategies, including positive self-talk, mindful observation of current thoughts and feelings, distraction (e.g., listening to music, watching a video, taking a walk), and talking with a supportive person.

The development of Action Plans to deal with situations in which overwhelmingly distressing feelings are experienced can initially be informed by the individual's Wellness Plan developed early in the CR for PTSD program. These Wellness Plans can in turn be modified to incorporate additional coping strategies identified and tested when making and following through on Action Plans. In this way, the Wellness Plan can become a kind of "living document" that continues to change and be modified over the course of the CR program.

UNSTABLE AND CONFLICT-RIDDEN INTERPERSONAL RELATIONSHIPS

Maintaining stable, mutually supportive, and satisfying relationships with other people is a frequent challenge for people with BPD. Conflict in close relationships (such as with intimate partners) can be fueled by a combination of the client's high dependency on the other person, impulsive and unpredictable behaviors (e.g., self-injury), intense displays of emotion, and dramatic swings in appraisals of the partner ranging from idealized and positive "overvaluation" to equally negative "devaluation," often leading the other person to feel bewildered, hurt, and/or angry (Manning & Linehan, 2011). Paradoxically, the fear of abandonment that is common in BPD is often reinforced when the strain of these challenging interpersonal behaviors reaches a breaking point and the other person ends the relationship or ceases contact. Helping clients better understand and modify these destructive dynamics in interpersonal relationships is crucial to enabling them to develop more stable and rewarding relationships with others.

Difficulties in interpersonal relationships in people with BPD are not limited to their day-to-day lives and can extend to the therapeutic relationship. For example, the client may sometimes espouse exaggerated perceptions of the therapist's skill and helpfulness and then at other times may believe and insist that they cannot be helped by the clinician (e.g., "No therapist has ever been able to help me, and so you can't either," "I can't trust you at all. You'll just abandon or traumatize me like everyone else in my life"). Addressing such relationship dynamics in therapy can be critical to maintaining a strong therapeutic alliance with the client and maximizing their chances of completing and fully benefiting from the CR program.

Effective Strategies

The therapist can help the client use cognitive restructuring to address negative feelings related to general relationship conflict in their lives. For example, the 5 Steps of CR could be used to examine a client's thought that "Person X doesn't give me enough attention or affirmation, and that means they're going to leave me or hurt me." Action Plans may be needed to deal with difficult or stressful relationships, especially those involving unhealthy or abusive behavior patterns, such as substance use, sexual exploitation, or interpersonal aggression.

For people with BPD, it is common for difficulties in interpersonal relationships to at times trigger feelings of anger, which can present special challenges to using cognitive restructuring to examine the thought and beliefs underlying those feelings. As we have discussed in previous chapters (Chapters 8 and 10, this volume), although anger is usually considered a "negative" emotion, it can also feel empowering and validating to the person, and thus people are often not as motivated to make their angry feelings go away (unlike anxiety, depression, or guilt/shame). There are three broad approaches to working with angry feelings in people with BPD and helping them reduce their negative effects on close relationships.

First, many clients with BPD recognize the tumultuous nature of their interpersonal relationships and want more stable, mutually rewarding, and peaceful relationships with others. Early during the CR for PTSD program, when exploring and the impact of PTSD on the client's life and potential goals for the client's participation in the program, the clinician should be alert to the client's interest in improving their relationships with others and seek to make this a goal of treatment when applicable. The client may want to improve their relationships in a variety of ways (e.g., improve the ability to get along better with others at work; enhance intimacy with a spouse or partner; improve relationships with other family members, such as children, siblings, or parents), and therefore, the more specific the therapist can be in helping the client articulate their particular goal, the easier it will be to track progress toward the goal over time. When improving relationships is an explicit goal of therapy, the clinician has more leeway in getting clients to examine their thoughts and beliefs underlying their angry feelings.

Second, anger is part of the fight-or-flight response to a perceived threat, and thus some degree of fear is implicit in any angry response to a situation. However, acknowledging and facing the fear underlying an angry reaction can make people feel uncomfortable and vulnerable. A strong therapeutic relationship with trust, transparency, and validation can provide clients with sufficient support to enable them to explore and be willing to fully experience these distressing emotions underlying their negative feelings. As their therapeutic relationship strengthens over the course of the CR for PTSD program, the ability of the therapist to assist clients in this way often grows over time as well.

Third, it is always important for the therapist to avoid getting into debates with the client when evaluating the evidence underlying angry feelings about another person during cognitive restructuring. Such debates can be perceived by clients with BPD as efforts to control them that may be experienced as reenactments of problematic relationships in the past, which undermine their sense of self-determination and may spark feelings of resentment and some intransience. Even when the evidence does not appear to the therapist to support the client's thought or belief underlying their angry feeling, if the therapist has done due diligence in helping them weigh the possible evidence for and against the belief, the clinician should yield to the client's decision that their belief is supported by the evidence and move onto making an Action Plan for dealing with the upsetting situation.

The collaborative nature of formulating an Action Plan can result in a dramatic change in the dynamic between the therapist and client (that can be associated with weighing the evidence for a belief), which can be a relief to both persons involved. In the long run, since Action Plans, by their very nature, involve implementing a solution to a problem and thus collecting more information about a situation (e.g., an important interpersonal relationship), formulating Action Plans often provides opportunities to revisit anger-related thoughts and feelings that may pervade close relationships at later points in time with a fresh perspective.

Minimizing or Addressing Conflict in the Therapeutic Relationship

The therapist can reduce the likelihood that difficulties the client has in establishing and maintaining good relationships will spill over and interfere with the therapeutic alliance by validating the client's efforts to learn the skills taught in the program and by remaining as neutral as possible during the sessions. Cognitive restructuring should not be presented to the client as a skill for "correcting cognitive errors or maladaptive thoughts" but rather as a useful tool for figuring out when a thought is not helpful, contributes needlessly to their emotional distress, or is simply not supported by the evidence. This includes upset feelings the client may have about the therapist. Rather than being defensive in response to these feelings, the therapist should encourage and help the client examine these types of thoughts together using the CR skills, just as they would do with any other negative feeling.

Following is an example of how the therapist uses the 5 Steps of CR with Leigh-Ann (who exhibits BPD traits that are also noted in her medical record) to address some of her recent behaviors that suggest a reduced engagement in therapy and possible negative feelings she may have about her therapist. The dialogue takes place in Session 9 of the CR for PTSD program and picks up after the review of Leigh-Ann's home assignment.

THERAPIST: Leigh-Ann, can we talk for a few minutes about our working together?

LEIGH-ANN: I guess so. What's up?

THERAPIST: I've noticed a few changes recently that I wanted to get your thoughts and perspective on.

LEIGH-ANN: OK. What type of changes are you talking about?

THERAPIST: A few things I've noticed. When we started working together a few months ago, you seemed really involved in our therapy sessions, including trying to follow through on most of the home assignments we came up with. And you made it to our sessions every week, so we were accomplishing a lot in the program. But the last few weeks have been a little different. It seems as though it's been harder for you to get around to practicing the skills on your own that we've been working on in the sessions, and there have been a few cancelled sessions. I bring this up because it is not uncommon for this sort of thing to crop up during the course of the program, but it is important to understand what it might be related to.

LEIGH-ANN: Well, I've had a lot going on recently, like starting a new job. Other things keep coming up, and I guess it's been hard to put the time into this.

THERAPIST: I understand that you have a lot going on, Leigh-Ann, and that it's hard to juggle these therapy sessions with everything else in your life. And I appreciate your willingness to talk with me about this kind of stuff, which I know can be hard. I also noticed that you seem a little less involved in our sessions than before—kind of like you're holding back your feelings or what's going on with you. Do you know what I mean?

LEIGH-ANN: I guess so. I know I haven't been quite as open when we meet. I just haven't felt like talking about things as much as before.

THERAPIST: I see. Can you tell me a little more about that?

LEIGH-ANN: At the beginning, it felt like there was a lot to talk about and learning about PTSD. But the more we've gotten into it, the more anxious I've felt, and I've begun to wonder what I should say, will any of this be helpful, is it all worth going into it? And then I just clam up.

THERAPIST: I can understand how hard that must be, and I'm so glad you are sharing this. When you think about talking with me and what you do or don't want to tell me, what are your concerns? What do you think might happen?

LEIGH-ANN: It's hard to talk about this stuff, and I wonder if I tell you about it, what are you going to do with it all? I mean, do you really care that much, or is this just your job? Do I really want to set myself up again with someone I don't know that well and take this risk?

THERAPIST: Does it feel maybe like it's hard for you to trust me—like you're not really sure if I have your best interests in mind?

LEIGH-ANN: Sort of. I mean, how can I know for sure?

THERAPIST: I think I know what you mean, and given what you've gone through in life, it makes a lot of sense, Leigh-Ann. If you

	haven't had many people in your life that you can trust and people have even abused and assaulted you, then it makes sense to wonder whether you can trust someone new in your life, like me.
LEIGH-ANN:	Yeah, I think that might be right.
THERAPIST:	This is really important, and I appreciate you being willing to talk it through. Feeling anxious about our therapy and our relationship and wondering how much trust you can have in me, in a way, is really like any other distressing situation that can be examined with the 5 Steps of CR. Do you see what I mean when I say that?
LEIGH-ANN:	Yes, I get that now that you explain it that way.
THERAPIST:	How about us working on this situation and going through the 5 Steps together and see where we land? Would that be OK?
LEIGH-ANN:	Yeah, I'm willing to give it a shot, I guess.

Following this initial discussion, the therapist began guiding Leigh-Ann through the 5 Steps of CR using the situation as described earlier (Step 1), and Leigh-Ann identified her strongest negative feeling as anxiety (Step 2). During Step 3, in line with her initial conversation with the therapist, Leigh-Ann identified her first distressing thought as "How can I know I can trust my therapist?" The therapist helped Leigh-Ann transform this thought into a more workable thought (i.e., statement of fact) that could be examined with CR: "I probably can't trust my therapist." With additional help from the therapist probing this thought further, Leigh-Ann identified several other distressing thoughts, including these: "My therapist probably doesn't care that much about me," "I'll probably be hurt again if I'm open about my feelings with my therapist," and "No one can really be trusted." The therapist asked a few more questions to see if Leigh-Ann's concerns could be linked with her traumatic experiences (sexual abuse as a child, sexual assault in adulthood), and Leigh-Ann identified one thought ("I was assaulted as a child and adult, and people have proved untrustworthy. I probably can't trust my therapist either"). After reviewing these different thoughts, Leigh-Ann selected the last thought as the most distressing one. At the end of Step 3 after selecting this thought, Leigh-Ann considered whether it might reflect a Common Style of Thinking. Despite the therapist's specific inquiry into whether the thought might be an example of overgeneralization or all-or-nothing thinking, Leigh-Ann was not convinced it was, so they went on to Step 4.

During Step 4, Leigh-Ann identified several pieces of evidence supporting her thought, including her traumatic experiences of being sexually abused and assaulted, several bad relationships she had had with men in which she had felt they had betrayed her, and several relationships with friends that had broken off because of things they had done that she felt made them untrustworthy. When asked, Leigh-Ann was not able to identify specific evidence suggesting that her CR for PTSD therapist could not be trusted. With probing from the therapist, Leigh-Ann also identified several additional pieces of evidence that did not support her distressing thought. First, Leigh-Ann identified a few professional people in her life whom she had been able to trust, including a teacher in school who took a special interest in her, her primary physician, and one of the case managers she had worked with. Second, with further exploration about Leigh-Ann's friendships and intimate relationships, the therapist was able to identify specific instances or periods of time in which another person had behaved in a trustworthy manner. Additional questioning about this matter also addressed whether Leigh-Ann had ever had a misunderstanding with someone else about trust, such as a time when she thought that the person had not been trustworthy about something when in fact they had been or a time when someone else thought that she had not been trustworthy about something when in fact she had been. Leigh-Ann could think of examples of both types of misunderstandings. This discussion helped Leigh-Ann begin to view trust in relationships as a quality that may change over time in relationships and that may be subject to misinterpretation, rather than an all-or-nothing characteristic of relationships.

After reviewing the evidence for and against her thought, Leigh-Ann concluded that the evidence did not support her thought that her therapist could not be trusted. She developed a new, more believable, and significantly less upsetting thought for the situation: "Although I experienced sexual abuse and assault in the past and some people in my life have violated my trust, some people have been trustworthy, and so far my therapist has been trustworthy as well."

CONCLUSION

BPD is characterized by a combination of difficulties regulating strong negative emotions, intense and unstable interpersonal relationships, disturbance in self-image, and impulsivity such as self-injurious behavior. People with BPD have a substantially increased likelihood of having PTSD, and their PTSD symptoms tend to be more severe than those in people with SMI without BPD. Despite these challenges, there is strong evidence that PTSD can be effectively treated using trauma-focused therapy in people with BPD, including the CR for PTSD program.

Some common challenges that arise when treating PTSD in people with BPD include difficulties with engagement and retention in therapy, intense distress and emotion regulation difficulties, and unstable and conflict-ridden relationships. Central to all effective treatment of PTSD in clients with BPD is a strong therapeutic relationship including clear agreement on the goals of treatment, validation and support for the distress experienced by the client, and honesty and transparency about the treatment methods used in the CR for PTSD program.

Breathing Retraining is a valuable skill to use throughout the CR for PTSD program, both within therapy sessions to manage intense and overwhelming emotions and outside of sessions to manage those feelings and to facilitate following through on home assignments to practice cognitive restructuring skills. The 5 Steps of CR can be used to address a broad range of challenges that occur during sessions, including therapy-interfering behaviors such as frequent cancelled appointments, distressing and inaccurate beliefs related to the therapeutic relationship, and other interpersonal problems (e.g., with partners, family, friends; at work/school). Action Plans can often be effective in helping clients identify additional coping strategies for dealing with intense emotions and for determining healthy next steps to take in problematic and stressful interpersonal relationships.

IV

CONCLUSION

14

The Role of the CR for PTSD Program in a Comprehensive System of Mental Health Care

Mental health systems of care have been evolving in recent years to become more recovery-oriented, based on the recognition that recovery from serious mental illness (SMI) is a deeply personal process of regaining meaning, sense of purpose, and autonomy in one's life beyond any psychiatric challenges the person experiences. Effective services are needed by individuals with SMI both to achieve greater mastery over their mental health challenges and to help them in pursuing functional and other personal recovery goals. This leads to the question of what the role is of the Cognitive Restructuring (CR) for posttraumatic stress disorder (PTSD) program in a comprehensive system of care. We argue that the primary case for providing the CR program is to honor the principle of client choice and self-determination in recovery-oriented systems of care.

IMPORTANCE OF CLIENT CHOICE

Central to the empowerment of people to gain control over their mental health conditions and their lives is for a system of care to provide active support for individuals' self-determination, autonomy, and choice. True support for self-determination includes respecting individuals' right to choose which treatment and rehabilitative services they want to engage in to aid in their recovery. For a comprehensive system of care to honor the principle of choice, clients must be provided with timely and accurate information about their conditions and the

https://doi.org/10.1037/0000423-014

Treatment of Posttraumatic Stress Disorder in Serious Mental Illness: The Cognitive Restructuring Program, by K. T. Mueser and J. D. Gottlieb

treatment options available to them, and a broad range of appropriate and effective services for SMI must be accessible. So which services should be provided by mental health systems and individual treatment providers?

Considering the ever-growing marketplace of interventions for the SMI population, systems of care need to judiciously choose which ones to invest in on behalf of the clients they serve. Given the assumption that as many clients as possible should have the right to access the most effective and state-of-the-art services possible for managing their mental health and achieving their goals, mental health facilities and individual practitioners need to select those interventions that (a) address the most common and pressing client needs or goals and (b) have the strongest scientific evidence (or promising evidence) supporting them.

Based on these two criteria, the CR for PTSD program deserves inclusion as a first-line treatment choice in a comprehensive system of care and by independent therapists. First, PTSD is a highly distressing and disabling disorder in the SMI population, with most estimates suggesting prevalence rates in the 30% to 35% range, indicating a high need for treatment among many individuals. Second, the CR program is now well standardized and flexible and has been shown to be effective for treating PTSD in people across a broad range of different psychiatric diagnoses and sociodemographic groups. Furthermore, strong research supports the effectiveness of the CR program for persons with SMI, and the program is based on well-established principles and methods of cognitive behavioral therapy that have been shown to be effective in treating PTSD in extensive research conducted with other trauma populations (ranging from sexual assault survivors, combat veterans, and victims of accidents, disasters, and mass violence).

Is PTSD already being treated effectively in most systems of care for persons with SMI? The advent of trauma-informed care might suggest that it is, but in fact it is not.

TRAUMA-INFORMED CARE IS NOT ENOUGH

The devastating impact of trauma on the lives of people with SMI is now widely accepted. It is also now recognized that treatment systems have often retraumatized the very people they are supposed to help, worsening their trauma symptoms and breeding distrust of the mental health profession. Trauma-informed services have emerged as a best practice in mental health systems aimed at rectifying the errors of the past (and present). Trauma-informed services entail broad-based education of mental health professionals aimed at creating an understanding of and sensitivity to the effects of trauma on people with SMI and at teaching skills and changing practices in order to minimize the chances of inadvertently retraumatizing individuals in these settings.

The development and growing dissemination of trauma-informed care has undoubtedly been an important step forward for mental health systems serving persons with SMI, one perhaps best summarized by the Hippocratic oath's promise to "First, do no harm." But having a trauma-informed system of care and "doing no harm" are not the same as having a system of care that is capable of directly treating PTSD and relieving the immense burden it imposes on the many individuals who have it. Trauma-informed care is a general approach to increasing awareness of trauma and reducing harmful practices in mental health providers. PTSD is a specific psychiatric disorder that has been intensively studied for over 40 years, and specific time-limited interventions for it have been shown to be remarkably effective at reducing symptom severity, often leading to permanent remission of the disorder. Trauma-informed care may avoid retraumatizing individuals with PTSD and facilitate retaining them in services generally, but there is no evidence that it alleviates PTSD symptoms. Providing trauma-informed services is not a substitute for providing a trauma-specific intervention that treats PTSD, such as the CR for PTSD program.

Based on the principle of respect for client choice and support for self-determination in recovery-oriented systems of care, people with SMI should have the right to access an evidence-based trauma-specific intervention for the treatment of their PTSD.

WHAT ARE THE CHOICES FOR TRAUMA-SPECIFIC SERVICES FOR PTSD IN PERSONS WITH SMI?

As reviewed in Chapter 2 in this volume, three trauma-specific psychotherapeutic interventions have been shown in extensive research to be most effective for treating PTSD in the general population: cognitive restructuring (which the CR program is based on), prolonged exposure (PE), and eye movement desensitization and reprocessing (EMDR). However, much less research has been conducted on these interventions in the SMI population. While it is possible for a comprehensive system of care or individual therapists serving people with SMI to offer more than one type of treatment for PTSD, there are both practical and empirical reasons for why priority should be given to providing the CR for PTSD program.

First, therapy interventions that require exposure to traumatic memories (such as PE and EMDR) may be less acceptable to people with PTSD (either with or without SMI) than programs that do not require such exposure—such as the CR program. This is to be expected given that one of the defining symptom clusters of PTSD is avoidance of trauma-related stimuli. While many individuals with PTSD agree to participate in a treatment program that requires exposure to their feared memories, some do not, and those individuals can be more readily encouraged to engage in an intervention based on cognitive restructuring. Since clients with SMI and PTSD are likely more willing to choose to participate in the CR program than PE or EMDR, this program has the greatest potential for reaching the most affected individuals.

Second, while PE, EMDR, and the CR program are effective at reducing PTSD symptoms, only the CR program teaches clients life skills that are useful beyond the treatment of their PTSD symptoms. The techniques used in PE and EMDR have less practical value beyond reducing PTSD symptoms. In contrast, most of the CR program focuses on teaching clients how to use cognitive restructuring as a self-management skill for dealing with all negative feelings (not just trauma-related or PTSD symptom-related ones) and for addressing any problematic situations that give rise to such feelings. As discussed throughout this volume, this powerful skill, which is embodied in the 5 Steps of CR, incorporates techniques for identifying, systematically evaluating, and changing inaccurate distressing thoughts and beliefs to more accurate ones and also presents strategies for developing practical Action Plans for addressing realistic concerns that call for effective problem solving (rather than changes in thoughts or beliefs). As experiencing all kinds of upsetting feelings is a part of everyday life (including both negative feelings related to the faulty appraisal of a situation as well as negative feelings due to genuine problems that require solutions), the 5 Steps of CR serves as a comprehensive and valuable skill clients can continue to use long after they have completed the CR for PTSD program.

Third, as reviewed in Chapter 2 in this volume, the two U.S. randomized controlled trials of the CR program were conducted with diagnostically hetero-geneous populations of people with SMI and PTSD, including clients with treatment-refractory major depression, bipolar disorder, schizophrenia, schi-zoaffective disorder, and borderline personality disorder. This is an important consideration as it demonstrates the higher level of generalizability to the overall SMI population compared to studies evaluating PE or EMDR which have focused more narrowly on psychotic disorders.

Based on the principles of respect for client choice of treatment and support for self-determination, the high prevalence of PTSD in the SMI population, and effective interventions for treating it, we have suggested that comprehensive and recovery-oriented systems of care (and other clinicians working with those with SMI) should provide access to effective treatment for PTSD, such as the CR for PTSD program. Trauma-informed care is not the same as trauma-specific inter-ventions that target PTSD, nor are trauma-informed services sufficient. Taking into account the different PTSD evidence-based intervention options for people with SMI (particularly those studied with heterogeneous client samples), the challenges of client acceptability of exposure-based interventions, and the inclusion of general lifelong skills to manage distress beyond just PTSD symptoms, the CR for PTSD program can be viewed the best option available.

NEXT STEPS FOR INCREASING ACCESS TO EFFECTIVE TREATMENT FOR PTSD, INCLUDING THE CR PROGRAM

While a compelling case can be made for making the CR for PTSD program broadly available to people with SMI receiving treatment in comprehensive, recovery-oriented systems of care and by independent practitioners, there are practical issues involved in how to do just that.

First, although effective and efficient methods for screening for trauma and PTSD in persons with SMI exist, they are not routinely utilized in most systems of care for this population, resulting in PTSD being overlooked and undertreated. While routine assessment of trauma and PTSD are not tantamount to treating PTSD impactfully, proper screening can be an important step toward recognizing the magnitude of the problem and considering the treatment options. As discussed in Chapter 3 in this volume, we strongly encourage clinicians to routinely screen for trauma and PTSD in the clients they personally treat and to advocate for similar routine screening within their work settings. Routine screening for PTSD within an entire system of care has the added advantages that it can identify particular subgroups of clients or (service programs) where the need for treatment is highest and can reveal important associations between PTSD and other important outcomes of concern (e.g., use or emergency or acute care services).

Second, there is a need for greater awareness of clinicians and other staff at mental health agencies to understand the nature of PTSD and effective interventions for treating it. Continuing education requirements or trauma-informed initiatives that are supplemented to include current and accurate information about PTSD and its treatment represent opportunities for increasing the knowledge of staff members.

Third, given the important effects of trauma and PTSD on their lives, those receiving mental health services with SMI who have PTSD have a need and right to accurate education about trauma and PTSD. Clinicians can play a vital role in routinely providing such information. Educating clients about PTSD should not be limited to the basic facts about prevalence, symptoms, and challenges associated with the disorder but should also include information about evidence-based treatment options. For the sake of honesty and transparency within a mental health system, clients have the right to know if effective treatments exist for a condition or challenge they have, even if those treatments are not available within their current system of care. This education can provide critical information that clients can then use to advocate for the availability of a noted effective intervention available (including the CR program) within their services setting or to explore availability of the treatment outside of their current system.

Fourth and last, education about the prevalence and correlates of trauma and PTSD and the CR program as an effective intervention for PTSD in persons with SMI needs to be shared with the broader range of stakeholders who are concerned with the welfare of the SMI population. At the grassroots level, this includes educating family members of persons with SMI who so often play an important role in advocating for critical services for their loved ones. At the organizational and policy levels, education campaigns are needed to inform mental health administrators and policymakers about the high prevalence of PTSD in persons with SMI and about the availability of effective programs for treating it, such as the CR program.

Tremendous advances have been made over the past 2 decades in our ability to recognize, assess, and treat PTSD in people with SMI. Clinicians now have improved access to the tools for alleviating PTSD in this population. However, those in the mental health field need to go an important step further beyond learning and mastering how to treat PTSD with the CR program. Clinicians also need to seek to raise awareness about this intervention—to other mental health professionals, to clients, to family members, and to administrators and policy-makers. It is only through broadscale and open education about PTSD and its effective treatment that the inertia and avoidance of the past can be overcome and PTSD can be seen for what it is—a highly distressing, commonly occurring, but very treatable disorder that needlessly compromises the lives of people with SMI.

We believe that the combination of our collective voices alongside reliable access to the CR for PTSD program and other evidence-based trauma-related services can demonstrate that the burden of trauma and PTSD on the lives of people with SMI can and should be systematically alleviated. Elevating the standard of care for people with SMI and PTSD must be a top societal priority.

Clinician Tools and Handouts

CLINICIAN TOOLS

1. CR for PTSD Session-By-Session Agenda for Clinicians
2. PTSD Assessment Tracking Sheet
3. Depression Assessment Tracking Sheet
4. Therapist Tracking Sheet for Client's Trauma-Related Cognitions

HANDOUTS FOR USE ACROSS ALL SESSIONS

1. CR for PTSD Agenda-Setting Worksheet
2. Home Practice/Outside Practice Plan

HANDOUTS FOR SESSIONS 1–3 (PRE-CR)

1. Orientation to the CR for PTSD Program
2. CR for PTSD Orientation and Session-By-Session Plan
3. Wellness Plan Worksheet
4. Learning Breathing Retraining
5. Practice Breathing Retraining Tracking Form 1: Nondistress Version
6. Breathing Retraining Tracking Form 2: Distress Version
7. Common Reactions to Trauma I: PTSD Symptoms
8. Common Reactions to Trauma II: Associated Problems
9. How Trauma Affects Thoughts and Feelings
10. Goal-Setting Worksheet for CR for PTSD Program

HANDOUTS FOR SESSIONS 4–16 (CR AND ONWARD)

1. Understanding the Thought–Feeling Model With the CBT Triangle
2. Common Styles of Thinking Information Sheet
3. Common Styles of Thinking Worksheet
4. Guide to Thoughts and Feelings Information Sheet
5. The 5 Steps of CR
6. The 5 Steps of CR (Alternate Worksheet With Ratings)
7. Tips for Finding Good Evidence Information Sheet
8. Action Plan Worksheet
9. Payoff Matrix
10. The 5 Steps of CR Notecard (2-sided)
11. Summing-Up Worksheet
12. Challenging My Most Distressing PTSD Symptoms and Thoughts

CR FOR PTSD SESSION-BY-SESSION AGENDA FOR CLINICIANS

Session no.	Topic covered	Sample session agenda	Handout/material needed
1	Overview Wellness Plan Breathing Retraining	1. Introductions/explain weekly agenda 2. Complete, score, discuss today's PCL and BDI 3. Program overview, review, questions, concerns 4. Complete Wellness Plan 5. Teach and practice BRT 6. Review session, preview next, plan and troubleshoot BRT home assignment	• CR for PTSD Orientation and Session-By-Session Plan • Wellness Plan Worksheet • Learning BRT • Practice BRT Tracking Form 1: Nondistress Version • PCL and BDI from screening • New blank PCL and BDI
2	Breathing Retraining Psychoeducation I	1. Review BRT home assignment practice, troubleshoot 2. Brief review and practice of BRT skill 3. Education about trauma and PTSD, Part I 4. Review session, preview next, plan and troubleshoot BRT home assignment	• Learning BRT • Practice BRT Tracking Form 1: Nondistress Version • BRT Tracking Form 2: Distress Version • Common Reactions to Trauma I: PTSD Symptoms
3	Breathing Retraining Psychoeducation II	1. Review BRT home assignment practice, troubleshoot 2. Brief practice of BRT skill 3. Education about trauma and PTSD, Part II 4. Wrapping up psychoeducation/goal setting 5. Review session, preview next, plan and troubleshoot BRT home assignment	• Learning BRT • BRT Tracking Form 2: Distress Version • Common Reactions to Trauma II: Associated Problems • How Trauma Affects Thoughts and Feelings • Goal-Setting Worksheet for CR for PTSD Program
4	Introduction to cognitive restructuring	1. Complete PCL and BDI (score, compare, discuss) 2. Review BRT home assignment practice, troubleshoot 3. Complete goal setting as needed 4. Teach Thought–Feeling Model 5. Introduction to CST 6. Brief CST practice 7. Review session, preview next, plan and troubleshoot CST home assignment	• Learning BRT • BRT Tracking Form 2: Distress Version • Goal-Setting Worksheet for CR for PTSD Program • CST Information Sheet • CST Worksheet • Prior PCLs and BDIs • New blank PCL and BDI

(continues)

Session no.	Topic covered	Sample session agenda	Handout/material needed
5	Introduction to cognitive restructuring	1. Review CST home assignment practice, troubleshoot 2. Continue teaching CST 3. CST practice 4. Review session, preview next, plan and troubleshoot CST home assignment	• CST Information Sheet • CST Worksheet • Guide to Thoughts and Feelings Information Sheet
6	The 5 Steps of CR	1. Review CST home assignment practice, troubleshoot 2. Additional brief CST practice as needed 3. Introduction to the 5 Steps of CR and Action Plan 4. Practice 5 Steps of CR 5. Review session, preview next, plan and troubleshoot 5 Steps of CR home assignment	• CST Information Sheet • CST Worksheet • The 5 Steps of CR • Action Plan Worksheet • Guide to Thoughts and Feelings Information Sheet • Tips for Finding Good Evidence Information Sheet
7–8/9	The 5 Steps of CR (basic)	1. Complete PCL and BDI (score, compare, discuss; Session 7) 2. Review 5 Steps of CR home assignment practice, troubleshoot 3. Continue with 5 Steps of CR and Action Plan teaching, trouble-shooting, and practice 4. Practice 5 Steps of CR (non-trauma-related) 5. Review session, preview next, plan and troubleshoot 5 Steps of CR home assignment	• CST Information Sheet • The 5 Steps of CR • Action Plan Worksheet • Guide to Thoughts and Feelings Information Sheet • Tips for Finding Good Evidence Information Sheet • For Session 7: Prior PCLs and BDIs • For Session 7: New blank PCL and BDI
8/9–14	The 5 Steps of CR (trauma-related)	1. Complete PCL and BDI (score, compare, discuss; Sessions 10 and 13) 2. Review 5 Steps of CR home assignment practice, troubleshoot 3. Continue with 5 Steps of CR and Action Plan teaching, trouble-shooting, and practice 4. Practice 5 Steps of CR. 5. Transition (Session 8/9) into 5 Steps of CR practice with trauma-related material 6. Review session, preview next, plan and troubleshoot 5 Steps of CR home assignment	• CST Information Sheet • The 5 Steps of CR • Action Plan Worksheet • Guide to Thoughts and Feelings Information Sheet • Tips for Finding Good Evidence Information Sheet • Payoff Matrix • For Sessions 10 and 13: Prior PCLs and BDIs • For Sessions 10 and 13: New blank PCL and BDI

15	Skill generalization	1. Review 5 Steps of CR home assignment practice, troubleshoot 2. Invite primary clinician to session (preplanned) 3. Collaborative program overview to primary clinician 4. Client leads primary clinician through 5 Steps of CR 5. Discuss skill generalization plan with primary clinician 6. Additional 5 Steps of CR practice for client if time 7. Review session, preview next/final session and termination, plan and troubleshoot 5 Steps of CR home assignment	• CST Information Sheet • The 5 Steps of CR • Action Plan Worksheet • Guide to Thoughts and Feelings Information Sheet • 5 Steps of CR Notecard
16	Skill generalization termination	1. <u>Complete final PCL and BDI (score, compare, discuss all measures from screening to present)</u> 2. Briefly review 5 Steps home assignment practice, troubleshoot 3. Brief debrief about Session 15 (primary clinician visit) 4. Discuss progress in program 5. Review previously set goals 6. Discuss continued skills practice 7. Provide additional blank copies of all handouts 8. Termination	• The 5 Steps of CR • Action Plan Worksheet • Challenging My Most Distressing PTSD Symptoms and Thoughts • Summing-Up Worksheet • 5 Steps of CR Notecard • All Prior PCLs and BDIs • New blank PCL and BDI (additional clean hardcopies of skill-based handouts for client to take home)

Note. All sessions, regardless of module, should include the agenda setting and outside practice/ home assignment review worksheets. CR = cognitive restructuring; PTSD = posttraumatic stress disorder; PCL = PTSD Checklist; BDI = Beck Depression Inventory; BRT = Breathing Retraining; Common Styles of Thinking.

PTSD ASSESSMENT TRACKING SHEET

Client name: _____

Therapist: _____

Index trauma: _____

Recommendation: Following the first administration of the PTSD Checklist (PCL-5) at the screening assessment, the PCL should be given at the beginning of Sessions 1, 4, 7, 10, 13, and 16 (or the last session). These scores can be tracked here, plotted into a graph below, and discussed with the client in session.

Session no.	Date administered	PCL score
Screening assessment		

Note. The cutoff score for "probable PTSD" is 33 or higher. PTSD Checklist data from Weathers et al. (2013).

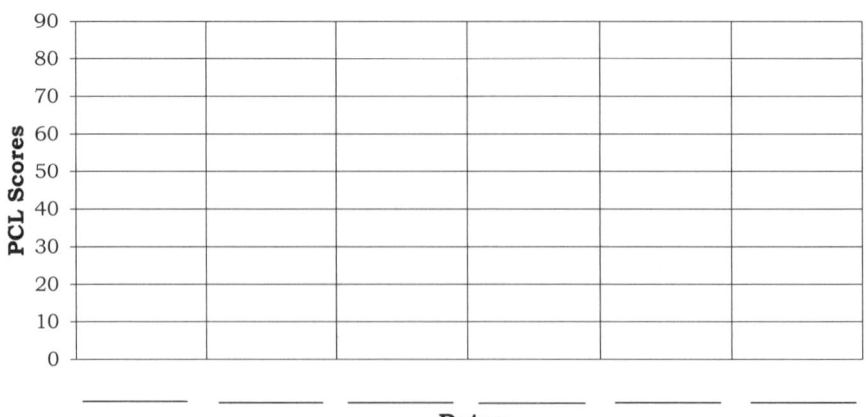

DEPRESSION ASSESSMENT TRACKING SHEET

Client name: _____

Therapist: _____

Recommendation: Following the first administration of the Beck Depression Inventory–II (BDI-II) at the screening assessment, the BDI-II should be given at the beginning of Sessions 1, 4, 7, 10, 13, and 16 (or the last session). These scores can be tracked here, plotted in the graph below, and discussed with the client in session.

Session no.	Date administered	BDI score
Screening assessment		

Note. Manual for the Beck Depression Inventory–II, by A. T. Beck, R. A. Steer, and G. K. Brown, 1996, Psychological Corporation.

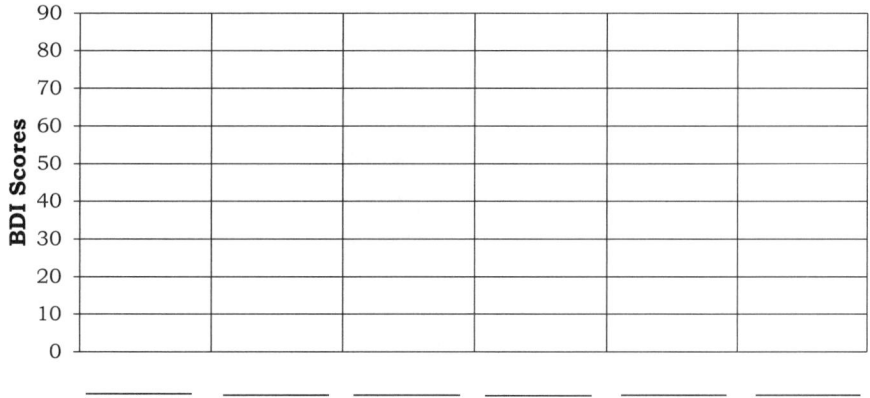

THERAPIST TRACKING SHEET FOR CLIENT'S TRAUMA-RELATED COGNITIONS

During the first six sessions of the CR for PTSD program, as you and the client are getting to know each other and work together, it is common for clients to mention some of their distressing thoughts and beliefs about their traumatic experience(s). This can occur quite naturally throughout the discussions and skill-building during orientation, BRT, psychoeducation, common styles of inaccurate thinking, or introducing the 5 Steps of CR. Many of these beliefs are either overtly trauma-related or are likely related to the impact of PTSD.

While you won't need to address or challenge these sorts of beliefs until you move into the more trauma-focused CR sessions, it can be helpful to make a note of these thoughts as they come up to keep in your records. That way you will have them later on as important and useful trauma-related material to help the client address in these later CR sessions. An example is given below:

Session date and topic	Client thought or belief mentioned (try to use client's own words when possible)	Other related notes
March 12, 2023, during Session 4 psychoeducation	*"I know I'll never be capable of having a romantic relationship ever again after what's happened to me. I am damaged goods forever."*	*Third time so far client has alluded to thoughts related to being faulty/defective/damaged as a result of the sexual assault.*

CR FOR PTSD AGENDA-SETTING WORKSHEET

In order to make the most of our time each session, it is helpful to set an agenda of the different important topics to make sure we cover them. This will help us figure out where to start and will also help us make sure that we save enough time for all of the topics that we need to work on today. Below, we will write out a list of what we want to cover for today's session.

Some tips:

- Keep the list manageable in length—not too long.
- Write just the brief, general topics below, and write out the whole list before starting to go into detail about any single item. There will be time for that later on.

Today's date: _____ Session no. (1–16): _____ Overall session topic: _____

Topics to cover (your therapist will likely have a list based on where you are in the CR intervention):

1. _____

2. _____

3. _____

4. _____

5. <u>Outside practice and plan for what will happen between now and the next meeting.</u>

Are there any other topics that you'd like to cover today that haven't already been listed out above? (Write down below any additional, specific topics that the client would like to talk about.)

1. _____

2. _____

HOME PRACTICE/OUTSIDE PRACTICE PLAN

As you've learned, putting aside some time to practice your skills is a VERY important part of this program. You can get the best results from this program if you practice the skills you are learning on a daily basis. Making a plan can help you remember to practice your skills over the following week.

Use this sheet to write down your plan for practicing your skills during the week:

Today's date: _____ Session no. (1–16): _____ Next session's date:_____

Overall session topic(s) covered:

_____

Based on today's session topics, here is what I will work on this week before our next session:

1. _____

2. _____

3. _____

Optional but encouraged: Now that you have a plan, can you think about what might get in the way of being able to complete this outside practice? You and your therapist can list any obstacles here and then list a possible solution next to each obstacle:

Possible obstacle: Possible solution:

_____   _____

_____   _____

_____   _____

Which handouts or worksheets do you need? Your therapist can give you extra copies.

_____

_____

_____

ORIENTATION TO THE CR FOR PTSD PROGRAM

The CR program for PTSD is a cognitive behavioral therapy program aimed at teaching people important information and skills for coping with and overcoming their PTSD symptoms in order to help get their lives back on track.

How the Program Works

The CR program for PTSD is provided over 12 to 16 sessions by an individual therapist. Sessions are usually conducted on a weekly basis, and each lasts about 1 hour.

The program includes three parts: (a) learning the skill of *Breathing Retraining (BRT)*, (b) education about *common reactions to trauma and PTSD*, and (c) developing *skills for dealing with upsetting thoughts and feelings*. These skills can help reduce PTSD symptoms like avoidance, anxiety, fear, distress, irritability, and high levels of body tension. Each of these parts is briefly described below:

- BRT: The Breathing Restraining skill involves learning a helpful new way to breathe that can help you to manage your anxiety and reduce other upsetting PTSD symptoms such as overarousal. Over time and with practice, you will learn how to use BRT to relax in stressful situations and lower your distress. By the end of the program, this skill will help you gain better control over your PTSD symptoms.

- Education: You will be taught about the common reactions people have to trauma, including PTSD symptoms. You will learn that you are not alone in how you reacted to the trauma in your life and that your PTSD symptoms that can be changed. This treatment program can teach you ways to respond differently to your PTSD distress to help you move forward in your life.

- CR: The Cognitive Restructuring skill involves learning how to identify and then challenge thoughts and beliefs that relate to your distress and PTSD symptoms. You will learn how to increase your awareness of these upsetting thoughts, how to examine those thoughts closely, and how to change them when they are inaccurate. You will see that challenging and changing inaccurate thinking that causes negative feelings can make you feel better.

Outside Practice ("Home Assignments")

The CR for PTSD program works by teaching people critical information and skills for overcoming their PTSD symptoms. In order to accomplish this, it is important to put aside some time every week to practice the skills taught in this program. At each session, you and your therapist will agree on a brief assignment to practice a skill you have learned over the next week (such as the BRT skill or the CR skill) to help you deal with your reactions to stressful things that happen during the week. During your sessions, you will go over how your outside practice went over the past week.

The more you practice the skills, the more you will benefit from this program. The goal is to practice them every day. Research on the CR for PTSD program shows that people who regularly do weekly home assignments outside of the sessions benefit more from the program than those who do not.

A Reminder

This program is designed to directly help you with your PTSD symptoms and upsetting thoughts related to the traumatic events and stressful things you have experienced. However, this treatment does not require that you describe or recount the details of those experiences. This program is very effective without the need to talk about those details.

This can feel reassuring to people who may have avoided other PTSD treatments in the past because they were anxious about having to relive their traumatic experiences. In this intervention, your therapist will be right by your side to help you learn about and work on your distressing PTSD symptoms and upsetting related thoughts and feelings.

CR FOR PTSD ORIENTATION AND SESSION-BY-SESSION PLAN

The CR for PTSD program is a cognitive behavioral therapy program aimed at teaching people important information and skills for coping with and overcoming their PTSD symptoms in order to help get their lives back on track.

How the Program Works

The CR for PTSD program is provided over 12 to 16 sessions by an individual therapist. Sessions are usually conducted on a weekly basis, and each lasts about 1 hour.

The program includes three parts: (a) learning the skill of *Breathing Retraining (BRT)*, (b) education about *common reactions to trauma and PTSD*, and (c) developing *skills for dealing with upsetting thoughts and feelings*. These skills can help reduce PTSD symptoms like avoidance, anxiety, fear, distress, irritability, and high levels of body tension. Each of these parts is briefly described below:

- BRT: The Breathing Retraining skill involves learning a helpful new way to breathe that can help you to manage your anxiety and reduce other upsetting PTSD symptoms such as overarousal. Over time and with practice, you will learn how to use BRT to relax in stressful situations and lower your distress. By the end of the program, this skill will help you gain better control over your PTSD symptoms.

- Education: You will be taught about the common reactions people have to trauma, including PTSD symptoms. You will learn that you are not alone in how you reacted to the trauma in your life and that your PTSD symptoms can be changed. This treatment program can teach you ways to respond differently to your PTSD distress to help you move forward in your life.

- CR: The Cognitive Restructuring skill involves learning how to identify and then challenge thoughts and beliefs that relate to your distress and PTSD symptoms. You will learn how to increase your awareness of these upsetting thoughts, how to examine them closely, and how to change them when they are inaccurate. You will see that challenging and changing inaccurate thinking that causes negative feelings can make you feel better.

Outside Practice ("Home Assignments")

The CR for PTSD program works by teaching people critical information and skills for overcoming their PTSD symptoms. In order to accomplish this, it is important to put aside some time every week to practice the skills taught in this program. At each session, you and your therapist will agree on a brief assignment to practice a skill you have learned over the next week (such as the BRT skill or the CR skill) to help you deal with your reactions to stressful things that happen during the week. During your sessions, you will go over how your outside practice went over the past week.

The more you practice the skills, the more you will benefit from this program. The goal is to practice them every day. Research on the CR for PTSD program shows that people who regularly do weekly home assignments outside of the sessions benefit more from the program than those who do not.

A Reminder

This program is designed to directly help you with your PTSD symptoms and upsetting thoughts related to the traumatic events and stressful things you have experienced. However, this treatment does not require that you describe or recount the details of those experiences. This program is very effective without the need to talk about those details.

This can feel reassuring to people who may have avoided other PTSD treatments in the past because they were anxious about having to relive their traumatic experiences. In this intervention, your therapist will be right by your side to help you learn about and work on your distressing PTSD symptoms and upsetting related thoughts and feelings.

Session-By-Session Overview

Here is what you can expect from each of the 16 sessions of this program. This will give you an idea of what will happen in each session and why:

Session no.	Topic	Purpose
1	Orientation Wellness Plan Breathing Retraining	• To learn about this program and what to expect • To make a plan to help you feel your best during this program • To teach a helpful skill right away that you can start to use to help with PTSD symptoms
2	Education about trauma and PTSD, Part I	• To learn about how trauma impacts people's lives • To learn about PTSD symptoms • To better understand how these have impacted your life directly
3	Education about trauma and PTSD, Part II	• To learn other common ways that trauma and PTSD affect people • To better understand how this has impacted your life directly • To set some personal goals related to having your PTSD symptoms decrease with this treatment

(continues)

Session no.	Topic	Purpose
4	The Thought–Feeling Model Common Styles of Thinking	• To learn about how our experiences impact our beliefs about the world • To learn how our thoughts can lead us to feel distressed • To understand how our thoughts are not always accurate and that this is common • To learn and practice a new skill to help pick out upsetting thoughts and feelings we have frequently
5	The 5 Steps of CR	• To learn and practice a new skill called Cognitive Restructuring to help with our upsetting thoughts and feelings that happen on a day-to-day basis
6–14	Continuing with the 5 Steps of CR	• To get comfortable with this new skill so that you can use it in many situations in your daily life • To practice this skill on your own for home assignments • To start to use this skill (with your therapist's help) to address some of your upsetting trauma-related thoughts • To directly help you deal with your PTSD symptoms
15	Postprogram support plan: inviting your primary clinician or other supportive person	• To share with your primary clinician (or other support) all that you have learned in the program • To show the 5 Steps of CR skill • To develop a solid plan with your primary clinician (or other support) for how to keep using these skills going forward
16	Ending the program and next steps	• To review what you learned in the program and what was helpful • To review progress toward goals made in Session 3 • To confirm plan for continuing to use the skills going forward to improve even more

WELLNESS PLAN WORKSHEET

Throughout this treatment program, we will be teaching skills to help you cope with PTSD symptoms or other upsetting feelings. It is helpful to have a clear plan in place for how to keep up your *wellness* while you are in this program. *Wellness* can include things like getting enough sleep, getting to your doctor appointments, and connecting with people who are supportive to you.

During stressful times in life or when PTSD symptoms are acting up, people often end up having an increase in other symptoms. And they may struggle to keep up with healthy coping skills. Having a good *Wellness Plan* can help keep you healthy.

Here are some important things to discuss with your CR for PTSD clinician:

1. *What types of stressful situations or crises would be difficult for you to handle? In what situations do you feel out of control, unsafe, or afraid—including being afraid of harming yourself or other people?*

   _____

   _____

   _____

2. *When you are under a lot of stress or when your PTSD symptoms are high, which of the following things do you notice about yourself?*
   - ❑ Suicidal thinking
   - ❑ Self-injurious behavior
   - ❑ Increased anxiety or depression
   - ❑ Increased other symptoms (such as voices)
   - ❑ Starting to use alcohol or drugs again, increasing use
   - ❑ Other: _____

3. *Who might you go to for help if you are under a lot of stress or having a crisis (e.g., friends, family, neighbors, mental health team members, support group, etc.)?*

   _____

   _____

   _____

4. *What are some healthy things that you already do to keep yourself well that are helpful? List them here:*

   _____

   _____

   _____

5. *What are a few healthy things to cope with stress or symptoms that you could try out that you haven't used already?*

_____

_____

_____

Now put it all together—your Wellness Plan

If I am feeling stress or PTSD or other symptoms, I will do the following (list the different steps below):
1. _____
2. _____
3. _____
4. _____
5. _____

Is there a supportive person(s) in your life who you would like to share a copy of this Wellness Plan with? List them here, and note when you will share with them:

Name(s): _____

When I will share: _____

LEARNING BREATHING RETRAINING

Breathing fast and taking deep breaths (*hyperventilating*) are common responses to feeling stressed. However, taking in too much extra air or breathing too fast increases the flow of oxygen to the brain. Taking deep breaths can actually lead to feeling lightheaded and feeling even more anxious. *Breathing Retraining (BRT)* is a skill that helps you slow down your breathing and decrease the amount of oxygen going to your brain, which can make you feel less anxious and distressed and help you think straight. The key to this skill is taking in a normal breath (not a deep one) and having a long, slow exhale. Try following the steps below:

Instructions for Breathing Retraining
1. Choose a word that you find relaxing, such as "calm" or "peace."
2. Take in a normal breath (*not a deep one*), and exhale slowly through your mouth.
3. While you exhale, very slowly say the relaxing word you have chosen ("calm" or "peace").
4. Pause briefly before taking your next breath. You can count to four before taking in each new breath.
5. Practice this exercise several times a day, taking 10 to 15 breaths at each practice.

Tips for Using Breathing Retraining

- It is easier to use a one-syllable word (e.g., "peace") than it is to use a two-syllable or longer word (e.g., "relax") during the exhale. This makes the exhalation much smoother.

- At first, while you are learning the skill, practice it only during times when you are feeling relatively calm and safe, *not* when you are feeling upset or anxious. This will help you master the skill so that you can then use it more easily in situations times when you are feeling anxious or distressed.

- It is best to learn and practice the skill by saying the relaxing word aloud. However, if you want to use Breathing Retraining in public, you can say the word in your head while exhaling instead.

Learning Breathing Retraining takes daily practice, but once you get good at it (usually after a few weeks), you can use it in any situation where you feel stressed or anxious or where your PTSD symptoms are getting in the way. It can be very helpful for getting to sleep. Track your progress on the Breathing Retraining Tracking Forms 1: Nondistress Version and 2: Distress Version.

PRACTICE BREATHING RETRAINING TRACKING FORM 1: NONDISTRESS VERSION

Now that you have been taught the Breathing Retraining (BRT) skill, the first step is to practice it every day until you get the hang of it. Try out this skill each day for a week (at least once per day), and use it only during times that you are ***not upset***. Why? You want to make sure that you really know how the skill works firsthand. That way, it will work better for you in the future when you really need it in situations where you feel upset.

Use this form whenever you use the BRT skill. Fill in the date you practiced, where you were and what you were doing, and the number that best describes your experience. There is a sample entry here to help guide you. The more you practice the skill, the easier it will be.

Date of practice	Where was I when I practiced, and what was I doing (brief description only)?	How did it go? 0 = *not well* 1 = *pretty well* 2 = *very well*
March 30, 2023	In bed, just after I woke up in the morning.	2

BREATHING RETRAINING TRACKING FORM 2: DISTRESS VERSION

Now that you have a little more practice with the Breathing Retraining (BRT) skill, you can start using it during stressful times to help you manage your anxiety or other PTSD symptoms. Use this form whenever you use BRT. Fill it out *right before* you use the skill and then *right after* you use the skill. That way you can see if the skill helped you feel better. There is a sample entry here to help guide you. The more you practice the skill and the more you record how it went on this form, the faster and better this skill will work for you.

Date and time	What situation made me upset (describe briefly)?	How upset was I before I practiced? 1 = *a little* 2 = *a lot* 3 = *extremely*	How upset was I after I practiced? 0 = *not at all* 1 = *a little* 2 = *a lot* 3 = *extremely*	Note or comment
April 7, 2023, 6 p.m.	Anxious in the very crowded grocery store; heart beating hard.	3	1	Using BRT before going into the store is a good idea for me.

COMMON REACTIONS TO TRAUMA I: PTSD SYMPTOMS

When people experience a traumatic event, it is common for them to have many distressing feelings as a result, even long after the event. Although each person responds to trauma in a unique way, there are also a number of common reactions. In order to learn how to manage these symptoms, it is helpful to first understand what they are and why they happen. This handout describes the symptoms of PTSD. These are the core symptoms of PTSD:

- *Reexperiencing* the traumatic event or events.
- *Avoiding* things that remind the person of the trauma.
- Being *overaroused or overreactive*.
- *Negative thoughts and mood*.

Reexperiencing the Trauma

A very common way that people reexperience traumatic events is by having unwanted *memories, images,* or *pictures* of part of the trauma suddenly pop into their mind. Sometimes a memory is so vivid that it temporarily feels like the event is actually happening again (a *flashback*). These memories may be triggered by external things (such as a smell, a noise, or a TV commercial) or internal things (such as a thought or feeling). Sometimes the memories seem to come out of nowhere. The person may also have *bad dreams* or *nightmares* about the trauma itself or other frightening situations. When these experiences happen, people may feel they have no control over what they are feeling, thinking, and experiencing.

Avoidance

People often *avoid other people, places,* or *things* that remind them of their traumatic events. Distressing thoughts and feelings about the events are also often avoided. This is quite natural, since thinking about traumatic experiences can be upsetting. However, the avoidance is usually only partially successful. It is difficult to avoid every possible reminder of trauma, and many people find that the more they try to avoid reminders, the more they encounter new triggers that can bring on their traumatic memories.

Sometimes people avoid memories and feelings about the trauma without even being aware of it, such as *forgetting important parts of what happened*. This is very common.

Overarousal and Overreactivity

Another common reaction to trauma is to be *overaroused or hyperalert*. People may feel *tense, agitated, jumpy,* or *hypervigilant*. The person may have a *racing heart* and *tense muscles* and *perspire easily*. People may also be *easily startled* and have *trouble sleeping.* These are all examples of *overreactivity.* All of these problems can lead to *irritable feelings* and *anger outbursts.*

These changes in your body are the result of fear. When people (and animals) are threatened by something, they react by fleeing or fighting—a normal response. This response requires a burst of adrenaline to get the body going and help it respond to danger. When people have experienced traumatic events, they may come to think of the world as dangerous and want to be ready for it. Their body may respond by being in a constant state of *arousal,* so they are ready to *react* right away to the sense of danger, even if there is no real threat. This response can happen quite a lot and can affect many areas of the person's life.

Negative Thoughts and Mood

People often have upsetting thoughts and feelings after traumatic experiences. These beliefs and feelings can be very strong and often overwhelming. Often, these thoughts are not accurate or true but can really feel that way to a person with PTSD. For example, people may have *exaggerated negative beliefs* about themselves, such as "I'm a bad person" or about other people, such as "No one can be trusted." They may also blame themselves for the trauma that happened.

As a result of having these sorts of thoughts, it is common for people with PTSD to have lots of *negative feelings* and *low mood.* They may very often or almost always feel fear, anxiety, anger, sadness or depression, guilt, or shame. And they may also have trouble feeling positive feelings. More information about upsetting feelings can be found in the Common Reactions to Trauma II: Associated Problems handout.

REEXPERIENCING SYMPTOMS WORKSHEET

Reexperiencing symptoms include the following:

- Frequent memories or images of the event.
- Distressing dreams/nightmares.
- Acting or feeling like the event is occurring again (flashbacks).
- Intense distress or feeling upset when reminded of event.
- Intense bodily reactions (heart racing, headache, stomachache, sweating) when reminded.

Instructions: Describe some of the reexperiencing symptoms that have troubled you in the space below:

Images:

Intrusive memories:

Nightmares:

Flashbacks:

Upsetting reminders and triggers:

Body reactions to memories and triggers:

Which of these reexperiencing symptoms is *most upsetting* to you?

Which is most *frequent?*

AVOIDANCE SYMPTOMS WORKSHEET

Avoidance symptoms include the following:

- Avoiding thoughts, feelings, or memories associated with the traumatic event.
- Avoiding talking with people about what happened to you.
- Avoiding activities, places, or people that remind you of the trauma.

Instructions: Describe some of the avoidance symptoms that have troubled you in the space below:

People I avoid:

Places I avoid:

Situations I avoid:

Feelings I avoid:

Thoughts I avoid:

Which of these avoidance symptoms is most *disruptive* or *upsetting* to you?

Which is most *frequent*?

OVERAROUSAL AND OVERREACTIVITY SYMPTOMS WORKSHEET

Instructions: In the space below, check off how your body reacts to stress:

_____ Heart pounding

_____ Trembling/shaking

_____ Sweating

_____ Hot flashes

_____ Trouble falling asleep

_____ Tense muscles

_____ Jitteriness

_____ Restlessness

_____ Feeling tense or uptight

_____ Dry mouth

_____ Lump in throat

_____ Chest pain or discomfort

_____ Nausea or stomachache

_____ Dizziness

_____ Jumpiness (exaggerated startle response)

_____ Difficulty concentrating

_____ Quick temper or anger outbursts

_____ Always on guard

_____ Irritability

_____ Risky, reckless or self-destructive behavior

_____ Other (describe): _____

Which of these overarousal signs is *most disruptive or upsetting* to you?

Which is most *frequent*?

NEGATIVE THOUGHTS AND MOOD WORKSHEET

Negative thoughts and mood symptoms include the following:

- Trouble remembering important parts of the traumatic event(s).
- Negative beliefs about yourself or others.
- Exaggerated or inaccurate thinking about the event(s) that lead you to blame yourself (or others).
- Frequent negative feelings and/or low mood, such as fear, sadness, guilt, shame, or anger.
- Losing interest in activities or people.
- Feeling detached or disconnected from others.
- Feeling numb or not being able to be happy or having a full range of feelings.
- Not seeing yourself as having a future.

Which of these symptoms do you currently experience?

Which is most *disruptive or upsetting* to you?

Which is most *frequent?*

COMMON REACTIONS TO TRAUMA II: ASSOCIATED PROBLEMS

Many people with PTSD also experience other reactions or problems that interfere with their lives, such as upsetting feelings and relationship problems. Understanding why these problems occur after traumatic events can prepare people for learning how to cope with these problems and eventually overcome them. This handout addresses some common associated problems for people who have PTSD:

- *Upsetting feelings*
- *Hearing voices* or other distressing experiences
- *Problems in relationships* with others
- Using too much *alcohol or other drugs*
- Problems with *work* life or *school*
- Challenges in managing with *physical health*

Upsetting Feelings

Common upsetting feelings include fear and anxiety, sadness and depression, guilt and shame, and anger.

1. Fear and anxiety: Anxiety and fear are common feelings after a traumatic event. As noted in the PTSD symptoms handout (Common Reactions to Trauma I: PTSD Symptoms), these feelings may come up when memories of traumatic events are triggered by something—like a certain place, smell, or thought.

   Another common symptom of PTSD is avoiding places, people, or other things that remind the person of their trauma and make them *feel afraid*. These feelings can spread to many different situations, even ones not clearly related to the trauma. This can get to the point where the person feels anxious and fearful much of the time. The person may view the world as a dangerous place and never feel comfortable and safe.

2. Sadness and depression: Another common reaction to experiencing a traumatic event is sadness. Sadness can be experienced as feeling blue, depressed, or hopeless about the future. When people are depressed, they sometimes cry, have thoughts about self-harm or death, and may even think about suicide. They may find it hard to concentrate, and their appetite and sleep patterns may be disturbed, either by eating or sleeping too much or too little. People often lose interest in activities they used to enjoy, so that nothing seems fun to them anymore.

   Sadness and depression may occur in people with PTSD because of the bad memories of their traumatic experiences that are stirred up or because of thoughts about their losses related to the trauma. Depression can also occur because their PTSD symptoms prevent them from being involved in or enjoying fun or meaningful activities—like close relationships, work, school, parenting, or leisure.

3. <u>Guilt and shame</u>: People often have feelings of guilt or shame related to something they did (or did not do) during or after their traumatic experiences. It is common for people to second-guess their reactions and blame themselves for what happened. For example, people who have been assaulted, either sexually or physically, may blame themselves for not having prevented the assault in the first place or for not having successfully fought off the attacker.

   People may also feel ashamed simply because they have PTSD. They may believe that having symptoms like frequent memories of the trauma or nightmares for a long time means they are weak or inferior because they should have "gotten over" the trauma by now.

4. <u>Anger</u>: Feelings of anger are also common reactions to trauma. The anger may be directed at someone who hurt the person. But it can be also stirred up in the presence of other people, such as loved ones or even strangers. The anger may be so strong that the person lashes out at others, either verbally or physically.

   Angry feelings may occur for a variety of reasons—feeling frustrated by having PTSD, misperceiving threats or insults from other people, or over-reacting to situations due to hypervigilance. Sometimes people get angry with themselves because of something they did or did not do during or after their traumatic experiences.

FEAR AND ANXIETY FEELINGS WORKSHEET

Instructions: Anxious and fearful feelings may come and go on their own. Or they may be triggered by thoughts, people, places, or other reminders of traumatic experiences. In the space below, write down the kinds of things that make you afraid.

Things that make me afraid or nervous:

1. *Places*

2. *People*

3. *Activities*

4. *Sounds, smells, sensations*

The way my body feels when I am afraid: _____

_____

My thoughts when I am afraid (check all that apply):

_____ Something terrible is going to happen.

_____ I am going to be attacked or hurt.

_____ I am going to be rejected or abandoned.

_____ I am going to lose control or go crazy.

_____ Other: _____

SADNESS AND DEPRESSION FEELINGS WORKSHEET

Common symptoms of depression include the following:

- Feeling "blue" or "down"
- Feeling worthless
- Feeling hopeless
- Feeling helpless
- Low self-esteem
- Thinking about death or life not being worth living
- Difficulty sleeping (either too little or too much)
- Loss of appetite or weight
- Difficulty concentrating
- Reduced energy level

Instructions: In the space below, write down any symptoms of depression you experience.

My symptoms of depression:

My thoughts when I am sad or depressed (check all that apply):

_____ I am worthless.

_____ I don't have anyone I can depend on.

_____ Nothing will ever get better.

_____ My life is not worth living.

_____ I have no future.

_____ Other: _____

GUILT AND SHAME FEELINGS WORKSHEET

Many people blame themselves for something they did or did not do to survive or cope with the trauma.

__Instructions__: In the space below, describe any feelings of guilt and/or shame you may have had.

Things I feel ashamed or guilty about:

My thoughts when I feel guilty or ashamed (check all that apply):

_____ I am weak or inadequate.

_____ I am a bad person.

_____ I am a failure.

_____ I am to blame for what happened to me.

_____ If only I hadn't done _____, this wouldn't have happened to me.

_____ Other: _____

ANGRY FEELINGS WORKSHEET

Angry feelings may be directed at a specific person involved in your traumatic experience. They can also be directed at people you love the most. Your anger may seem too intense or seem like an overreaction to the situation.

Instructions: In the space below, describe difficulties with anger you have had, including the situations, events, and people that trigger your anger:

Things that trigger my anger:

Situations/events:

People:

My thoughts when I am angry (check all that apply):

_____ I am being treated unfairly.

_____ I am being taken advantage of.

_____ This situation is unfair.

_____ Other: _____

Hearing Voices and Other Distressing Experiences

Hearing voices or noises that other people do not hear is more common when someone has experienced a trauma. In addition, seeing, tasting, smelling, or feeling things that other people do not perceive can also happen when one has had a trauma and as a result of PTSD symptoms.

Sometimes the voice(s) heard are directly related to the traumatic event or memories of the trauma, like hearing the voice of a relative who harmed you. Sometimes the voices say upsetting or blaming things about your experience with the trauma or with having PTSD. They may tell you that the trauma was all your fault or that you deserved to be hurt.

The voices may not seem to be directly related to the trauma but may be negative or critical in general. They may insult you or tell you specific things to do or to not do in your daily life.

These kinds of experiences can be frightening. They can also make someone feel even more fear, sadness, guilt, or anger. When voices or other sensory experiences happen frequently or loudly, they can be very distracting. This can cause even more anxiety and get in the way of living a normal life.

HEARING VOICES AND OTHER DISTRESSING EXPERIENCES WORKSHEET

<u>Instructions</u>: In the space below, check off the types of experiences you have had:

- ❑ Hearing voices
- ❑ Seeing things that others do not see in the moment
- ❑ Unusual scents
- ❑ Unusual tastes
- ❑ Feeling things that others do not report feeling in the moment
- ❑ Seeing another person who is not there or sensing their presence
- ❑ Other unusual experiences? Describe: _____

_____

Which of these is most distressing or upsetting to you?

Which is most frequent?

How do you think this has anything to do with the trauma you experienced or your PTSD symptoms? In which ways?

My thoughts when I am hearing voices or having these other experiences (check all that apply):

_____ I am in danger. I will be harmed by this experience.

_____ I am not able to control my own actions. I have to do what the voice(s) says.

_____ The voice(s) is correct about the negative things they are saying about me.

_____ Other: _____

Note. Data from Amy Hardy, PhD.

Relationship Difficulties

People with PTSD often have difficulty with relationships. These problems may be a result of strong feelings of depression, anxiety, sadness, or anger, which can get in the way of getting along with others. People who have been victimized by another person (like being attacked, raped, or abused) may find it very *hard to trust people* or allow themselves to feel close to someone else. Situations that involve intimacy and closeness can stir up distressing emotions and memories. This can lead people to withdraw and avoid spending time with other people.

Traumatic experiences and PTSD symptoms can also lead to *sexual difficulties* for people who have intimate relationships. They may be less interested in sex because of depression, or they may avoid it because it reminds them of their trauma or makes them feel vulnerable. Sexual relations may also be uncomfortable because they bring on feelings of shame or guilt.

Family relationships can provide joy and support, but they can also be affected when a family member has had trauma. For example, *family relationships may be strained* or *cut off* when one member victimizes another or when a child or adolescent reports being abused to a parent but is not believed.

In general, family members often do not know how to support a relative with PTSD. They may be unable or unwilling to listen to them talk about their traumatic experiences. People with PTSD may also feel inferior around their family because they have not accomplished what they hoped to. It is common for people with PTSD to think their relatives do not understand why they have not yet "gotten over" what happened to them.

RELATIONSHIP DIFFICULTIES WORKSHEET

Problems in your relationships may be related to upsetting feelings you have, such as fear, sadness, guilt, or anger. It may be difficult for you to trust other people or feel close to them. People who love you may have a hard time hearing about your experiences.

Instructions: In the space below, check the types of relationship problems that you are having:

_____ Conflict with spouse/partner/significant other

_____ Conflict with other family members

_____ Violence in relationships/fear for safety

_____ Difficulty developing relationships or friendships

_____ Difficulty keeping relationships or friendships

_____ Difficulty being emotionally close to others

_____ Difficulty trusting others

_____ Sexual difficulties

_____ Other: _____

My thoughts related to relationships with others (check all that apply):

_____ No one can really be trusted.

_____ I don't deserve to have a healthy or happy relationship.

_____ If people found out about my traumatic experiences, they wouldn't want anything to do with me.

_____ Other: _____

Work or School Difficulties

It is common for people with PTSD to have problems working or going to school. People may have fear about going to work or school because it reminds them of their trauma. Or they may believe that they are not capable of working or performing as a student because of what happened to them or due to their PTSD symptoms.

At work, it may be hard to follow directions and perform job tasks because of difficulties concentrating or not getting enough sleep. These same difficulties can interfere with the ability to focus during class, to study for tests, and to complete course assignments.

Problems getting along with other people can also interfere with work or school. Difficulties with trust and feeling comfortable around others can prevent people from forming good relationships with coworkers or other students. If the person was victimized by someone who was an authority figure (such as parent, stepparent, teacher, or coach), it may be hard to listen to and follow instructions from a supervisor, boss, or teacher. Having a lot of angry feelings or a "short fuse" resulting in outbursts of anger can make it hard to cope with the challenges of work or school. This can result in people impulsively quitting a job or dropping out of school when they feel frustrated about something.

WORK AND SCHOOL DIFFICULTIES WORKSHEET

People with trauma may believe they are not capable of working or studying, or they may avoid these activities because of worries they will be reminded about these experiences. People with PTSD may also find it hard to work or go to school due to difficulties such as problems with concentrating, getting along with others, and getting frustrated easily.

Are you currently working or going to school, or have you recently worked or gone to school?

_____ No.

_____ Yes, I am working, or I recently worked.

_____ Yes, I am going to school, or I recently went to school.

If no, would you like to work or go to school?

_____ No.

_____ Yes, I would like to work.

_____ Yes, I would like to go to school.

Instructions: In the space below, check the types of difficulties related to work or school that you are having or have recently had (or think you might have in the future):

_____ Upsetting reminders of trauma

_____ Difficulty concentrating/easily distracted

_____ Uncomfortable around other people

_____ Getting frustrated easily

_____ Conflicts with other people

_____ Feels difficult to be told what to do by boss/supervisor/teacher

_____ Other: _____

My thoughts related to work or school difficulties (check all that apply):

_____ I'm not capable of working or going to school because of my trauma.

_____ People should give me more of a break because of all I have been through.

_____ Work/school is too stressful. I can't handle it.

_____ Other: _____

Drug and Alcohol Problems

Sometimes people with traumatic experiences use alcohol or drugs to avoid thinking about their traumatic experiences or to sleep better. This is very common. Although drinking or using drugs can provide a temporary escape from distressing thoughts and feelings, using substances to cope with PTSD symptoms usually ends up making them worse.

Alcohol or drugs may help people get to sleep faster, but they disrupt the natural sleep cycle, so people end up having more sleep problems in the long run.

The CR for PTSD program teaches people helpful skills for dealing with distressing feelings and traumatic experiences so that they can reduce their need to use drugs or alcohol to cope. However, in order to learn these skills, it is important that you practice them each day and only while sober. If you use substances to cope with your PTSD symptoms, your therapist can help you make a plan for how to not use them before your weekly CR for PTSD sessions or during your practice of the skills on your own between sessions.

DRUGS AND ALCOHOL PROBLEMS WORKSHEET

Alcohol or drugs may be used to try to avoid thinking about trauma, to escape upsetting feelings, or to try to sleep better. While this is a very common and understandable coping strategy, using these substances usually makes things worse in the long run.

Instructions: Describe your use of alcohol and drugs by completing the questions below:

Has there ever been a period of time when the following happened (circle your answer)?

You felt that you used too much.   No   Yes

Your use led to problems (such as relationships, work, legal, health).   No   Yes

Your use was out of your own control.   No   Yes

Someone else was concerned about your use.   No   Yes

If you answered "Yes" to any of these questions, indicate which substances you were using:

_____ Alcohol

_____ Marijuana

_____ Cocaine/crack

_____ Amphetamines/MDMA (meth, molly, ecstasy)

_____ Heroin or other narcotics/opioids (such as oxycodone, fentanyl, Vicodin)

_____ Sedatives (such as Ambien, Ativan, Benzos, Xanax)

_____ Other: _____

Do you use any of these substances on a regular basis?   No   Yes

Do you use more of any of these substances when your PTSD symptoms   No   Yes
are worse?

If so, what happens? Does it help, or does it make your symptoms worse?

_____

_____

_____

My thoughts related to my drug or alcohol use (check all that apply):

_____ This is the only way I can get any relief from my distress/PTSD.

_____ I can't cope or handle it when the traumatic memories come back, so I have to numb myself with substances.

_____ Drugs or alcohol are the only things that bring me any peace or enjoyment.

_____ Other: _____

Managing Physical Health Difficulties

Trauma can take a heavy toll on our bodies and our wellness. People who have experienced trauma are more likely to have physical conditions as a result. Because of their PTSD symptoms, people may not take care of their physical health. People who have been victimized by others may avoid going to the doctor or seeing other healthcare professionals because they feel uncomfortable with the attention to their body. They may not take care of chronic medical conditions because they are preoccupied with their PTSD symptoms.

People may also not live as healthy a lifestyle as they would like to because of their traumatic experiences. Avoiding things that remind them of their trauma can interfere with getting out of their homes for regular exercise. Rather than eating a healthier diet, people may tend to eat less healthy foods that are higher in fat and sweet content because they are comforting and distract them from upsetting memories. Similarly, smoking is also common among people with PTSD and often is used as a comforting coping strategy.

MANAGING PHYSICAL HEALTH DIFFICULTIES WORKSHEET

Trauma can take a heavy toll on our bodies and our wellness. People who have experienced trauma may be more likely to have physical conditions as a result. Because of PTSD symptoms, people may not take care of their physical health and not live as healthy a lifestyle as they would like to.

Instructions: In the space below, check the types of challenges that you are having with managing your physical health:

_____ Not seeing the doctor regularly for routine checkups

_____ Not taking medication regularly for health condition

_____ Not getting enough exercise

_____ Not maintaining a healthy diet

_____ Not taking good care of a medical condition (such as diabetes)

_____ Smoking too much

_____ Other: _____

My thoughts related to managing my physical health (check all that apply):

_____ I have enough problems. It's too much effort to take care of my health.

_____ It's not worth the effort to exercise or eat healthily. Nothing will ever change.

_____ I can't handle a doctor examining me because of my trauma and PTSD symptoms.

_____ I feel judged when I see a healthcare professional.

_____ Other: _____

HOW TRAUMA AFFECTS THOUGHTS AND FEELINGS

Trauma and PTSD often lead to negative thoughts about oneself, other people, and the world in general. Thoughts related to traumatic experiences are very common and can have very personal meanings to us, but they are often not truly accurate. In this treatment program, you will learn more about how to challenge and change distressing thoughts that are not helpful or accurate. The first step, though, is to identify what these thoughts are. How do the traumatic events you've experienced affect how you think about yourself?

Do you tend to *blame yourself*, or are you very *critical of yourself*?

Yes   **No**

If yes, give examples of these types of thoughts:

_____

_____

_____

Do you tend to *distrust other people*?

Yes   **No**

If yes, give examples of these types of thoughts:

_____

_____

_____

Are you generally very fearful, or do you think that *the world is an unsafe place*?

Yes   **No**

If yes, give examples of these types of thoughts:

_____

_____

_____

GOAL-SETTING WORKSHEET FOR THE CR FOR PTSD PROGRAM

Let's say you hadn't ever experienced these traumatic events and you didn't have PTSD. What would be different in your life today? In what ways is your life most impacted by PTSD? If you were able to not be as bothered by your PTSD symptoms, what would your life look like? What are the sorts of things you want for yourself?

Complete this goal-setting sheet to lay out the kinds of goals that you'd like to aim for. This CR for PTSD intervention can help you move toward or achieve these goals.

Some common goals that people have are related to family, friends and romantic relationships, socializing and leisure activities, increasing their activity level, taking better care of their physical health, and pursuing work or school.

Area	Example of goals
1. *Close relationships*	Having friends, seeing friends more often Having a girlfriend, boyfriend, or intimate partner Enjoying sexual relations Spending more time with a family member or friend Improving your relationship with your child
Your goal: _____	
2. *Work and school*	Working at a part-time or full-time job Pursuing a more interesting or demanding job Getting a volunteer job Returning to school or taking a class
Your goal: _____	
3. *Leisure and recreation*	Being able to concentrate while reading Pursuing a fun activity outside the home Developing a hobby or pastime Pursuing a form of self-expression such as art, music, poetry
Your goal: _____	
4. *Self-care and independent living*	Improving care of personal hygiene Doing more household tasks Stopping or reducing the use of alcohol Attending to medical and dental needs Reducing hospitalizations Doing grocery or other household shopping Improving diet and exercise
Your goal: _____	

Now choose your top two or three goals from the above, and briefly describe them below. You and your clinician can work together during the course of the CR for PTSD program to help you take steps toward these goals.

Goal 1: _____

_____

Goal 2: _____

_____

Goal 3: _____

_____

Note. Data from the collective CR for PTSD clinical work of Barent Walsh, PhD, Andrea Wolloff, LMHC, Melissa Jadhav, LMHC, and Angela Bellville, LMHC.

UNDERSTANDING THE THOUGHT–FEELING MODEL WITH THE CBT TRIANGLE

Our feelings don't come from out of nowhere, even though it may seem as though they sometimes do. And our reactions to our feelings (or behaviors) don't come out of nowhere either. In fact, our feelings and how we react to a particular situation are usually caused by the thoughts and beliefs we are having in that situation. That means that if we are feeling sad, we are probably having a thought that is making us feel that way, such as "I'm a worthless person" or "I have no future to look forward to." And if we keep believing that this thought is accurate, rather than challenging and changing it, we will continue to be stuck feeling sad. This is called the *Thought–Feeling Model*.

The same goes for other emotions like anxiety, fear, anger, guilt, or shame. All of these feelings are related to certain thoughts or beliefs we have. But not all of the thoughts and beliefs we have are accurate. In fact, if we closely examine the thoughts and beliefs underlying these negative feelings, we often find they are *not* true.

Where do our thoughts and beliefs come from? We develop thoughts and beliefs about ourselves, other people, and the world based on our personal life experiences, both growing up and in adulthood, including past traumatic experiences. We usually continue to believe our thoughts are true unless we learn how to carefully and critically examine them and change them when they are inaccurate. Learning how to catch and change inaccurate and untrue thoughts and beliefs can reduce or eliminate the distress associated with this thinking.

The first step in learning how to deal with upsetting thoughts and feelings is to better understand what our own patterns of thinking are and what they lead to. The CBT Triangle can help us figure out and learn more about these patterns.

Instructions: To try this out, think of an upsetting situation you had recently. Starting with the "emotions" section of the triangle, write in the blank space the distressing feeling you felt as a result of that situation. In the "thoughts" section, write down the thought you had in that situation that led to the emotion. From there, you can fill in the "behaviors" section by noting how you reacted to that upsetting thought and feeling. There is space on this worksheet for three different upsetting situations.

THE CBT TRIANGLE

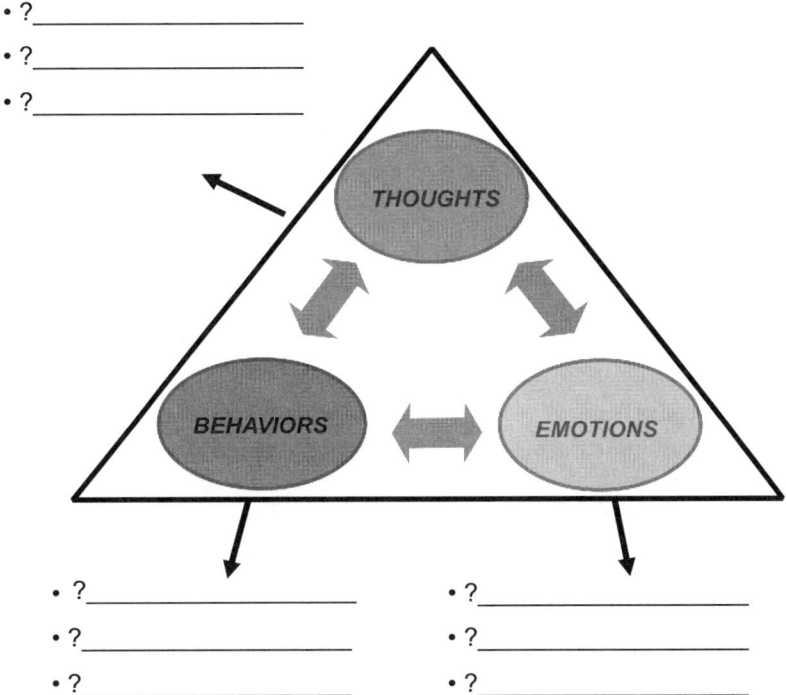

- ?_____
- ?_____
- ?_____

- ?_____
- ?_____
- ?_____

- ?_____
- ?_____
- ?_____

COMMON STYLES OF THINKING INFORMATION SHEET

The Thought–Feeling Model teaches us that our feelings and our thoughts are related to each other and that negative feelings are often caused by thoughts and beliefs. These thoughts and beliefs can be about ourselves, other people, or the world in general, and they come from our past experiences, including traumatic ones.

It is important to understand that not *all* of our thoughts and beliefs are accurate or true. Some are definitely *not accurate*. It is common for people to have inaccurate thinking from time to time. This is especially common for people who have had stressful life events, trauma, and PTSD. Their thoughts and beliefs can be very intense and seem (and feel) very true, and they can lead them to feel a lot of distress. But not all of these thoughts and beliefs *are* true. Catching and changing inaccurate thinking can often reduce or even eliminate the negative feelings associated with them.

It is useful to learn how to take a closer look at your thoughts when you are feeling upset so that you don't end up *jumping to conclusions* in your thinking. Your thought may not actually be accurate or true. Because this is a common problem, it can be helpful to know that there are a number of different categories that most inaccurate beliefs fall into, called *Common Styles of Thinking* (CSTs). Being able to recognize that an upsetting thought you are having is one of these CSTs and therefore is not accurate can help you change the thought to make it more accurate.

Review the list below, and note if you (or someone you know) has had thoughts that fall into these categories.

Common Styles of Thinking Categories

<u>All-or-nothing thinking</u>	The world is seen in extremes with nothing in between. For example: • "Either I'm a perfect student/employee/parent/partner, or I'm a failure." • "The world is a totally dangerous place." Your example:
<u>Catastrophizing</u>	These thoughts occur when people focus on the most extreme and most negative possible outcome. The thoughts often come out of the blue or after a minor problem when the person assumes the very worst will happen. • "I'm probably going to be attacked on the way to work." • "I didn't do well on this exam, so I'm sure I'm going to flunk the class." Your example:

(continues)

Mind reading	This happens when people assume that they know what someone else is thinking without finding out from that person directly. For example: • "She's just being nice because she thinks I am pathetic." • "Everyone is always going think that I am an absolute mess of a person." Your example:
Overgeneralization	A single distressing event is seen as a never-ending pattern. When something bad happens, it is assumed that it will happen again and again. • "Once a victim, always a victim." • "I was unable to keep myself safe before; therefore, I will always be unable to protect myself in the future." Your example:
"Must," "should," or "never" statements	These are unwritten rules or expectations for how people think they should behave that are not based on facts. These "rules" may have been learned when growing up, and they may seem unchangeable. When they cannot be followed, they are distressing. • "I never should have let it happen." • "I should have gotten over this by now." • "I must stop thinking about my abusive experiences." Your example:
Emotional reasoning	This occurs when a person's feelings determine what they think or believe, even though there is no hard evidence to support the belief. Just because a person feels something is true, it doesn't mean that it really is true. • "I feel anxious and afraid, so I must be in danger." • "I feel ashamed, so I must be a bad person." • "I feel down and can't see a future, so my life must be hopeless." • "I feel angry, so somebody must have wronged me." Your example:
Overestimation of risk	The person thinks the risk of something is much greater than evidence supports. • "I'm not going to take a walk because I'll probably be attacked." • "I'm not going to drive because I might get into a car accident." Your example:

(continues)

Inaccurate or excessive self-blame	The person blames themselves for something they had little or no control over or responsibility for. • "It's my fault that I let the abusive relationship go on for so long." • "I'm completely responsible because my child got into a fight at school." Your example: _____
Mental filter	These thoughts occur when the person focuses only on negative aspects of something and ignores the positive aspects. By focusing on the negative, the person does not see the whole picture and feels worse than necessary. • After fumbling for words in a conversation, you tell yourself, "I'm such a screw-up. I made a total fool of myself." • Your boss gives you positive feedback about your work but then recommends improving one area. You think, "My boss is unhappy with my performance." Your example: _____

COMMON STYLES OF THINKING WORKSHEET

<u>Directions</u>: When you begin to feel distressed or upset in any way, ask yourself, "What am I thinking right now that is causing this feeling?" Identify whether the upsetting thought is a Common Style of Thinking, and try to come up with a more helpful or realistic thought. You can use the Common Styles of Thinking Information Sheet handout to guide you. Use this sheet to write down your thoughts.

Situation	Upsetting thought and feeling	Common Style of Thinking[a]	More ACCURATE or realistic thought
Example: On Friday at noon, I was walking down the street when I saw a friend across the street. I called out to say, "Hello," but she did not say anything back to me.	*She must not like me anymore.* *Sad*	*Mind reading*	*Maybe she did not really see me. Maybe she was distracted and was thinking about something else.*

[a] More than one Common Style of Thinking may be related to the distressing thought.

GUIDE TO THOUGHTS AND FEELINGS INFORMATION SHEET

Feeling	Ask yourself	Related thought
Fear or anxiety	What bad things do I expect to happen? What am I scared is going to happen?	Thoughts that something bad will happen, such as these: • Some terrible thing is going to happen. • I am going to be attacked or hurt. • I am going to be rejected or abandoned. • I am going to lose control or go crazy.
Sadness or depression	What have I lost? What is missing in me or in my life?	Thoughts of loss, such as these: • I am worthless. • I don't have anyone I can depend on. • Nothing will ever get better.
Guilt or shame	What bad thing have I done? What is wrong with me?	Thoughts of having done something wrong or lacking in some way, such as these: • I am a failure. • I am to blame for what happened to me. • I am a bad person.
Anger	What is unfair about this situation? Who has wronged me?	Thoughts of being treated unfairly or having been wronged, such as these: • I am being treated unfairly. • I am being taken advantage of. • Someone has done something wrong to me.

THE 5 STEPS OF CR

1. Situation

Ask yourself: "What happened that made me upset?" Write down a *brief* description of the situation, including just the facts:

Situation:

_____

_____

_____

2. Feeling

Circle your strongest feeling. If you have more than one, that's OK (if none of these fit, you can write one in.):

Fear/anxiety   Sadness/depression   Guilt/shame   Anger

3. Thought

Ask yourself: "What am I thinking that is leading me to feel this way?" You can use your *Guide to Thoughts and Feelings Information Sheet* to identify thoughts related to the feeling(s) circled above.

  You may have more than one thought related to the upsetting feeling(s). Write down your thoughts below, but then choose ONE thought to work on. Choose the thought that is *most distressing to you right now, and circle that thought*.

Thoughts:

_____

_____

_____

Is this thought a Common Style of Thinking? If yes, circle the style:

All-or-nothing   Mind reading   Overgeneralization

Must/should/never   Catastrophizing   Emotional reasoning

Overestimation of risk   Self-blame   Mental filter

Write the thought you chose from Step 3 here:

Upsetting thought:

_____

_____

_____

4. Evaluate Your Thought

Now ask yourself: "What evidence do I have *for and against* this thought?" First, write down all the evidence that <u>DOES</u> support your thought. Then, write down all the evidence that <u>DOES</u> <u>NOT</u> support your thought. You can use your *Tips for Finding Good Evidence Information Sheet* to help come up with evidence that DOES NOT support your thought.

Things that <u>DO</u> support my thought:

1. _____

2. _____

3. _____

4. _____

5. _____

6. _____

7. _____

Things that <u>DO NOT</u> support my thought:

1. _____

2. _____

3. _____

4. _____

5. _____

6. _____

7. _____

5. Take Action!

Now, ask yourself: "Do things mostly *support* my thought, or do things mostly *NOT support* my thought?"

❑ **NO**, the evidence *does not* support my thought.

If the evidence does NOT support your thought, come up with a new thought that is supported by the evidence. These thoughts are usually more balanced and accurate (and helpful).

Write your new thought in the space below. Remember, when you think of this upsetting situation in the future or when a similar situation happens, replace your unhelpful thought with this new and more accurate thought.

My new thought:

_____

_____

_____

❑ **YES**, the evidence *does* support my thought.

If the evidence DOES support your thought, decide what you need to do next in order to deal with the situation. Ask yourself, "Do I need to get more information about what to do?" "Do I need to get some help?" "Do I need to take steps to make sure I am safe?" Complete the *Action Plan Worksheet* to help you answer these questions and create a solid plan to deal with the situation.

Note. In some cases, you may decide that the evidence *does not* support your upsetting thought and change it to a more accurate and helpful one. If so, you may also find it helpful to make an Action Plan to deal with that situation. Thus, in some situations, you may find that doing both things—coming up with a new and more accurate thought AND ALSO creating an Action Plan—can be very helpful.

THE 5 STEPS OF CR (ALTERNATE WORKSHEET WITH RATINGS)

1. Situation

Ask yourself: "What happened that made me upset?" Write down a *brief* description of the situation, including just the facts:

Situation:

_____

_____

_____

2. Feeling

Circle your strongest feeling. If you have more than one, that's OK (if none of these fit, you can write one in.):

Fear/anxiety   Sadness/depression   Guilt/shame   Anger

3. Thought

Ask yourself: "What am I thinking that is leading me to feel this way?" You can use your *Guide to Thoughts and Feelings Information Sheet* to identify thoughts related to the feeling(s) circled above.

You may have more than one thought related to the upsetting feeling(s). Write down your thoughts below, but then choose ONE thought to work on. Choose the thought that is *most distressing to you right now, and circle that thought.*

Thoughts:

_____

_____

_____

Write the thought you chose from Step 3 here:

Upsetting thought:

_____

_____

_____

Belief rating: How accurate is this thought? (0 = *completely untrue*, 100 = completely true)

_____

Distress rating: How upsetting is this thought? (0 = *not upsetting*, 100 = *extremely upsetting*)

_____

Is this thought a Common Style of Thinking? If yes, circle the style:

All-or-nothing	Mind reading	Overgeneralization
Must/should/never	Catastrophizing	Emotional reasoning
Overestimation of risk	Self-blame	Mental filter

4. Evaluate Your Thought

Now ask yourself: "What evidence do I have *for and against* this thought?" First, write down all the evidence that <u>DOES</u> support your thought. Then, write down all the evidence that <u>DOES NOT</u> support your thought. You can use your *Tips for Finding Good Evidence Information Sheet* to help come up with evidence that DOES NOT support your thought.

Things that <u>DO</u> support my thought:

1. _____
2. _____
3. _____
4. _____
5. _____
6. _____
7. _____

Things that <u>DO NOT</u> support my thought:

1. _____
2. _____
3. _____
4. _____
5. _____
6. _____
7. _____

5. Take Action!

Considering all the evidence FOR and AGAINST your thought, now how accurate do you think this thought is?

Belief rating: How accurate is the thought? _____ (0 = *completely untrue*, 100 = *completely true*)

NOW, ask yourself: "Do things mostly *support* my thought, or do things mostly *NOT support* my thought?"

❑ **NO**, the evidence *does not* completely support my thought. My belief rating is lower than before.

If the evidence does NOT support your thought, come up with a new thought that is supported by the evidence. These thoughts are usually more balanced and accurate (and helpful).

Write your new thought in the space below. Remember, when you think of this upsetting situation in the future or when a similar situation happens, replace your unhelpful thought with this new and more accurate thought.

My new thought:

_____

_____

_____

New belief rating: _____ (0 = *completely untrue*, 100 = *completely true*)

How much distress do you feel when you think of this new thought? Most people find replacing incorrect, unhelpful thoughts with more accurate and helpful ones reduces their distress.

New distress rating: _____ (0 = *not upsetting*, 100 = *extremely upsetting*)

❑ **YES**, the evidence *does completely* support my thought. My belief rating is the same as before.

If the evidence DOES support your thought, decide what you need to do next in order to deal with the situation. Ask yourself, "Do I need to get more information about what to do?" "Do I need to get some help?" "Do I need to take steps to make sure I am safe?"

Complete the *Action Plan Worksheet* to help you answer these questions and create a solid plan to deal with the situation.

Note. In some cases, you may decide that the evidence *does not* support your upsetting thought and change it to a more accurate and helpful one. If so, you may also find it helpful to make an Action Plan to deal with that situation. Thus, in some situations, you may find that doing both things—coming up with a new and more accurate thought AND ALSO creating an Action Plan—can be very helpful.

TIPS FOR FINDING GOOD EVIDENCE INFORMATION SHEET

You are now learning how to use the *5 Steps of CR*, which is a very important skill. It is the heart of this treatment. One of the most important parts of the *5 Steps of CR* is Step 4: "Evaluate Your Thought." In this step, you first try to think of evidence that supports your upsetting thought. And then you try to think of evidence that *does not* support your upsetting thought.

Sometimes it is difficult to come up with evidence that *does not* support your thought. This is a common challenge when you are learning this skill. It is completely normal to have some trouble with this at first. Some of these upsetting thoughts you have had for many years (maybe since you were a child), and so it can be hard to think of ways that these thoughts may not be true or accurate.

When you are working on Step 4, there are some simple questions you can ask yourself. These will help you come up with some good evidence against your upsetting thought. And they will also aid you in making sure that the evidence you do come up with in both parts of Step 4 is solid and strong. This can assist you greatly as you move through the *5 Steps of CR* so that you feel less upset at the end—which is the goal of the skill and this program.

1. <u>Review the list of questions below, and ask yourself the following:</u>

   - Is there another way to look at this situation?

   - Has there *ever* been *any* time where this thought was not true? When?

   - Can you think of any specific examples of when this thought is not *completely* true?

   - If you decided this thought was a Common Style of Thinking (CST) and is therefore inaccurate, what about the thought makes it a CST? What is the evidence against the thought?

   - Is this thought (or this piece of evidence) really a fact, or is it actually an *opinion*?

   - If you presented this piece of evidence in court, would it hold up? Why or why not?

   - Is this "hard" evidence (based on facts), or is it actually "soft" evidence (based on feelings or thoughts that might seem true but are not necessarily true)?

   If the upsetting thought is so personal that it makes it hard to be balanced in your evaluation of the evidence, ask yourself the following:

   - Do you think other people would see the situation this way? If not, how would they see it?

   - What would someone who was not in the situation say about it? How would they look at it?

   - What would someone else (a friend or supportive person) think about this situation?

- If you presented this to _____, what would they say?
- If a friend was in the same situation, what would *you* say to them?
- What would you say to _____ if this happened to them?
- How would any person in that same situation be expected to respond?
- How do most people tend to react when they are really afraid?

If the upsetting thought is related to something that happened <u>in the past</u>, ask yourself the following:

- What is different about you now versus back then?
- What was going on in your life back when the situation happened?
- What do you think is age-appropriate for a child?
- Does a child have the knowledge of what to do in this type of situation?
- What do we know about how a child should be treated?
- What were you expected to do in that situation? Does that make sense given your age or circumstances?

2. <u>Which of the above questions do you find most helpful? Choose three to five from the list above, and write them below. You can also add one or two of your own questions too.</u>

<u>These are the key questions to ask yourself when you are doing the 5 Steps of CR in the future.</u>

1. _____

2. _____

3. _____

4. _____

5. _____

ACTION PLAN WORKSHEET

Instructions: Follow the steps below to develop a helpful Action Plan.

1. **Define the goal**: What situation requires action?

   Think about what change you would like to see in this situation. Be as specific as possible.

   _____

   _____

   _____

2. **Brainstorm possible strategies**: What can you do to change the situation?

   Use your creative problem-solving skills to think of all the possible things you could do to reduce your distress or address the problem in this situation. When you have made a list of different strategies, think carefully about each one, and place a star (*) next to the best one or ones.

   _____

   _____

   _____

3. **Plan how to put into practice the strategy (or strategies) you chose**: What steps can you take to make this happen?

   Consider these questions: What information do you need to have? Do you need to get some help? Who can support you in taking this action? What obstacles or challenges could interfere with the plan? How could you prevent or deal with these obstacles or challenges? Write down the plan below. Be specific about the actions you will take.

   _____

   _____

   _____

4. **Set a time or a situation to follow up your plan**: When and how are you going to take this action?

   Ask yourself: When do you want to begin your plan? Is there a specific situation or type of situation where you want to use your plan? When is that situation likely to come up again next?

   _____

   _____

   _____

PAYOFF MATRIX

Instructions: This is the thought or belief I am having trouble letting go:

_____

_____

List the advantages and disadvantages of keeping this thought or belief *versus* changing it to a more accurate one. Be as specific as possible.

Advantages of <u>keeping</u> this thought or belief:	**Advantages of <u>changing</u> this thought or belief:**
How does *holding onto* your thought or belief make your life seem more manageable, safer, or easier to handle? Does the thought or belief provide you with a sense of control, security, or predictability of the future?	How could *changing* your thought or belief improve your life? Consider whether changing your thought or belief would reduce distressing feelings and free you of concerns about past events.
Disadvantages of <u>keeping</u> this thought or belief:	**Disadvantages of <u>changing</u> this thought or belief:**
How does *holding onto* your thought or belief make your life more difficult? Consider the role of the thought or belief in causing upsetting feeling for you and preventing you from doing the things you would like to do.	What are the possible disadvantages of *changing* your thought or belief? Would changing the thought or belief lead to you feeling less control, security, or an inability to predict what is going to happen?

The 5 Steps of CR Notecard (2-sided)

The 5 Steps of CR	The 5 Steps of CR

What is
 	
 1. the <u>situation</u>?
 	
 2. my upsetting <u>feeling</u>?
 	
 3. my upsetting <u>thought</u>?
 	
 4. <u>evidence</u> **FOR** the thought? <u>evidence</u> **AGAINST** the thought?
 	
————————————
 	
 5. **Take <u>action</u>! Does the evidence support the thought?**
 	
   NO: What is a more **<u>accurate thought</u>**?
 	
   YES: Make an **Action Plan** for situation.
	What is
	
	 1. the <u>situation</u>?
	
	 2. my upsetting <u>feeling</u>?
	
	 3. my upsetting <u>thought</u>?
	
	 4. <u>evidence</u> **FOR** the thought? <u>evidence</u> **AGAINST** the thought?
	
	————————————
	
	 5. **Take <u>action</u>! Does the evidence support the thought?**
	
	   NO: What is a more **<u>accurate thought</u>**?
	
	   YES: Make an **Action Plan** for situation.

The 5 Steps of CR	The 5 Steps of CR

What is
 	
 1. the <u>situation</u>?
 	
 2. my upsetting <u>feeling</u>?
 	
 3. my upsetting <u>thought</u>?
 	
 4. <u>evidence</u> **FOR** the thought? <u>evidence</u> **AGAINST** the thought?
 	
————————————
 	
 5. **Take <u>action</u>! Does the evidence support the thought?**
 	
   NO: What is a more **<u>accurate thought</u>**?
 	
   YES: Make an **Action Plan** for situation.
	What is
	
	 1. the <u>situation</u>?
	
	 2. my upsetting <u>feeling</u>?
	
	 3. my upsetting <u>thought</u>?
	
	 4. <u>evidence</u> **FOR** the thought? <u>evidence</u> **AGAINST** the thought?
	
	————————————
	
	 5. **Take <u>action</u>! Does the evidence support the thought?**
	
	   NO: What is a more **<u>accurate thought</u>**?
	
	   YES: Make an **Action Plan** for situation.

Tips for finding evidence	Tips for finding evidence
Ask yourself the following: • If this is a Common Style of Thinking, why? • Is there any other way to look at this? • What would you say to a friend in this situation? • Is this a feeling, an opinion or feeling, or a fact? • Do you think other people would see it this way? • Can you think of a time when there has been an exception to this being true? • What is different about you now than before? • How would any person in this situation be expected to respond? • Looking back, what were you supposed to do in that situation given your age and circumstances?	*Ask yourself the following:* • If this is a Common Style of Thinking, why? • Is there any other way to look at this? • What would you say to a friend in this situation? • Is this a feeling, an opinion or feeling, or a fact? • Do you think other people would see it this way? • Can you think of a time when there has been an exception to this being true? • What is different about you now than before? • How would any person in this situation be expected to respond? • Looking back, what were you supposed to do in that situation given your age and circumstances?
Tips for finding evidence	**Tips for finding evidence**
Ask yourself the following: • If this is a Common Style of Thinking, why? • Is there any other way to look at this? • What would you say to a friend in this situation? • Is this a feeling, an opinion or feeling, or a fact? • Do you think other people would see it this way? • Can you think of a time when there has been an exception to this being true? • What is different about you now than before? • How would any person in this situation be expected to respond? • Looking back, what were you supposed to do in that situation given your age and circumstances?	*Ask yourself the following:* • If this is a Common Style of Thinking, why? • Is there any other way to look at this? • What would you say to a friend in this situation? • Is this a feeling, an opinion or feeling, or a fact? • Do you think other people would see it this way? • Can you think of a time when there has been an exception to this being true? • What is different about you now than before? • How would any person in this situation be expected to respond? • Looking back, what were you supposed to do in that situation given your age and circumstances?

SUMMING-UP WORKSHEET

Now that you are nearing completion of the CR for PTSD intervention, it can be helpful to review what you have learned and how to use those skills going forward from here. You and your therapist can discuss the topics below to help you come up with a plan to make sure you are continuing to make progress in the areas of your life that are most important to you.

Skills covered in CR for PTSD program:

- Education about PTSD and related symptoms
- Breathing Retraining for anxiety and PTSD symptom management
- Cognitive restructuring for general and trauma-related distress

What things have gotten better since I started the CR for PTSD program?

1. _____
2. _____
3. _____
4. _____
5. _____

What things do I still want to work on after the program ends?

1. _____
2. _____
3. _____
4. _____
5. _____

Which skills from the CR for PTSD program will help me to work on these things?

1. _____
2. _____
3. _____
4. _____
5. _____

What (and/or who) can help me to remember to use my new skills in these situations?

1. _____

2. _____

3. _____

CHALLENGING MY MOST DISTRESSING PTSD SYMPTOMS AND THOUGHTS

You have worked very hard in this CR for PTSD program to overcome your PTSD symptoms and difficulties. Now that you are close to completing the program, it will be helpful to review the most upsetting situations, feelings, and thoughts related to trauma you have experienced and the ways you have examined them closely. That way, if you have upsetting thoughts and feelings in similar situations in the future, you can remember how you challenged those thoughts and reduced your distress, either by making the thought more accurate or by developing an Action Plan to deal with the situation.

You and your therapist can complete this in your last session(s). An example is provided below to help you.

Upsetting trauma-related situation or reaction	Related distressing feeling(s)	Upsetting thought and Common Style of Thinking	New, more accurate thought and/or Action Plan
Having a hard time with friendships and avoiding other people	*Anxiety Shame*	*No one can be trusted (over-generalization). I'm damaged goods because of what happened to me, and I'm not worth loving (self-blame).*	*There are some people over the years who have shown me kindness who I can trust. Even though I went through something horrible, it was not my fault, and I am worthy of being loved again at some point. Action Plan: Join survivors' support group and one social activity per month.*

REFERENCES

Aas, M., Andreassen, O. A., Aminoff, S. R., Færden, A., Romm, K. L., Nesvåg, R., Berg, A. O., Simonsen, C., Agartz, I., & Melle, I. (2016). A history of childhood trauma is associated with slower improvement rates: Findings from a one-year follow-up study of patients with a first-episode psychosis. *BMC Psychiatry, 16*(1), Article 126. https://doi.org/10.1186/s12888-016-0827-4

Abdelghaffar, W., Ouali, U., Jomli, R., Zgueb, Y., & Nacef, F. (2018). Posttraumatic stress disorder in first-episode psychosis: Prevalence and related factors. *Clinical Schizophrenia & Related Psychoses, 12*(3), 105–112B. https://doi.org/10.3371/CSRP. ABOU.123015

Alameda, L., Christy, A., Rodriguez, V., Salazar de Pablo, G., Thrush, M., Shen, Y., Alameda, B., Spinazzola, E., Iacoponi, E., Trotta, G., Carr, E., Ruiz Veguilla, M., Aas, M., Morgan, C., & Murray, R. M. (2021). Association between specific childhood adversities and symptom dimensions in people with psychosis: Systematic review and meta-analysis. *Schizophrenia Bulletin, 47*(4), 975–985. https://doi.org/10.1093/schbul/sbaa199

Allen, J. G. (2005). *Coping with trauma: A guide to understanding* (2nd ed.). American Psychiatric Association.

Allness, D. J., & Knoedler, W. H. (1998). *The PACT model of community-based treatment for persons with severe and persistent mental illness: A manual for PACT start-up.* National Alliance on Mental Illness.

Álvarez, M. J., Roura, P., Foguet, Q., Osés, A., Solà, J., & Arrufat, F. X. (2012). Posttraumatic stress disorder comorbidity and clinical implications in patients with severe mental illness. *Journal of Nervous and Mental Disease, 200*(6), 549–552. https://doi.org/10.1097/NMD.0b013e318257cdf2

American Psychiatric Association. (1980). *Diagnostic and statistical manual of mental disorders* (3rd ed.).

American Psychiatric Association. (2013). *Diagnostic and statistical manual of mental disorders* (5th ed.).

American Psychological Association. (2017). *Clinical practice guideline for the treatment of posttraumatic stress disorder (PTSD) in adults.* https://doi.org/10.1037/e501872017-001

Anderson, C. M., Reiss, D. J., & Hogarty, G. E. (1986). *Schizophrenia and the family.* Guilford Press.

Anthony, W. A. (1993). Recovery from mental illness: The guiding vision of the mental health service system in the 1990s. *Psychosocial Rehabilitation Journal, 16*(4), 11–23. https://doi.org/10.1037/h0095655

Arata, C. M. (2002). Child sexual abuse and sexual revictimization. *Clinical Psychology: Science and Practice, 9*(2), 135–164. https://doi.org/10.1093/clipsy.9.2.135

Ascher-Svanum, H., & Krause, A. A. (1991). *Psychoeducational groups for patients with schizophrenia: A guide for practitioners.* Aspen Publishers.

Ashcraft, L., & Anthony, W. (2008). Eliminating seclusion and restraint in recovery-oriented crisis services. *Psychiatric Services, 59*(10), 1198–1202. https://doi.org/10.1176/ps.2008.59.10.1198

Avison, W. R., & Gotlib, I. H. (Eds.). (1994). *Stress and mental health: Contemporary issues and prospects for the future.* Plenum. https://doi.org/10.1007/978-1-4899-1106-3

Baethge, C. (2002). Grief hallucinations: True or pseudo? Serious or not? An inquiry into psychopathological and clinical features of a common phenomenon. *Psychopathology, 35*(5), 296–302. https://doi.org/10.1159/000067067

Baldessarini, R. J., Faedda, G. L., Offidani, E., Vázquez, G. H., Marangoni, C., Serra, G., & Tondo, L. (2013). Antidepressant-associated mood-switching and transition from unipolar major depression to bipolar disorder: A review. *Journal of Affective Disorders, 148*(1), 129–135. https://doi.org/10.1016/j.jad.2012.10.033

Barbuti, M., Pacchiarotti, I., Vieta, E., Azorin, J.-M., Angst, J., Bowden, C. L., Mosolov, S., Young, A. H., Perugi, G., & the BRIDGE-II-Mix Study Group. (2017). Antidepressant-induced hypomania/mania in patients with major depression: Evidence from the BRIDGE-II-MIX study. *Journal of Affective Disorders, 219*, 187–192. https://doi.org/10.1016/j.jad.2017.05.035

Barrowclough, C., Meier, P., Beardmore, R., & Emsley, R. (2010). Predicting therapeutic alliance in clients with psychosis and substance misuse. *Journal of Nervous and Mental Disease, 198*(5), 373–377. https://doi.org/10.1097/NMD.0b013e3181da4d4e

Bebbington, P. E., & Kuipers, L. (1992). Life events and social factors. In D. J. Kavanagh (Ed.), *Schizophrenia: An overview and practical handbook* (pp. 126–144). Chapman & Hall. https://doi.org/10.1007/978-1-4899-4457-3_9

Beck, A. T., Rector, N. A., Stolar, N., & Grant, P. (2009). *Schizophrenia: Cognitive theory, research, and therapy.* Guilford Press.

Beck, A. T., Rush, A. J., Shaw, B. F., & Emery, G. (1979). *Cognitive therapy of depression.* Guilford Press.

Beck, A. T., Steer, R. A., & Brown, G. K. (1996). *Manual for the Beck Depression Inventory–II.* Psychological Corporation.

Beck, A. T., Steer, R. A., & Garbin, M. G. (1988). Psychometric properties of the Beck Depression Inventory: Twenty-five years of evaluation. *Clinical Psychology Review, 8*(1), 77–100. https://doi.org/10.1016/0272-7358(88)90050-5

Beevers, C. G., Mullarkey, M. C., Dainer-Best, J., Stewart, R. A., Labrada, J., Allen, J. J. B., McGeary, J. E., & Shumake, J. (2019). Association between negative cognitive bias and depression: A symptom-level approach. *Journal of Abnormal Psychology, 128*(3), 212–227. https://doi.org/10.1037/abn0000405

Bendall, S., Jackson, H. J., Hulbert, C. A., & McGorry, P. D. (2008). Childhood trauma and psychotic disorders: A systematic, critical review of the evidence. *Schizophrenia Bulletin, 34*(3), 568–579. https://doi.org/10.1093/schbul/sbm121

Bentall, R. P., Wickham, S., Shevlin, M., & Varese, F. (2012). Do specific early-life adversities lead to specific symptoms of psychosis? A study from the 2007 The Adult Psychiatric Morbidity Survey. *Schizophrenia Bulletin, 38*(4), 734–740. https://doi.org/10.1093/schbul/sbs049

Berenbaum, H., & Oltmanns, T. F. (1992). Emotional experience and expression in schizophrenia and depression. *Journal of Abnormal Psychology, 101*(1), 37–44. https://doi.org/10.1037/0021-843X.101.1.37

Besser, A., Weinberg, M., Zeigler-Hill, V., & Neria, Y. (2014). Acute symptoms of posttraumatic stress and dissociative experiences among female Israeli civilians exposed to war: The roles of intrapersonal and interpersonal sources of resilience. *Journal of Clinical Psychology, 70*(12), 1227–1239. https://doi.org/10.1002/jclp.22083

Bisson, J. I., Roberts, N. P., Andrew, M., Cooper, R., & Lewis, C. (2013). Psychological treatment of post-traumatic stress disorder (PTSD). *Cochrane Database of Systematic Reviews, 12*, Article CD003388. https://doi.org/10.1002/14651858. CD003388.pub3

Blake, D. D., Weathers, F. W., Nagy, L. M., Kaloupek, D. G., Charney, D. S., & Keane, T. M. (1995). *Clinician Administered PTSD Scale for DSM-IV*. National Center for Posttraumatic Stress Disorder.

Blanchard, E. P., Jones-Alexander, J., Buckley, T. C., & Forneris, C. A. (1996). Psychometric properties of the PTSD Checklist (PCL). *Behaviour Research and Therapy, 34*(8), 669–673. https://doi.org/10.1016/0005-7967(96)00033-2

Blanchard, J. J., Bellack, A. S., & Mueser, K. T. (1994). Affective and social–behavioral correlates of physical and social anhedonia in schizophrenia. *Journal of Abnormal Psychology, 103*(4), 719–728. https://doi.org/10.1037/0021-843X.103.4.719

Blanchard, J. J., Savage, C. L. G., Orth, R. D., Jacome, A. M., & Bennett, M. E. (2020). Sleep problems and social impairment in psychosis: A transdiagnostic study examining multiple social domains. *Frontiers in Psychiatry, 11*, Article 486. https://doi.org/10.3389/fpsyt.2020.00486

Bohus, M., Dyer, A. S., Priebe, K., Krüger, A., Kleindienst, N., Schmahl, C., Niedtfeld, I., & Steil, R. (2013). Dialectical behaviour therapy for post-traumatic stress disorder after childhood sexual abuse in patients with and without borderline personality disorder: A randomised controlled trial. *Psychotherapy and Psychosomatics, 82*(4), 221–233. https://doi.org/10.1159/000348451

Bolton, E. E., Mueser, K. T., & Rosenberg, S. D. (2006). Symptom correlates of posttraumatic stress disorder in clients with borderline personality disorder. *Comprehensive Psychiatry, 47*(5), 357–361. https://doi.org/10.1016/j.comppsych. 2005.12.002

Bovin, M. J., Marx, B. P., Weathers, F. W., Gallagher, M. W., Rodriguez, P., Schnurr, P. P., & Keane, T. M. (2016). Psychometric properties of the PTSD Checklist for *Diagnostic and Statistical Manual of Mental Disorders–Fifth Edition* (PCL-5) in veterans. *Psychological Assessment, 28*(11), 1379–1391. https://doi.org/10.1037/pas0000254

Braakman, M. H., Kortmann, F. A. M., & van den Brink, W. (2009). Validity of 'post-traumatic stress disorder with secondary psychotic features': A review of the evidence. *Acta Psychiatrica Scandinavica, 119*(1), 15–24. https://doi.org/10.1111/j.1600-0447.2008.01252.x

Brady, S., Rierdan, J., Penk, W., Losardo, M., & Meschede, T. (2003). Post-traumatic stress disorder in adults with serious mental illness and substance abuse. *Journal of Trauma & Dissociation, 4*(4), 77–90. https://doi.org/10.1300/J229v04n04_06

Braga, R. J., Mendlowicz, M. V., Marrocos, R. P., & Figueira, I. L. (2005). Anxiety disorders in outpatients with schizophrenia: Prevalence and impact on the subjective quality of life. *Journal of Psychiatric Research, 39*(4), 409–414. https://doi.org/10.1016/j.jpsychires.2004.09.003

Brand, R. M., McEnery, C., Rossell, S., Bendall, S., & Thomas, N. (2018). Do trauma-focussed psychological interventions have an effect on psychotic symptoms? A systematic review and meta-analysis. *Schizophrenia Research, 195*, 13–22. https://doi.org/10.1016/j.schres.2017.08.037

Brandes, D., Ben-Schachar, G., Gilboa, A., Bonne, O., Freedman, S., & Shalev, A. Y. (2002). PTSD symptoms and cognitive performance in recent trauma survivors. *Psychiatry Research, 110*(3), 231–238. https://doi.org/10.1016/S0165-1781(02)00125-7

Brehm, J. W. (1966). *A theory of psychological reactance*. Academic Press.

Breslau, N., Davis, G. C., Peterson, E. L., & Schultz, L. R. (2000). A second look at comorbidity in victims of trauma: The posttraumatic stress disorder-major depression connection. *Biological Psychiatry, 48*(9), 902–909. https://doi.org/10.1016/S0006-3223(00)00933-1

Briere, J. (1992). *Child abuse trauma: Theory and treatment of the lasting effects*. Sage Publications.

Brooker, C., Tocque, K., Kennedy, A., & Brown, M. (2016). The Care Programme Approach, sexual violence and clinical practice in mental health. *Journal of Forensic and Legal Medicine, 43*, 97–101. https://doi.org/10.1016/j.jflm.2016.07.011

Brown, L. A., & Foa, E. B. (2022). Empirically supported psychological treatments: Prolonged exposure. In J. G. Beck & D. M. Sloan (Eds.), *The Oxford handbook of traumatic stress disorders* (2nd ed., pp. 754–770). Oxford University Press.

Brown, V. M., Strauss, J. L., LaBar, K. S., Gold, A. L., McCarthy, G., & Morey, R. A. (2014). Acute effects of trauma-focused research procedures on participant safety and distress. *Psychiatry Research, 215*(1), 154–158. https://doi.org/10.1016/j.psychres.2013.10.038

Browne, J., Cather, C., & Mueser, K. T. (2021). Common factors in psychotherapy. In T. Wykes (Ed.), *Oxford research encyclopedia of psychology* (pp. 1–13). Oxford University Press. https://doi.org/10.1093/acrefore/9780190236557.013.79

Browne, J., Nagendra, A., Kurtz, M., Berry, K., & Penn, D. L. (2019). The relationship between the therapeutic alliance and client variables in individual treatment for schizophrenia spectrum disorders and early psychosis: Narrative review. *Clinical Psychology Review, 71*, 51–62. https://doi.org/10.1016/j.cpr.2019.05.002

Browne, J., Wright, A. C., Berry, K., Mueser, K. T., Cather, C., Penn, D. L., & Kurtz, M. M. (2021). The alliance–outcome relationship in individual psychosocial treatment for schizophrenia and early psychosis: A meta-analysis. *Schizophrenia Research, 231*, 154–163. https://doi.org/10.1016/j.schres.2021.04.002

Burger, S. R., van der Linden, T., Hardy, A., de Bont, P., van der Vleugel, B., Staring, A. B. P., de Roos, C., van Zelst, C., Gottlieb, J. D., Mueser, K. T., van

Minnen, A., de Jongh, A., Marcelis, M., van der Gaag, M., & van den Berg, D. (2022). Trauma-focused therapies for post-traumatic stress in psychosis: Study protocol for the RE.PROCESS randomized controlled trial. *Trials, 23*(1), Article 851. https://doi.org/10.1186/s13063-022-06808-6

Burns, D. D. (1999). *Feeling good: The new mood therapy* (Rev. ed.). Avon.

Butler, R. W., Mueser, K. T., Sprock, J., & Braff, D. L. (1996). Positive symptoms of psychosis in posttraumatic stress disorder. *Biological Psychiatry, 39*(10), 839–844. https://doi.org/10.1016/0006-3223(95)00314-2

Byrne, S., Birchwood, M., Trower, P. E., & Meaden, A. (2006). *A casebook of cognitive behaviour therapy for command hallucinations: A social rank theory approach.* Routledge.

Cackowski, S., Neubauer, T., & Kleindienst, N. (2016). The impact of posttraumatic stress disorder on the symptomatology of borderline personality disorder. *Borderline Personality Disorder and Emotion Dysregulation, 3*, Article 7. https://doi.org/10.1186/s40479-016-0042-4

Calhoun, P. S., Bosworth, H. B., Stechuchak, K. A., Strauss, J., & Butterfield, M. I. (2006). The impact of posttraumatic stress disorder on quality of life and health service utilization among veterans who have schizophrenia. *Journal of Traumatic Stress, 19*(3), 393–397. https://doi.org/10.1002/jts.20114

Calsyn, R. J., Klinkenberg, W. D., Morse, G. A., & Lemming, M. R. (2006). Predictors of the working alliance in assertive community treatment. *Community Mental Health Journal, 42*(2), 161–175. https://doi.org/10.1007/s10597-005-9022-7

Carr, S., Hardy, A., & Fornells-Ambrojo, M. (2018). The Trauma and Life Events (TALE) checklist: Development of a tool for improving routine screening in people with psychosis. *European Journal of Psychotraumatology, 9*(1), Article 1512265. https://doi.org/10.1080/20008198.2018.1512265

Catone, G., Marwaha, S., Kuipers, E., Lennox, B., Freeman, D., Bebbington, P., & Broome, M. (2015). Bullying victimisation and risk of psychotic phenomena: Analyses of British national survey data. *The Lancet Psychiatry, 2*(7), 618–624. https://doi.org/10.1016/S2215-0366(15)00055-3

Cella, M., & Wykes, T. (2019). The nuts and bolts of cognitive remediation: Exploring how different training components relate to cognitive and functional gains. *Schizophrenia Research, 203*, 12–16. https://doi.org/10.1016/j.schres.2017.09.012

Chadwick, P. (2006). *Person-based cognitive therapy for distressing psychosis.* Wiley. https://doi.org/10.1002/9780470713075

Chadwick, P., & Birchwood, M. (1994). The omnipotence of voices. A cognitive approach to auditory hallucinations. *The British Journal of Psychiatry, 164*(2), 190–201. https://doi.org/10.1192/bjp.164.2.190

Chadwick, P., Birchwood, M., & Trower, P. (1996). *Cognitive therapy for delusions, voices and paranoia.* Wiley.

Chemtob, C. M., Novaco, R. W., Hamada, R. S., Gross, D. M., & Smith, G. (1997). Anger regulation deficits in combat-related posttraumatic stress disorder. *Journal of Traumatic Stress, 10*(1), 17–36. https://doi.org/10.1002/jts.2490100104

Clark, D. M. (1989). Anxiety states: Panic and generalized anxiety. In K. Hawton, P. Salkovskis, J. Kirk, & D. M. Clark (Eds.), *Cognitive behavioural therapy for psychiatric problems: A practical guide* (pp. 52–96). Oxford University Press. https://doi.org/10.1093/med:psych/9780192615879.003.0003

Cloitre, M. (2020). *ICD-11* complex post-traumatic stress disorder: Simplifying diagnosis in trauma populations. *The British Journal of Psychiatry, 216*(3), 129–131. https://doi.org/10.1192/bjp.2020.43

Cloitre, M., Koenen, K. C., Cohen, L. R., & Han, H. (2002). Skills training in affective and interpersonal regulation followed by exposure: A phase-based treatment for PTSD related to childhood abuse. *Journal of Consulting and Clinical Psychology, 70*(5), 1067–1074. https://doi.org/10.1037/0022-006X.70.5.1067

Cloitre, M., Stovall-McClough, K. C., Miranda, R., & Chemtob, C. M. (2004). Therapeutic alliance, negative mood regulation, and treatment outcome in child abuse-related posttraumatic stress disorder. *Journal of Consulting and Clinical Psychology, 72*(3), 411–416. https://doi.org/10.1037/0022-006X.72.3.411

Copeland, M. E. (2011). *Wellness recovery action plan* (Rev. ed.). Peach Press.

Corbière, M., Lecomte, T., Reinharz, D., Kirsh, B., Goering, P., Menear, M., Berbiche, D., Genest, K., & Goldner, E. M. (2017). Predictors of acquisition of competitive employment for people enrolled in supported employment programs. *Journal of Nervous and Mental Disease, 205*(4), 275–282. https://doi.org/10.1097/NMD.0000000000000612

Cougle, J. R., Resnick, H., & Kilpatrick, D. G. (2009). Does prior exposure to interpersonal violence increase risk of PTSD following subsequent exposure? *Behaviour Research and Therapy, 47*(12), 1012–1017. https://doi.org/10.1016/j.brat.2009.07.014

Courtois, C. A., & Ford, J. D. (Eds.). (2009). *Treating complex traumatic stress disorders: An evidence-based guide.* Guilford Press.

Coverdale, J. H., & Grunebaum, H. (1998). Sexuality and family planning. In K. T. Mueser & N. Tarrier (Eds.), *Handbook of social functioning in schizophrenia* (pp. 224–237). Allyn & Bacon.

Craske, M. G., & Lewin, M. R. (1998). Cognitive-behavioral treatment of panic disorders. In V. E. Caballo (Ed.), *International handbook of cognitive and behavioural treatments for psychological disorders* (pp. 105–128). Pergamon. https://doi.org/10.1016/B978-008043433-9/50006-7

Cristofaro, S. L., Cleary, S. D., Ramsay Wan, C., Broussard, B., Chapman, C., Haggard, P. J., Jananeh, S., Myers, N. L., & Compton, M. T. (2013). Measuring trauma and stressful events in childhood and adolescence among patients with first-episode psychosis: Initial factor structure, reliability, and validity of the Trauma Experiences Checklist. *Psychiatry Research, 210*(2), 618–625. https://doi.org/10.1016/j.psychres.2013.06.015

Cusack, K., Jonas, D. E., Forneris, C. A., Wines, C., Sonis, J., Middleton, J. C., Feltner, C., Brownley, K. A., Olmsted, K. R., Greenblatt, A., Weil, A., & Gaynes, B. N. (2016). Psychological treatments for adults with posttraumatic stress disorder: A systematic review and meta-analysis. *Clinical Psychology Review, 43*, 128–141. https://doi.org/10.1016/j.cpr.2015.10.003

Cusack, K. J., Grubaugh, A. L., Knapp, R. G., & Frueh, B. C. (2006). Unrecognized trauma and PTSD among public mental health consumers with chronic and severe mental illness. *Community Mental Health Journal, 42*(5), 487–500. https://doi.org/10.1007/s10597-006-9049-4

Cusack, K. J., Herring, A. H., & Steadman, H. J. (2013). PTSD as a mediator between lifetime sexual abuse and substance use among jail diversion participants. *Psychiatric Services, 64*(8), 776–781. https://doi.org/10.1176/appi.ps.000052012

Dalgleish, T. (2004). Cognitive approaches to posttraumatic stress disorder: The evolution of multirepresentational theorizing. *Psychological Bulletin, 130*(2), 228–260. https://doi.org/10.1037/0033-2909.130.2.228

Davidson, L., Tondora, J., Lawless, M. S., O'Connell, M. J., & Rowe, M. (2009). *A practical guide to recovery-oriented practice: Tools for transforming mental health care.* Oxford University Press.

Davison, G. C. (2000). Stepped care: Doing more with less? *Journal of Consulting and Clinical Psychology, 68*(4), 580–585. https://doi.org/10.1037/0022-006X.68.4.580

de Bont, P. A., van den Berg, D. P., van der Vleugel, B. M., de Roos, C., de Jongh, A., van der Gaag, M., & van Minnen, A. (2015). Predictive validity of the Trauma Screening Questionnaire in detecting post-traumatic stress disorder in patients with psychotic disorders. *The British Journal of Psychiatry, 206*(5), 408–416. https://doi.org/10.1192/bjp.bp.114.148486

de Jongh, A., Resick, P. A., Zoellner, L. A., van Minnen, A., Lee, C. W., Monson, C. M., Foa, E. B., Wheeler, K., Broeke, E. T., Feeny, N., Rauch, S. A. M., Chard, K. M., Mueser, K. T., Sloan, D. M., van der Gaag, M., Rothbaum, B. O., Neuner, F., de Roos, C., Hehenkamp, L. M. J., ... Bicanic, I. A. E. (2016). A critical analysis of the current treatment guidelines for complex PTSD in adults. *Depression and Anxiety, 33*(5), 359–369. https://doi.org/10.1002/da.22469

de Jongh, A., ten Broeke, E., Farrell, D. W., & Maxfield, L. (2022). Empirically supported psychological treatments: EMDR therapy. In J. G. Beck & D. M. Sloan (Eds.), *The Oxford handbook of traumatic stress disorders* (2nd ed., pp. 789–803). Oxford University Press.

de Moraes Costa, G., Zanatta, F. B., Ziegelmann, P. K., Soares Barros, A. J., & Mello, C. F. (2020). Pharmacological treatments for adults with post-traumatic stress disorder: A network meta-analysis of comparative efficacy and acceptability. *Journal of Psychiatric Research, 130*, 412–420. https://doi.org/10.1016/j.jpsychires.2020.07.046

de Vries, B., van Busschbach, J. T., van der Stouwe, E. C. D., Aleman, A., van Dijk, J. J. M., Lysaker, P. H., Arends, J., Nijman, S. A., & Pijnenborg, G. H. M. (2019). Prevalence rate and risk factors of victimization in adult patients with a psychotic disorder: A systematic review and meta-analysis. *Schizophrenia Bulletin, 45*(1), 114–126. https://doi.org/10.1093/schbul/sby020

Dean, K., Laursen, T. M., Pedersen, C. B., Webb, R. T., Mortensen, P. B., & Agerbo, E. (2018). Risk of being subjected to crime, including violent crime, after onset of mental illness: A Danish national registry study using police data. *JAMA Psychiatry, 75*(7), 689–696. https://doi.org/10.1001/jamapsychiatry.2018.0534

Dean, K., Moran, P., Fahy, T., Tyrer, P., Leese, M., Creed, F., Burns, T., Murray, R., & Walsh, E. (2007). Predictors of violent victimization amongst those with psychosis. *Acta Psychiatrica Scandinavica, 116*(5), 345–353. https://doi.org/10.1111/j.1600-0447.2007.01078.x

Deegan, P. E. (1988). Recovery: The lived experience of rehabilitation. *Psychosocial Rehabilitation Journal, 11*(4), 11–19. https://doi.org/10.1037/h0099565

Deegan, P. E. (1990). Spirit breaking: When the helping professions hurt. *The Humanistic Psychologist, 18*(3), 301–313. https://doi.org/10.1080/08873267.1990.9976897

DeTore, N. R., Gottlieb, J. D., & Mueser, K. T. (2021). Prevalence and correlates of PTSD in first episode psychosis: Findings from the RAISE-ETP study. *Psychological Services, 18*(2), 147–153. https://doi.org/10.1037/ser0000380

DeVylder, J. E., Lukens, E. P., Link, B. G., & Lieberman, J. A. (2015). Suicidal ideation and suicide attempts among adults with psychotic experiences: Data from the Collaborative Psychiatric Epidemiology Surveys. *JAMA Psychiatry*, *72*(3), 219–225. https://doi.org/10.1001/jamapsychiatry.2014.2663

Dube, S. R., Cook, M. L., & Edwards, V. J. (2010). Health-related outcomes of adverse childhood experiences in Texas, 2002. *Preventing Chronic Disease*, *7*(3), Article A52. https://www.ncbi.nlm.nih.gov/pmc/articles/PMC2879984/pdf/PCD73A52.pdf

Duke, L. A., Allen, D. N., Ross, S. A., Strauss, G. P., & Schwartz, J. (2010). Neurocognitive function in schizophrenia with comorbid posttraumatic stress disorder. *Journal of Clinical and Experimental Neuropsychology*, *32*(7), 737–751. https://doi.org/10.1080/13803390903512660

Dunkley, J. E., Bates, G. W., & Findlay, B. M. (2015). Understanding the trauma of first-episode psychosis. *Early Intervention in Psychiatry*, *9*(3), 211–220. https://doi.org/10.1111/eip.12103

Edwards, V. J., Holden, G. W., Felitti, V. J., & Anda, R. F. (2003). Relationship between multiple forms of childhood maltreatment and adult mental health in community respondents: Results from the adverse childhood experiences study. *The American Journal of Psychiatry*, *160*(8), 1453–1460. https://doi.org/10.1176/appi.ajp.160.8.1453

Ehlers, A., & Clark, D. M. (2000). A cognitive model of posttraumatic stress disorder. *Behaviour Research and Therapy*, *38*(4), 319–345. https://doi.org/10.1016/S0005-7967(99)00123-0

Ehlers, A., Clark, D. M., Hackmann, A., McManus, F., & Fennell, M. (2005). Cognitive therapy for post-traumatic stress disorder: Development and evaluation. *Behaviour Research and Therapy*, *43*(4), 413–431. https://doi.org/10.1016/j.brat.2004.03.006

Ehlers, A., Ehring, T., & Kleim, B. (2012). Information processing in posttraumatic stress disorder. In J. G. Beck & D. M. Sloan (Eds.), *The Oxford handbook of traumatic stress disorders* (pp. 191–218). Guilford Press. https://doi.org/10.1093/oxfordhb/9780195399066.013.0014

Ehlers, A., Ehring, T., Wittekind, C. E., & Kleim, B. (2022). Information processing in posttraumatic stress disorder. In J. G. Beck & D. M. Sloan (Eds.), *The Oxford handbook of traumatic stress disorders* (Vol. 2, pp. 367–414). Oxford University Press.

Ehring, T., Welboren, R., Morina, N., Wicherts, J. M., Freitag, J., & Emmelkamp, P. M. G. (2014). Meta-analysis of psychological treatments for posttraumatic stress disorder in adult survivors of childhood abuse. *Clinical Psychology Review*, *34*(8), 645–657. https://doi.org/10.1016/j.cpr.2014.10.004

El Jabiry, S.-E., Barrimi, M., Oneib, B., & El Ghazouani, F. (2022). Post-traumatic stress disorder in patients treated for schizophrenia: A cross-sectional study in the psychiatric department of Oujda, Morocco. *Annals of Medicine and Surgery*, *77*, Article 103651. https://doi.org/10.1016/j.amsu.2022.103651

Enright, R. D. (2001). *Forgiveness is a choice: A step-by-step process for resolving anger and restoring hope*. American Psychological Association.

Fan, X., Henderson, D. C., Nguyen, D. D., Cather, C., Freudenreich, O., Evins, A. E., Borba, C. P., & Goff, D. C. (2008). Posttraumatic stress disorder, cognitive function and quality of life in patients with schizophrenia. *Psychiatry Research*, *159*(1–2), 140–146. https://doi.org/10.1016/j.psychres.2007.10.012

Farkas, M. (2007). The vision of recovery today: What it is and what it means for services. *World Psychiatry, 6*(2), 68–74. https://www.ncbi.nlm.nih.gov/pmc/articles/PMC2219905/pdf/wpa060068.pdf

Feiring, C., Taska, L., & Chen, K. (2002). Trying to understand why horrible things happen: Attribution, shame, and symptom development following sexual abuse. *Child Maltreatment, 7*(1), 26–41. https://doi.org/10.1177/1077559502007001003

Felitti, V. J., Anda, R. F., Nordenberg, D., Williamson, D. F., Spitz, A. M., Edwards, V., Koss, M. P., & Marks, J. S. (1998). Relationship of childhood abuse and household dysfunction to many of the leading causes of death in adults: The Adverse Childhood Experiences (ACE) Study. *American Journal of Preventive Medicine, 14*(4), 245–258. https://doi.org/10.1016/S0749-3797(98)00017-8

First, M. B., Williams, J. B. W., Karg, R. S., & Spitzer, R. L. (2015). *Structured Clinical Interview for DSM-5 Disorders: Research Version (SCID-5-RV)*. American Psychiatric Association.

Flory, J. D., & Yehuda, R. (2015). Comorbidity between post-traumatic stress disorder and major depressive disorder: Alternative explanations and treatment considerations. *Dialogues in Clinical Neuroscience, 17*(2), 141–150. https://doi.org/10.31887/DCNS.2015.17.2/jflory

Foa, E. B., Ehlers, A., Clark, D. M., Tolin, D. F., & Orsillo, S. M. (1999). The Posttraumatic Cognitions Inventory (PTCI): Development and validation. *Psychological Assessment, 11*(3), 303–314. https://doi.org/10.1037/1040-3590.11.3.303

Foa, E. B., Hembree, E. A., Cahill, S. P., Rauch, S. A. M., Riggs, D. S., Feeny, N. C., & Yadin, E. (2005). Randomized trial of prolonged exposure for posttraumatic stress disorder with and without cognitive restructuring: Outcome at academic and community clinics. *Journal of Consulting and Clinical Psychology, 73*(5), 953–964. https://doi.org/10.1037/0022-006X.73.5.953

Foa, E. B., Hembree, E. A., Rothbaum, B. O., & Rauch, S. A. A. (2019). *Prolonged exposure therapy for PTSD: Emotional processing of traumatic experiences—Therapist guide* (2nd ed.). Oxford University Press. https://doi.org/10.1093/med-psych/9780190926939.001.0001

Foa, E. B., & Kozak, M. J. (1986). Emotional processing of fear: Exposure to corrective information. *Psychological Bulletin, 99*(1), 20–35. https://doi.org/10.1037/0033-2909.99.1.20

Foa, E. B., McLean, C. P., Zang, Y., Zhong, J., Powers, M. B., Kauffman, B. Y., Rauch, S., Porter, K., & Knowles, K. (2016). Psychometric properties of the Posttraumatic Diagnostic Scale for *DSM-5* (PDS-5). *Psychological Assessment, 28*(10), 1166–1171. https://doi.org/10.1037/pas0000258

Foa, E. B., Riggs, D. S., Dancu, C. V., & Rothbaum, B. O. (1993). Reliability and validity of a brief instrument for assessing post-traumatic stress disorder. *Journal of Traumatic Stress, 6*(4), 459–473. https://doi.org/10.1002/jts.2490060405

Foa, E. B., Riggs, D. S., Massie, E., & Yarczower, M. (1995). The impact of fear activation and anger on the efficacy of exposure treatment for posttraumatic stress disorder. *Behavior Therapy, 26*(3), 487–499. https://doi.org/10.1016/S0005-7894(05)80096-6

Foa, E. B., & Rothbaum, B. O. (1998). *Treating the trauma of rape: Cognitive-behavioral therapy for PTSD*. Guilford Press.

Fowler, D., Garety, P., & Kuipers, E. (1995). *Cognitive behaviour therapy for psychosis: Theory and practice*. Wiley.

Freedman, S. R., & Enright, R. D. (1996). Forgiveness as an intervention goal with incest survivors. *Journal of Consulting and Clinical Psychology, 64*(5), 983–992. https://doi.org/10.1037/0022-006X.64.5.983

Freeman, D., Waite, F., Startup, H., Myers, E., Lister, R., McInerney, J., Harvey, A. G., Geddes, J., Zaiwalla, Z., Luengo-Fernandez, R., Foster, R., Clifton, L., & Yu, L.-M. (2015). Efficacy of cognitive behavioural therapy for sleep improvement in patients with persistent delusions and hallucinations (BEST): A prospective, assessor-blind, randomised controlled pilot trial. *The Lancet Psychiatry, 2*(11), 975–983. https://doi.org/10.1016/S2215-0366(15)00314-4

Frueh, B. C., Grubaugh, A. L., Cusack, K. J., Kimble, M. O., Elhai, J. D., & Knapp, R. G. (2009). Exposure-based cognitive-behavioral treatment of PTSD in adults with schizophrenia or schizoaffective disorder: A pilot study. *Journal of Anxiety Disorders, 23*(5), 665–675. https://doi.org/10.1016/j.janxdis.2009.02.005

Fukui, S., Rollins, A. L., & Salyers, M. P. (2020). Characteristics and job stressors associated with turnover and turnover intention among community mental health providers. *Psychiatric Services, 71*(3), 289–292. https://doi.org/10.1176/appi.ps.201900246

Garety, P. A., & Hemsley, D. R. (1994). *Delusions: Investigations into the psychology of delusional reasoning.* Oxford University Press.

Gearon, J. S., & Bellack, A. S. (1999). Women with schizophrenia and co-occurring substance use disorders: An increased risk for violent victimization and HIV. *Community Mental Health Journal, 35*(5), 401–419. https://doi.org/10.1023/A:1018778310859

Gehrs, M., & Goering, P. (1994). The relationship between the working alliance and rehabilitation outcomes of schizophrenia. *Psychosocial Rehabilitation Journal, 18*(2), 43–54. https://doi.org/10.1037/h0095517

Gershuny, B. S., Cloitre, M., & Otto, M. W. (2003). Peritraumatic dissociation and PTSD severity: Do event-related fears about death and control mediate their relation? *Behaviour Research and Therapy, 41*(2), 157–166. https://doi.org/10.1016/S0005-7967(01)00134-6

Gilbert, P., & Choden. (2014). *Mindful compassion: How the science of compassion can help you understand your emotions, live in the present, and connect deeply with others.* New Harbinger.

Gilbert, P., & Irons, C. (2005). Focused therapies and compassionate mind training for shame and self-attacking. In P. Gilbert (Ed.), *Compassion: Conceptualisations, research and use in psychotherapy* (pp. 263–325). Routledge. https://doi.org/10.4324/9780203003459-15

Gilbertson, M. W., Paulus, L. A., Williston, S. K., Gurvits, T. V., Lasko, N. B., Pitman, R. K., & Orr, S. P. (2006). Neurocognitive function in monozygotic twins discordant for combat exposure: Relationship to posttraumatic stress disorder. *Journal of Abnormal Psychology, 115*(3), 484–495. https://doi.org/10.1037/0021-843X.115.3.484

Gingerich, S., & Mueser, K. T. (2011). *Illness management and recovery: Personalized skills and strategies for those with mental illness* (3rd ed.). Hazelden.

Goldberg, J. F., & Ernst, C. L. (2016). What to do when your depressed patient develops mania. *Federal Practitioner, 33*(Suppl. 2), 26S–33S. https://www.ncbi.nlm.nih.gov/pmc/articles/PMC6375439/pdf/fp-33-3s-26s.pdf

Goldstein, R. B., Smith, S. M., Chou, S. P., Saha, T. D., Jung, J., Zhang, H., Pickering, R. P., Ruan, W. J., Huang, B., & Grant, B. F. (2016). The epidemiology of *DSM-5* posttraumatic stress disorder in the United States: Results from the National Epidemiologic Survey on Alcohol and Related Conditions-III. *Social Psychiatry and Psychiatric Epidemiology, 51*(8), 1137–1148. https://doi.org/10.1007/s00127-016-1208-5

Goodman, C., Finkel, B., Naser, M., Andreyev, P., Segev, Y., Kurs, R., Melamed, Y., & Bleich, A. (2007). Neurocognitive deterioration in elderly chronic schizophrenia patients with and without PTSD. *Journal of Nervous and Mental Disease, 195*(5), 415–420. https://doi.org/10.1097/NMD.0b013e31802c1424

Goodman, L. A., Corcoran, C., Turner, K., Yuan, N., & Green, B. L. (1998). Assessing traumatic event exposure: General issues and preliminary findings for the Stressful Life Events Screening Questionnaire. *Journal of Traumatic Stress, 11*(3), 521–542. https://doi.org/10.1023/A:1024456713321

Goodman, L. A., Dutton, M. A., & Harris, M. (1995). Physical and sexual assault prevalence among episodically homeless women with serious mental illness. *American Journal of Orthopsychiatry, 65*(4), 468–478. https://doi.org/10.1037/h0079669

Goodman, L. A., Salyers, M. P., Mueser, K. T., Rosenberg, S. D., Swartz, M., Essock, S. M., Osher, F. C., Butterfield, M. I., Swanson, J., Lamb-Pagone, J., Burns, B. J., Meador, K. G., Swanson, J. W., Becker, M. E., Bosworth, H. B., Frothingham, R., Horner, R. D., McIntyre, L. M., Spivey, P. M., . . . Vidaver, R. M. (2001). Recent victimization in women and men with severe mental illness: Prevalence and correlates. *Journal of Traumatic Stress, 14*(4), 615–632. https://doi.org/10.1023/A:1013026318450

Goodman, L. A., Thompson, K. M., Weinfurt, K., Corl, S., Acker, P., Mueser, K. T., & Rosenberg, S. D. (1999). Reliability of reports of violent victimization and PTSD among men and women with SMI. *Journal of Traumatic Stress, 12*(4), 587–599. https://doi.org/10.1023/A:1024708916143

Goodwin, F. K., & Jamison, K. R. (2007). *Manic depressive illness* (2nd ed.). Oxford University Press.

Gottlieb, J. D., Poyato, N., Valiente, C., Perdigón, A., & Vázquez, C. (2018). Trauma and posttraumatic stress disorder in Spanish public mental health system clients with severe psychiatric conditions: Clinical and demographic correlates. *Psychiatric Rehabilitation Journal, 41*(3), 234–242. https://doi.org/10.1037/prj0000318

Gould, F., Harvey, P. D., Hodgins, G., Jones, M. T., Michopoulos, V., Maples-Keller, J., Rothbaum, B. O., Rothbaum, A. O., Ressler, K. J., & Nemeroff, C. B. (2021). Prior trauma-related experiences predict the development of posttraumatic stress disorder after a new traumatic event. *Depression and Anxiety, 38*(1), 40–47. https://doi.org/10.1002/da.23084

Gradus, J. L., Qin, P., Lincoln, A. K., Miller, M., Lawler, E., Sørensen, H. T., & Lash, T. L. (2010). Posttraumatic stress disorder and completed suicide. *American Journal of Epidemiology, 171*(6), 721–727. https://doi.org/10.1093/aje/kwp456

Granholm, E., Ben-Zeev, D., & Link, P. C. (2009). Social disinterest attitudes and group cognitive-behavioral social skills training for functional disability in schizophrenia. *Schizophrenia Bulletin, 35*(5), 874–883. https://doi.org/10.1093/schbul/sbp072

Granholm, E., Holden, J., Link, P. C., & McQuaid, J. R. (2014). Randomized clinical trial of cognitive behavioral social skills training for schizophrenia: Improvement in functioning and experiential negative symptoms. *Journal of Consulting and Clinical Psychology, 82*(6), 1173–1185. https://doi.org/10.1037/a0037098

Granholm, E., Holden, J., & Worley, M. (2018). Improvement in negative symptoms and functioning in cognitive-behavioral social skills training for schizophrenia: Mediation by defeatist performance attitudes and asocial beliefs. *Schizophrenia Bulletin, 44*(3), 653–661. https://doi.org/10.1093/schbul/sbx099

Granholm, E. L., McQuaid, J. R., & Holden, J. L. (2016). *Cognitive-behavioral social skills training for schizophrenia: A practical treatment guide.* Guilford Press.

Grant, P. M., & Beck, A. T. (2009). Defeatist beliefs as a mediator of cognitive impairment, negative symptoms, and functioning in schizophrenia. *Schizophrenia Bulletin, 35*(4), 798–806. https://doi.org/10.1093/schbul/sbn008

Grant, P. M., Huh, G. A., Perivoliotis, D., Stolar, N. M., & Beck, A. T. (2012). Randomized trial to evaluate the efficacy of cognitive therapy for low-functioning patients with schizophrenia. *Archives of General Psychiatry, 69*(2), 121–127. https://doi.org/10.1001/archgenpsychiatry.2011.129

Grubaugh, A. L., Brown, W. J., Wojtalik, J. A., Myers, U. S., & Eack, S. M. (2021). Meta-analysis of the treatment of posttraumatic stress disorder in adults with comorbid severe mental illness. *Journal of Clinical Psychiatry, 82*(2), Article 20r13584. https://doi.org/10.4088/JCP.20r13584

Grubaugh, A. L., Clapp, J. D., Frueh, B. C., Tuerk, P. W., Knapp, R. G., & Egede, L. E. (2016). Open trial of exposure therapy for PTSD among patients with severe and persistent mental illness. *Behaviour Research and Therapy, 78*, 1–12. https://doi.org/10.1016/j.brat.2015.12.006

Grubaugh, A. L., Cusack, K. J., & Zinzow, H. M. (2008). "Trumping rules" affect diagnoses of persons with severe mental illness. *Psychiatric Services, 59*(10), 1219–1220. https://doi.org/10.1176/ps.2008.59.10.1219

Grubaugh, A. L., Elhai, J. D., Cusack, K. J., Wells, C., & Frueh, B. C. (2007). Screening for PTSD in public-sector mental health settings: The diagnostic utility of the PTSD checklist. *Depression and Anxiety, 24*(2), 124–129. https://doi.org/10.1002/da.20226

Grubaugh, A. L., Zinzow, H. M., Paul, L., Egede, L. E., & Frueh, B. C. (2011). Trauma exposure and posttraumatic stress disorder in adults with severe mental illness: A critical review. *Clinical Psychology Review, 31*(6), 883–899. https://doi.org/10.1016/j.cpr.2011.04.003

Halász, I., Levy-Gigi, E., Kelemen, O., Benedek, G., & Kéri, S. (2013). Neuropsychological functions and visual contrast sensitivity in schizophrenia: The potential impact of comorbid posttraumatic stress disorder (PTSD). *Frontiers in Psychology, 4*, Article 136. https://doi.org/10.3389/fpsyg.2013.00136

Hamblen, J. L., Jankowski, M. K., Rosenberg, S. D., & Mueser, K. T. (2004). Cognitive-behavioral treatment for PTSD in people with severe mental illness: Three case studies. *American Journal of Psychiatric Rehabilitation, 7*(2), 147–170. https://doi.org/10.1080/15487760490476192

Hardy, K. V., & Mueser, K. T. (2017). Trauma, psychosis and posttraumatic stress disorder. *Frontiers in Psychiatry, 8*, Article 220. https://doi.org/10.3389/fpsyt.2017.00220

Harned, M. S., Korslund, K. E., & Linehan, M. M. (2014). A pilot randomized controlled trial of dialectical behavior therapy with and without the dialectical behavior therapy prolonged exposure protocol for suicidal and self-injuring women with borderline personality disorder and PTSD. *Behaviour Research and Therapy, 55*, 7–17. https://doi.org/10.1016/j.brat.2014.01.008

Harvey, P. D., Siever, L. J., Huang, G. D., Muralidhar, S., Zhao, H., Miller, P., Aslan, M., Mane, S., McNamara, M., Gleason, T., Brophy, M., Przygodszki, R., O'Leary, T. J., Gaziano, M., & Concato, J. (2014). The genetics of functional disability in schizophrenia and bipolar illness: Methods and initial results for VA cooperative study #572. *American Journal of Medical Genetics Part B: Neuropsychiatric Genetics, 165*(4), 381–389. https://doi.org/10.1002/ajmg.b.32242

Havens, J. F., Ford, J., Grasso, D., & Marr, M. (2012). Opening Pandora's box: The importance of trauma identification and intervention in hospitalized and incarcerated adolescent populations. *Adolescent Psychiatry, 2*(4), 309–312. https://doi.org/10.2174/2210676611202040309

Hayes, S. C., Strosahl, K. D., & Wilson, K. G. (2012). *Acceptance and commitment therapy: An experiential approach to behavior change* (2nd ed.). Guilford Press. https://doi.org/10.1037/17335-000

Herman, J. L. (1992). Complex PTSD: A syndrome in survivors of prolonged and repeated trauma. *Journal of Traumatic Stress, 5*(3), 377–391. https://doi.org/10.1002/jts.2490050305

Ho, F. Y.-Y., Yeung, W.-F., Ng, T. H. Y., & Chan, C. S. (2016). The efficacy and cost-effectiveness of stepped care prevention and treatment for depressive and/or anxiety disorders: A systematic review and meta-analysis. *Scientific Reports, 6*(1), Article 29281. https://doi.org/10.1038/srep29281

Hoffmann, H., Jäckel, D., Glauser, S., Mueser, K. T., & Kupper, Z. (2014). Long-term effectiveness of supported employment: 5-year follow-up of a randomized controlled trial. *The American Journal of Psychiatry, 171*(11), 1183–1190. https://doi.org/10.1176/appi.ajp.2014.13070857

Horowitz, M. J. (1975). Intrusive and repetitive thoughts after stress. *Archives of General Psychiatry, 32*(11), 1457–1463. https://doi.org/10.1001/archpsyc.1975.01760290125015

Horowitz, M. J. (1986). *Stress response syndromes* (2nd ed.). Jason Aronson.

Horvath, A. O., & Greenberg, L. S. (1989). Development and validation of the Working Alliance Inventory. *Journal of Counseling Psychology, 36*(2), 223–233. https://doi.org/10.1037/0022-0167.36.2.223

Hoskins, M. D., Bridges, J., Sinnerton, R., Nakamura, A., Underwood, J. F. G., Slater, A., Lee, M. R. D., Clarke, L., Lewis, C., Roberts, N. P., & Bisson, J. I. (2021). Pharmacological therapy for post-traumatic stress disorder: A systematic review and meta-analysis of monotherapy, augmentation and head-to-head approaches. *European Journal of Psychotraumatology, 12*(1), Article 1802920. https://doi.org/10.1080/20008198.2020.1802920

Howes, O. D., & Murray, R. M. (2014). Schizophrenia: An integrated sociodevelopmental-cognitive model. *Lancet, 383*(9929), 1677–1687. https://doi.org/10.1016/S0140-6736(13)62036-X

Huang, Z.-D., Zhao, Y.-F., Li, S., Gu, H.-Y., Lin, L.-L., Yang, Z.-Y., Niu, Y.-M., Zhang, C., & Luo, J. (2020). Comparative efficacy and acceptability of pharmaceutical management for adults with post-traumatic stress disorder: A systematic review and meta-analysis. *Frontiers in Pharmacology, 11*, Article 559. https://doi.org/10.3389/fphar.2020.00559

Huckshorn, K., & Lebel, J. L. (2013). Trauma-informed care. In K. Yeager, D. Cutler, D. Svendsen, & G. Sills (Eds.), *Modern community mental health: An interdisciplinary approach* (pp. 62–83). Oxford University Press.

Ibáñez, A. F., Sevillano, C. P., Serven, E. G., & Sánchez, E. A. (2014). Trauma, posttraumatic stress disorder and psychosis: Etiopathogenic and nosological implications. *European Journal of Psychiatry, 28*(1), 27–38. https://doi.org/10.4321/S0213-61632014000100003

International Society for Traumatic Stress Studies. (2018). *ISTSS PTSD prevention and treatment guidelines: Methodology and recommendations.* https://istss.org/getattachment/Treating-Trauma/New-ISTSS-Prevention-and-Treatment-Guidelines/ISTSS_PreventionTreatmentGuidelines_FNL.pdf.aspx

Janoff-Bulman, R. (1989). Assumptive worlds and the stress of traumatic events: Applications of the schema construct. *Social Cognition, 7*(2), 113–136. https://doi.org/10.1521/soco.1989.7.2.113

Janoff-Bulman, R. (1992). *Shattered assumptions: Towards a new psychology of trauma.* The Free Press.

Jennings, A. (1994). On being invisible in the mental health system. *Journal of Mental Health Administration, 21*(4), 374–387. https://doi.org/10.1007/BF02521356

Jennings, A. (1995). Retraumatizing victims of sexual abuse. In M. Pritchard (Ed.), *Dare to vision: Shaping the national agenda for women, abuse and mental health services* (pp. 16–18). Human Resource Association of the Northeast.

Jiang, W.-J., Zhong, B.-L., Liu, L.-Z., Zhou, Y.-J., Hu, X.-H., & Li, Y. (2018). Reliability and validity of the Chinese version of the Childhood Trauma Questionnaire–Short Form for inpatients with schizophrenia. *PLOS ONE, 13*(12), Article e0208779. https://doi.org/10.1371/journal.pone.0208779

Johnsen, G. E., & Asbjørnsen, A. E. (2008). Consistent impaired verbal memory in PTSD: A meta-analysis. *Journal of Affective Disorders, 111*(1), 74–82. https://doi.org/10.1016/j.jad.2008.02.007

Kahn, R. S., & Keefe, R. S. (2013). Schizophrenia is a cognitive illness: Time for a change in focus. *JAMA Psychiatry, 70*(10), 1107–1112. https://doi.org/10.1001/jamapsychiatry.2013.155

Kane, J. M., Robinson, D. G., Schooler, N. R., Mueser, K. T., Penn, D. L., Rosenheck, R. A., Addington, J., Brunette, M. F., Correll, C. U., Estroff, S. E., Marcy, P., Robinson, J., Meyer-Kalos, P. S., Gottlieb, J. D., Glynn, S. M., Lynde, D. W., Pipes, R., Kurian, B. T., Miller, A. L., . . . Heinssen, R. K. (2016). Comprehensive versus usual care for first episode psychosis: Two-year outcomes from the NIMH RAISE Early Treatment Program. *The American Journal of Psychiatry, 173*(4), 362–372. https://doi.org/10.1176/appi.ajp.2015.15050632

Kaplan, B. (Ed.). (1964). *The inner world of mental illness.* Harper & Row.

Karatzias, T., McGlanaghy, E., & Cloitre, M. (2023). Enhanced skills training in affective and interpersonal regulation (ESTAIR): A new modular treatment for *ICD-11* complex posttraumatic stress disorder (CPTSD). *Brain Sciences, 13*(9), Article 1300. https://doi.org/10.3390/brainsci13091300

Karatzias, T., Murphy, P., Cloitre, M., Bisson, J., Roberts, N., Shevlin, M., Hyland, P., Maercker, A., Ben-Ezra, M., Coventry, P., Mason-Roberts, S., Bradley, A., & Hutton, P. (2019). Psychological interventions for *ICD-11* complex PTSD symptoms: Systematic review and meta-analysis. *Psychological Medicine, 49*(11), 1761–1775. https://doi.org/10.1017/S0033291719000436

Kaulkstein, S., Hurford, I., & Gur, R. C. (2010). Neurocognition in schizophrenia. In N. R. Swerdlow (Ed.), *Behavioral neurobiology of schizophrenia and its treatment* (Vol. 4, pp. 373–390). Springer. https://doi.org/10.1007/7854_2010_42

Kendler, K. S., Ohlsson, H., Mezuk, B., Sundquist, J. O., & Sundquist, K. (2016). Observed cognitive performance and deviation from familial cognitive aptitude at age 16 years and ages 18 to 20 years and risk for schizophrenia and bipolar illness in a Swedish national sample. *JAMA Psychiatry, 73*(5), 465–471. https://doi.org/10.1001/jamapsychiatry.2016.0053

Kennedy, A. C., & Prock, K. A. (2018). "I still feel like i am not normal": A review of the role of stigma and stigmatization among female survivors of child sexual abuse, sexual assault, and intimate partner violence. *Trauma, Violence & Abuse, 19*(5), 512–527. https://doi.org/10.1177/1524838016673601

Kessler, R. C., Benjet, C., Bromet, E. J., & Rosellini, A. J. (2022). The epidemiology of PTSD among adults. In J. G. Beck & D. M. Sloan (Eds.), *The Oxford handbook of traumatic stress disorders* (2nd ed., pp. 126–154). Oxford University Press.

Kessler, R. C., Chiu, W. T., Demler, O., Merikangas, K. R., & Walters, E. E. (2005). Prevalence, severity, and comorbidity of 12-month *DSM-IV* disorders in the National Comorbidity Survey Replication. *Archives of General Psychiatry, 62*(6), 617–627. https://doi.org/10.1001/archpsyc.62.6.617

Kessler, R. C., Rose, S., Koenen, K. C., Karam, E. G., Stang, P. E., Stein, D. J., Heeringa, S. G., Hill, E. D., Liberzon, I., McLaughlin, K. A., McLean, S. A., Pennell, B. E., Petukhova, M., Rosellini, A. J., Ruscio, A. M., Shahly, V., Shalev, A. Y., Silove, D., Zaslavsky, A. M., . . . Carmen Viana, M. (2014). How well can post-traumatic stress disorder be predicted from pre-trauma risk factors? An exploratory study in the WHO World Mental Health Surveys. *World Psychiatry, 13*(3), 265–274. https://doi.org/10.1002/wps.20150

Kessler, R. C., Sonnega, A., Bromet, E., Hughes, M., & Nelson, C. B. (1995). Posttraumatic stress disorder in the National Comorbidity Survey. *Archives of General Psychiatry, 52*(12), 1048–1060. https://doi.org/10.1001/archpsyc.1995.03950240066012

Khalifeh, H., Johnson, S., Howard, L. M., Borschmann, R., Osborn, D., Dean, K., Hart, C., Hogg, J., & Moran, P. (2015). Violent and non-violent crime against adults with severe mental illness. *The British Journal of Psychiatry, 206*(4), 275–282. https://doi.org/10.1192/bjp.bp.114.147843

Kilpatrick, D. G., Resnick, H. S., Milanak, M. E., Miller, M. W., Keyes, K. M., & Friedman, M. J. (2013). National estimates of exposure to traumatic events and PTSD prevalence using *DSM-IV* and *DSM-5* criteria. *Journal of Traumatic Stress, 26*(5), 537–547. https://doi.org/10.1002/jts.21848

Kim, D., Bae, H., Han, C., Oh, H. Y., & Macdonald, K. (2013). Psychometric properties of the Childhood Trauma Questionnaire–Short Form (CTQ-SF) in Korean patients with schizophrenia. *Schizophrenia Research, 144*(1–3), 93–98. https://doi.org/10.1016/j.schres.2012.12.020

Kingdon, D. G., & Turkington, D. (1994). *Cognitive-behavioral therapy of schizophrenia.* Guilford Press.

Kingdon, D. G., & Turkington, D. (2004). *Cognitive therapy of schizophrenia.* Guilford Press.

Kopelovich, S. L., Strachan, E., Sivec, H., & Kreider, V. (2019). Stepped care as an implementation and service delivery model for cognitive behavioral therapy for psychosis. *Community Mental Health Journal, 55*(5), 755–767. https://doi.org/10.1007/s10597-018-00365-6

Kredlow, M. A., Szuhany, K. L., Lo, S., Xie, H., Gottlieb, J. D., Rosenberg, S. D., & Mueser, K. T. (2017). Cognitive behavioral therapy for posttraumatic stress disorder in individuals with severe mental illness and borderline personality disorder. *Psychiatry Research, 249,* 86–93. https://doi.org/10.1016/j.psychres.2016.12.045

Kremen, W. S., Koenen, K. C., Boake, C., Purcell, S., Eisen, S. A., Franz, C. E., Tsuang, M. T., & Lyons, M. J. (2007). Pretrauma cognitive ability and risk for posttraumatic stress disorder: A twin study. *Archives of General Psychiatry, 64*(3), 361–368. https://doi.org/10.1001/archpsyc.64.3.361

Kring, A. M., & Elis, O. (2013). Emotion deficits in people with schizophrenia. *Annual Review of Clinical Psychology, 9*(1), 409–433. https://doi.org/10.1146/annurev-clinpsy-050212-185538

Kring, A. M., Gur, R. E., Blanchard, J. J., Horan, W. P., & Reise, S. P. (2013). The Clinical Assessment Interview for Negative Symptoms (CAINS): Final development and validation. *The American Journal of Psychiatry, 170*(2), 165–172. https://doi.org/10.1176/appi.ajp.2012.12010109

Kubany, E. S., Haynes, S. N., Leisen, M. B., Owens, J. A., Kaplan, A. S., Watson, S. B., & Burns, K. (2000). Development and preliminary validation of a brief broad-spectrum measure of trauma exposure: The Traumatic Life Events Questionnaire. *Psychological Assessment, 12*(2), 210–224. https://doi.org/10.1037/1040-3590.12.2.210

Kukla, M., & Bond, G. R. (2009). The working alliance and employment outcomes for people with severe mental illness enrolled in vocational programs. *Rehabilitation Psychology, 54*(2), 157–163. https://doi.org/10.1037/a0015596

Kukla, M., Bond, G. R., & Xie, H. (2012). A prospective investigation of work and nonvocational outcomes in adults with severe mental illness. *Journal of Nervous and Mental Disease, 200*(3), 214–222. https://doi.org/10.1097/NMD.0b013e318247cb29

Landy, M. S. H., Wagner, A. C., Brown-Bowers, A., & Monson, C. M. (2015). Examining the evidence for complex posttraumatic stress disorder as a clinical diagnosis. *Journal of Aggression, Maltreatment & Trauma, 24*(3), 215–236. https://doi.org/10.1080/10926771.2015.1002649

Le Boutillier, C., Leamy, M., Bird, V. J., Davidson, L., Williams, J., & Slade, M. (2011). What does recovery mean in practice? A qualitative analysis of international recovery-oriented practice guidance. *Psychiatric Services, 62*(12), 1470–1476. https://doi.org/10.1176/appi.ps.001312011

Leamy, M., Bird, V., Le Boutillier, C., Williams, J., & Slade, M. (2011). Conceptual framework for personal recovery in mental health: Systematic review and narrative synthesis. *The British Journal of Psychiatry, 199*(6), 445–452. https://doi.org/10.1192/bjp.bp.110.083733

Lecomte, T., Paquin, K., Mueser, K. T., MacEwan, W., Goldner, E., Thornton, A. E., Brink, J., Lang, D., Kang, S., Barr, A. M., & Honer, W. G. (2013). Relationships among depression, PTSD, methamphetamine abuse, and psychosis. *Journal of Dual Diagnosis, 9*(2), 115–122. https://doi.org/10.1080/15504263.2013.778930

Lee, D. A. (2005). The perfect nurturer: A model to develop a compassionate mind within the context of cognitive therapy. In P. Gilbert (Ed.), *Compassion: Conceptualisations, research and use in psychotherapy* (pp. 326–351). Routledge.

Levy-Frank, I., Hasson-Ohayon, I., Kravetz, S., & Roe, D. (2011). Family psychoeducation and therapeutic alliance focused interventions for parents of a daughter or son with a severe mental illness. *Psychiatry Research, 189*(2), 173–179. https://doi.org/10.1016/j.psychres.2011.02.012

Lewis-Fernández, R., Garrido-Castillo, P., Bennasar, M. C., Parrilla, E. M., Laria, A. J., Ma, G., & Petkova, E. (2002). Dissociation, childhood trauma, and ataque de nervios among Puerto Rican psychiatric outpatients. *The American Journal of Psychiatry*, *159*(9), 1603–1605. https://doi.org/10.1176/appi.ajp.159.9.1603

Lieb, K., Zanarini, M. C., Schmahl, C., Linehan, M. M., & Bohus, M. (2004). Borderline personality disorder. *Lancet*, *364*(9432), 453–461. https://doi.org/10.1016/S0140-6736(04)16770-6

Linehan, M. M. (1993). *Cognitive-behavioral treatment of borderline personality disorder*. Guilford Press.

Liu, H., Petukhova, M. V., Sampson, N. A., Aguilar-Gaxiola, S., Alonso, J., Andrade, L. H., Bromet, E. J., de Girolamo, G., Haro, J. M., Hinkov, H., Kawakami, N., Koenen, K. C., Kovess-Masfety, V., Lee, S., Medina-Mora, M. E., Navarro-Mateu, F., O'Neill, S., Piazza, M., Posada-Villa, J., . . . the World Health Organization World Mental Health Survey Collaborators. (2017). The association of *DSM-IV* post-traumatic stress disorder with traumatic experience type and history in the World Health Organization World Mental Health Surveys. *JAMA Psychiatry*, *74*(3), 270–281. https://doi.org/10.1001/jamapsychiatry.2016.3783

Lommen, M. J., & Restifo, K. (2009). Trauma and posttraumatic stress disorder (PTSD) in patients with schizophrenia or schizoaffective disorder. *Community Mental Health Journal*, *45*(6), 485–496. https://doi.org/10.1007/s10597-009-9248-x

Lovallo, W. R. (2005). *Stress and health: Biological and psychological interactions* (2nd ed.). Sage Publications.

Lu, W., Fite, R., Kim, E., Hyer, L., Yanos, P. T., Mueser, K. T., & Rosenberg, S. D. (2009). Cognitive-behavioral treatment of PTSD in severe mental illness: Pilot study replication in an ethnically diverse population. *American Journal of Psychiatric Rehabilitation*, *12*(1), 73–91. https://doi.org/10.1080/15487760802615863

Lu, W., Mueser, K. T., Rosenberg, S. D., & Jankowski, M. K. (2008). Correlates of adverse childhood events in adults with major mood disorders. *Psychiatric Services*, *59*(9), 1018–1026. https://doi.org/10.1176/ps.2008.59.9.1018

Lu, W., Mueser, K. T., Rosenberg, S. D., Yanos, P. T., & Mahmoud, N. (2017). Post-traumatic reactions to psychosis: A qualitative analysis. *Frontiers in Psychiatry*, *8*, Article 129. https://doi.org/10.3389/fpsyt.2017.00129

Lu, W., Mueser, K. T., Shami, A., Siglag, M., Petrides, G., Schoepp, E., Putts, M., & Saltz, J. (2011). Post-traumatic reactions to psychosis in people with multiple psychotic episodes. *Schizophrenia Research*, *127*(1–3), 66–75. https://doi.org/10.1016/j.schres.2011.01.006

Lu, W., Mueser, K. T., Yanos, P. T., Siriram, A., Jia, Y., Leong, A., Silverstein, S. M., Gottlieb, J., & Jankowski, M. K. (2023). Post-Traumatic Cognitions Inventory (PTCI): Psychometric properties in clients with serious mental illness and co-occurring PTSD. *Behavioural and Cognitive Psychotherapy*, *51*(5), 459–474. https://doi.org/10.1017/S1352465823000140

Lu, W., Silverstein, S. M., Mueser, K. T., Minsky, S., Bullock, D., Buchbinder, S., Chen, Q., Eubanks, R., & Guillaume-Salvant, A. (2023). Undocumented PTSD among African American clients with serious mental illness in a statewide mental health system. *Psychological Trauma: Theory, Research, Practice, and Policy*, *15*(5), 781–790. https://doi.org/10.1037/tra0001243

Lu, W., Srijeyanthan, J., Mueser, K. T., Yanos, P. T., Parrot, J. S., Siriram, A., Gottlieb, J. D., Marcello, S., & Silverstein, S. M. (2022). Predictors of undocumented PTSD among persons diagnosed with serious mental illness. *Psychiatry Research, 317*, Article 114892. https://doi.org/10.1016/j.psychres. 2022.114892

Lu, W., Waynor, W., Yanos, P. T., Reilly, A., Stone, B., Bazan, C., & Giocobbe, G. R. (2017). The hidden barrier to employment: Untreated and undiagnosed post-traumatic stress disorder. *Journal of Rehabilitation, 83*(2), 11–16. https://link.gale.com/apps/doc/A503309636/AONE?u=anon~ 34ce011&sid=googleScholar&xid=da8c9f9d

Lu, W., Yanos, P. T., Gottlieb, J. D., Duva, S. M., Silverstein, S. M., Xie, H., Rosenberg, S. D., & Mueser, K. T. (2012). Use of fidelity assessments to train clinicians in the CBT for PTSD program for clients with serious mental illness. *Psychiatric Services, 63*(8), 785–792. https://doi.org/10.1176/appi.ps. 201000458

Lu, W., Yanos, P. T., Silverstein, S. M., Mueser, K. T., Rosenberg, S. D., Gottlieb, J. D., Duva, S. M., Kularatne, T., Dove-Williams, S., Paterno, D., Hawthorne, D., & Giacobbe, G. (2013). Public mental health clients with severe mental illness and probable posttraumatic stress disorder: Trauma exposure and correlates of symptom severity. *Journal of Traumatic Stress, 26*(2), 266–273. https://doi.org/ 10.1002/jts.21791

Lu, W., Yanos, P. T., Waynor, W., Jia, Y., Siriram, A., Leong, A., Gill, K., & Mueser, K. T. (2022). Psychometric properties of post-traumatic stress disorder (PTSD) checklist for *DSM-5* in persons with serious mental illness. *European Journal of Psychotraumatology, 13*(1), Article 2038924. https://doi.org/10.1080/20008198. 2022.2038924

Lysaker, P. H., & Lysaker, J. T. (2008). *Schizophrenia and the fate of the self.* Oxford University Press.

MacCabe, J. H., Wicks, S., Löfving, S., David, A. S., Berndtsson, Å., Gustafsson, J.-E., Allebeck, P., & Dalman, C. (2013). Decline in cognitive performance between ages 13 and 18 years and the risk for psychosis in adulthood: A Swedish longitudinal cohort study in males. *JAMA Psychiatry, 70*(3), 261–270. https://doi.org/10.1001/ 2013.jamapsychiatry.43

Maniglio, R. (2009). Severe mental illness and criminal victimization: A systematic review. *Acta Psychiatrica Scandinavica, 119*(3), 180–191. https://doi.org/10.1111/ j.1600-0447.2008.01300.x

Manning, S. Y., & Linehan, M. M. (2011). *Loving someone with borderline personality disorder: How to keep out-of-control emotions from destroying your relationship.* Guilford Press.

Marks, I., Lovell, K., Noshirvani, H., Livanou, M., & Thrasher, S. (1998). Treatment of posttraumatic stress disorder by exposure and/or cognitive restructuring: A controlled study. *Archives of General Psychiatry, 55*(4), 317–325. https://doi.org/ 10.1001/archpsyc.55.4.317

Martin, D. J., Garske, J. P., & Davis, M. K. (2000). Relation of the therapeutic alliance with outcome and other variables: A meta-analytic review. *Journal of Consulting and Clinical Psychology, 68*(3), 438–450. https://doi.org/10.1037/ 0022-006X.68.3.438

Martínez-Martínez, C., Richart-Martínez, M., & Ramos-Pichardo, J. D. (2020). Operational definition of serious mental illness: Heterogeneity in a review of the research on quality-of-life interventions. *Journal of the American Psychiatric Nurses Association, 26*(3), 229–244. https://doi.org/10.1177/1078390320902823

Matheson, S. L., Shepherd, A. M., Pinchbeck, R. M., Laurens, K. R., & Carr, V. J. (2013). Childhood adversity in schizophrenia: A systematic meta-analysis. *Psychological Medicine, 43*(2), 225–238. https://doi.org/10.1017/S0033291712000785

Mauritz, M. W., Goossens, P. J. J., Draijer, N., & van Achterberg, T. (2013). Prevalence of interpersonal trauma exposure and trauma-related disorders in severe mental illness. *European Journal of Psychotraumatology, 4*(1), Article 19985. https://doi.org/10.3402/ejpt.v4i0.19985

Mavranezouli, I., Megnin-Viggars, O., Daly, C., Dias, S., Welton, N. J., Stockton, S., Bhutani, G., Grey, N., Leach, J., Greenberg, N., Katona, C., El-Leithy, S., & Pilling, S. (2020). Psychological treatments for post-traumatic stress disorder in adults: A network meta-analysis. *Psychological Medicine, 50*(4), 542–555. https://doi.org/10.1017/S0033291720000070

McCabe, P. J., Christopher, P. P., Druhn, N., Roy-Bujnowski, K. M., Grudzinskas, A. J., Jr., & Fisher, W. H. (2012). Arrest types and co-occurring disorders in persons with schizophrenia or related psychoses. *The Journal of Behavioral Health Services & Research, 39*(3), 271–284. https://doi.org/10.1007/s11414-011-9269-4

McCauley, J. L., Killeen, T., Gros, D. F., Brady, K. T., & Back, S. E. (2012). Posttraumatic stress disorder and co-occurring substance use disorders: Advances in assessment and treatment. *Clinical Psychology: Science and Practice, 19*(3), 283–304. https://doi.org/10.1111/cpsp.12006

McFarlane, A. C. (1996). Resilience, vulnerability, and the course of posttraumatic reactions. In B. A. van der Kolk, A. C. McFarlane, & L. Weisaeth (Eds.), *Traumatic stress: The effects of overwhelming experience on mind, body, and society* (pp. 155–181). Guilford Press.

McFarlane, A. C., Bookless, C., & Air, T. (2001). Posttraumatic stress disorder in a general psychiatric inpatient population. *Journal of Traumatic Stress, 14*(4), 633–645. https://doi.org/10.1023/A:1013077702520

McGorry, P. D., Chanen, A., McCarthy, E., Van Riel, R., McKenzie, D., & Singh, B. S. (1991). Posttraumatic stress disorder following recent-onset psychosis. An unrecognized postpsychotic syndrome. *Journal of Nervous and Mental Disease, 179*(5), 253–258. https://doi.org/10.1097/00005053-199105000-00002

McGovern, M. P., Mueser, K. T., Hamblen, J. L., & Jankowski, M. K. (2010). *Cognitive-behavioral therapy for PTSD: A program for addiction professionals.* Hazelden.

McGrath, J. J., McLaughlin, K. A., Saha, S., Aguilar-Gaxiola, S., Al-Hamzawi, A., Alonso, J., Bruffaerts, R., de Girolamo, G., de Jonge, P., Esan, O., Florescu, S., Gureje, O., Haro, J. M., Hu, C., Karam, E. G., Kovess-Masfety, V., Lee, S., Lepine, J. P., Lim, C. C. W., . . . Kessler, R. C. (2017). The association between childhood adversities and subsequent first onset of psychotic experiences: A cross-national analysis of 23 998 respondents from 17 countries. *Psychological Medicine, 47*(7), 1230–1245. https://doi.org/10.1017/S0033291716003263

McLean, C. P., Levy, H. C., Miller, M. L., & Tolin, D. F. (2022). Exposure therapy for PTSD: A meta-analysis. *Clinical Psychology Review, 91*, Article 102115. https://doi.org/10.1016/j.cpr.2021.102115

McNally, R. J., & Shin, L. M. (1995). Association of intelligence with severity of posttraumatic stress disorder symptoms in Vietnam combat veterans. *The American Journal of Psychiatry, 152*(6), 936–938. https://doi.org/10.1176/ajp.152.6.936

McNeill, S. A., & Galovski, T. E. (2015). Coping styles among individuals with severe mental illness and comorbid PTSD. *Community Mental Health Journal, 51*(6), 663–673. https://doi.org/10.1007/s10597-015-9887-z

Meyer, I. H., Muenzenmaier, K., Cancienne, J., & Struening, E. (1996). Reliability and validity of a measure of sexual and physical abuse histories among women with serious mental illness. *Child Abuse & Neglect, 20*(3), 213–219. https://doi.org/10.1016/S0145-2134(95)00137-9

Meyer-Kalos, P. S., Gottlieb, J. D., Penn, D. L., Mueser, K. T., & Gingerich, S. (2015). Individual resiliency training: An early intervention approach to enhance well-being in people with first-episode psychosis. *Psychiatric Annals, 45*(11), 554–560. https://doi.org/10.3928/00485713-20151103-06

Millet, K. (1991). *The Loony Bin trip*. Virago Press.

Minsky, S. K., Lu, W., Silverstein, S. M., Gara, M., Gottlieb, J. D., & Mueser, K. T. (2015). Service use and self-reported symptoms among persons with positive PTSD screens and serious mental illness. *Psychiatric Services, 66*(8), 845–850. https://doi.org/10.1176/appi.ps.201400192

Mohamed, S. (2013). Adaptation of intensive mental health intensive case management to rural communities in the Veterans Health Administration. *Psychiatric Quarterly, 84*(1), 103–114. https://doi.org/10.1007/s11126-012-9231-5

Molebatsi, K., Ng, L. C., & Chiliza, B. (2021). A culturally adapted brief intervention for post-traumatic stress disorder in people with severe mental illness in Botswana: Protocol for a randomised feasibility trial. *Pilot and Feasibility Studies, 7*(1), Article 170. https://doi.org/10.1186/s40814-021-00904-1

Mollon, J., David, A. S., Zammit, S., Lewis, G., & Reichenberg, A. (2018). Course of cognitive development from infancy to early adulthood in the psychosis spectrum. *JAMA Psychiatry, 75*(3), 270–279. https://doi.org/10.1001/jamapsychiatry.2017.4327

Monahan, J., Vesselinov, R., Robbins, P. C., & Appelbaum, P. S. (2017). Violence to others, violent self-victimization, and violent victimization by others among persons with a mental illness. *Psychiatric Services, 68*(5), 516–519. https://doi.org/10.1176/appi.ps.201600135

Monson, C. M. (2005). PTSD and intimate relationships. *PTSD Research Quarterly, 16*(4), 1–8.

Morgan, C., Gayer-Anderson, C., Beards, S., Hubbard, K., Mondelli, V., Di Forti, M., Murray, R. M., Pariante, C., Dazzan, P., Craig, T. J., Reininghaus, U., & Fisher, H. L. (2020). Threat, hostility and violence in childhood and later psychotic disorder: Population-based case–control study. *The British Journal of Psychiatry, 217*(4), 575–582. https://doi.org/10.1192/bjp.2020.133

Morrison, A. P., Renton, J. C., Dunn, H., Williams, S., & Bentall, R. P. (2004). *Cognitive therapy for psychosis: A formulation-based approach*. Routledge. https://doi.org/10.4324/9780203493465

Morrison, A. P., Renton, J. C., French, P., & Bentall, R. P. (2008). *Think you're crazy? Think again: A resource book for cognitive therapy for psychosis*. Routledge.

Mueser, K. T., Becker, D. R., Torrey, W. C., Xie, H., Bond, G. R., Drake, R. E., & Dain, B. J. (1997). Work and nonvocational domains of functioning in persons with severe mental illness: A longitudinal analysis. *Journal of Nervous and Mental Disease, 185*(7), 419–426. https://doi.org/10.1097/00005053-199707000-00001

Mueser, K. T., Bellack, A. S., & Brady, E. U. (1990). Hallucinations in schizophrenia. *Acta Psychiatrica Scandinavica, 82*(1), 26–29. https://doi.org/10.1111/j.1600-0447.1990.tb01350.x

Mueser, K. T., Bellack, A. S., Gingerich, S., Agresta, J., & Fulford, D. (2024). *Social skills training for schizophrenia: A step-by-step guide* (3rd ed.). Guilford Press.

Mueser, K. T., Bolton, E. E., Carty, P. C., Bradley, M. J., Ahlgren, K. F., DiStaso, D. R., Gilbride, A., & Liddel, C. (2007). The trauma recovery group: A cognitive-behavioral program for PTSD in persons with severe mental illness. *Community Mental Health Journal, 43*, 281–304. https://doi.org/10.1007/s10597-006-9075-2

Mueser, K. T., & Butler, R. W. (1987). Auditory hallucinations in combat-related chronic posttraumatic stress disorder. *The American Journal of Psychiatry, 144*(3), 299–302. https://doi.org/10.1176/ajp.144.3.299

Mueser, K. T., Corrigan, P. W., Hilton, D., Tanzman, B., Schaub, A., Gingerich, S., Essock, S. M., Tarrier, N., Morey, B., Vogel-Scibilia, S., & Herz, M. I. (2002). Illness management and recovery for severe mental illness: A review of the research. *Psychiatric Services, 53*(10), 1272–1284. https://doi.org/10.1176/appi.ps.53.10.1272

Mueser, K. T., Davis, K., Burke-Miller, J. K., Marcello, S., Gottlieb, J. D., Fraser, V., & Razzano, L. A. (in press). Implementation of a brief treatment program for PTSD in persons with serious mental illness in a large mental health agency: The BREATHE program. *Psychiatric Rehabilitation Journal.*

Mueser, K. T., Deavers, F., Penn, D. L., & Cassisi, J. E. (2013). Psychosocial treatments for schizophrenia. *Annual Review of Clinical Psychology, 9*(1), 465–497. https://doi.org/10.1146/annurev-clinpsy-050212-185620

Mueser, K. T., Essock, S. M., Haines, M., Wolfe, R., & Xie, H. (2004). Posttraumatic stress disorder, supported employment, and outcomes in people with severe mental illness. *CNS Spectrums, 9*(12), 913–925. https://doi.org/10.1017/S1092852900009779

Mueser, K. T., Goodman, L. B., Trumbetta, S. L., Rosenberg, S. D., Osher, C., Vidaver, R., Auciello, P., & Foy, D. W. (1998). Trauma and posttraumatic stress disorder in severe mental illness. *Journal of Consulting and Clinical Psychology, 66*(3), 493–499. https://doi.org/10.1037/0022-006X.66.3.493

Mueser, K. T., Gottlieb, J. D., Xie, H., Lu, W., Yanos, P. T., Rosenberg, S. R., Silverstein, S. M., Duva, S. M., Minsky, S., Wolfe, R., & McHugo, G. J. (2015). Evaluation of cognitive restructuring for PTSD in people with severe mental illness. *The British Journal of Psychiatry, 206*(6), 501–508. https://doi.org/10.1192/bjp.bp.114.147926

Mueser, K. T., Lu, W., Rosenberg, S. D., & Wolfe, R. (2010). The trauma of psychosis: Posttraumatic stress disorder and recent onset psychosis. *Schizophrenia Research, 116*(2–3), 217–227. https://doi.org/10.1016/j.schres.2009.10.025

Mueser, K. T., McGurk, S. R., Xie, H., Bolton, E. E., Jankowski, M. K., Lu, W., Rosenberg, S. D., & Wolfe, R. (2018). Neuropsychological predictors of response to cognitive behavioral therapy for posttraumatic stress disorder in persons with severe mental illness. *Psychiatry Research, 259*, 110–116. https://doi.org/10.1016/j.psychres.2017.10.016

Mueser, K. T., Penn, D. L., Addington, J., Brunette, M. F., Gingerich, S., Glynn, S. M., Lynde, D. W., Gottlieb, J. D., Meyer-Kalos, P., Cather, C., McGurk, S. R., Saade, S., Robinson, D. G., Schooler, N. R., Rosenheck, R. A., & Kane, J. M. (2015). The NAVIGATE program for first episode psychosis: Rationale, overview, and description of psychosocial components. *Psychiatric Services, 66*(7), 680–690. https://doi.org/10.1176/appi.ps.201400413

Mueser, K. T., & Rosenberg, S. D. (2003). Treating the trauma of first episode psychosis: A PTSD perspective. *Journal of Mental Health, 12*(2), 103–108. https://doi.org/10.1080/09638230021000583371

Mueser, K. T., Rosenberg, S. D., Goodman, L. A., & Trumbetta, S. L. (2002). Trauma, PTSD, and the course of schizophrenia: An interactive model. *Schizophrenia Research, 53*(1–2), 123–143. https://doi.org/10.1016/S0920-9964(01)00173-6

Mueser, K. T., Rosenberg, S. D., Jankowski, M. K., Hamblen, J. L., & Descamps, M. (2004). A cognitive-behavioral treatment program for posttraumatic stress disorder in severe mental illness. *American Journal of Psychiatric Rehabilitation, 7*(2), 107–146. https://doi.org/10.1080/15487760490476183

Mueser, K. T., Rosenberg, S. D., & Rosenberg, H. J. (2009). *Treatment of posttraumatic stress disorder in special populations: A cognitive restructuring program.* American Psychological Association. https://doi.org/10.1037/11889-000

Mueser, K. T., Rosenberg, S. D., Xie, H., Jankowski, M. K., Bolton, E. E., Lu, W., Hamblen, J. L., Rosenberg, H. J., McHugo, G. J., & Wolfe, R. (2008). A randomized controlled trial of cognitive-behavioral treatment for posttraumatic stress disorder in severe mental illness. *Journal of Consulting and Clinical Psychology, 76*(2), 259–271. https://doi.org/10.1037/0022-006X.76.2.259

Mueser, K. T., Salyers, M. P., Rosenberg, S. D., Ford, J. D., Fox, L., & Carty, P. (2001). A psychometric evaluation of trauma and PTSD assessments in persons with severe mental illness. *Psychological Assessment, 13*(1), 110–117. https://doi.org/10.1037/1040-3590.13.1.110

Mueser, K. T., Salyers, M. P., Rosenberg, S. D., Goodman, L. A., Essock, S. M., Osher, F. C., Swartz, M. S., Butterfield, M. I., & the 5 Site Health and Risk Study Research Committee. (2004). Interpersonal trauma and posttraumatic stress disorder in patients with severe mental illness: Demographic, clinical, and health correlates. *Schizophrenia Bulletin, 30*(1), 45–57. https://doi.org/10.1093/oxfordjournals.schbul.a007067

Mueser, K. T., & Taub, J. (2008). Trauma and PTSD among adolescents with severe emotional disorders involved in multiple service systems. *Psychiatric Services, 59*(6), 627–634. https://doi.org/10.1176/ps.2008.59.6.627

Mueser, K. T., Valentiner, D. P., & Agresta, J. (1997). Coping with negative symptoms of schizophrenia: Patient and family perspectives. *Schizophrenia Bulletin, 23*(2), 329–339. https://doi.org/10.1093/schbul/23.2.329

Murphy, J., Shevlin, M., Adamson, G., & Houston, J. E. (2013). From sexual abuse to psychosis: A pilot study exploring the social deafferentation hypothesis and the mediating role of avoidance. *Psychosis, 5*(1), 36–47. https://doi.org/10.1080/17522439.2011.622781

Murray, R. M., Bhavsar, V., Tripoli, G., & Howes, O. (2017). 30 years on: How the neurodevelopmental hypothesis of schizophrenia morphed into the developmental risk factor model of psychosis. *Schizophrenia Bulletin, 43*(6), 1190–1196. https://doi.org/10.1093/schbul/sbx121

Naim, R., Abend, R., Wald, I., Eldar, S., Levi, O., Fruchter, E., Ginat, K., Halpern, P., Sipos, M. L., Adler, A. B., Bliese, P. D., Quartana, P. J., Pine, D. S., & Bar-Haim, Y. (2015). Threat-related attention bias variability and posttraumatic stress. *The American Journal of Psychiatry, 172*(12), 1242–1250. https://doi.org/10.1176/appi.ajp.2015.14121579

Najavits, L. M. (2002). *Seeking safety: A treatment manual for PTSD and substance abuse.* Guilford Press.

Najavits, L. M., & Hien, D. (2013). Helping vulnerable populations: A comprehensive review of the treatment outcome literature on substance use disorder and PTSD. *Journal of Clinical Psychology, 69*(5), 433–479. https://doi.org/10.1002/jclp.21980

National Institute for Health and Care Excellence. (2018). *Guideline for post-traumatic stress disorder.*

Neff, K. (2011). *Self-compassion: The proven power of being kind to oneself.* William Morrow.

Nelson, H. (1997). *Cognitive behavioural therapy with schizophrenia: A practice manual.* Nelson Thornes.

Neria, Y., Bromet, E. J., Sievers, S., Lavelle, J., & Fochtmann, L. J. (2002). Trauma exposure and posttraumatic stress disorder in psychosis: Findings from a first-admission cohort. *Journal of Consulting and Clinical Psychology, 70*(1), 246–251. https://doi.org/10.1037/0022-006X.70.1.246

Newman, C. F., Leahy, R. L., Beck, A. T., Reilly-Harrington, N. A., & Gyulai, L. (2002). *Bipolar disorder: A cognitive therapy approach.* American Psychological Association. https://doi.org/10.1037/10442-000

Newman, J. M., Turnbull, A., Berman, B. A., Rodrigues, S., & Serper, M. R. (2010). Impact of traumatic and violent victimization experiences in individuals with schizophrenia and schizoaffective disorder. *Journal of Nervous and Mental Disease, 198*(10), 708–714. https://doi.org/10.1097/NMD.0b013e3181f49bf1

Ng, L. C., Miller, A. N., Bowers, G., Cheng, Y., Brigham, R., Tai, M. H., Smith, A. M., Mueser, K. T., Fortuna, L. R., & Coles, M. (2023). A pragmatic feasibility trial of the primary care intervention for PTSD: A health service delivery model to reduce health disparities for low-income and BIPOC youth. *Behaviour Research and Therapy, 165*, Article 104310. https://doi.org/10.1016/j.brat.2023.104310

Ng, L. C., Petruzzi, L. J., Greene, M. C., Mueser, K. T., Borba, C. P. C., & Henderson, D. C. (2016). Posttraumatic stress disorder symptoms and social and occupational functioning of people with schizophrenia. *Journal of Nervous and Mental Disease, 204*(8), 590–598. https://doi.org/10.1097/NMD.0000000000000523

Ng, L. C., Serba, E. G., Dubale, B. W., Fekadu, A., & Hanlon, C. (2021). Posttraumatic stress disorder intervention for people with severe mental illness in a low-income country primary care setting: A randomized feasibility trial protocol. *Pilot and Feasibility Studies, 7*(1), Article 149. https://doi.org/10.1186/s40814-021-00883-3

Nishith, P., Huang, J., Morse, G. A., Dell, N., Murphy, A., & Mueser, K. T. (2022). A test of self-medication hypothesis for drug use in homeless persons: The role of severe mental illness. *Journal of Social Distress and Homelessness, 32*(2), 255–262. https://doi.org/10.1080/10530789.2022.2025704

Nishith, P., Mechanic, M. B., & Resick, P. A. (2000). Prior interpersonal trauma: The contribution to current PTSD symptoms in female rape victims. *Journal of Abnormal Psychology, 109*(1), 20–25. https://doi.org/10.1037/0021-843X.109.1.20

Nishith, P., Mueser, K. T., & Morse, G. A. (2015). A brief intervention for posttraumatic stress disorder in persons with a serious mental illness. *Psychiatric Rehabilitation Journal, 38*(4), 314–319. https://doi.org/10.1037/prj0000158

Nishith, P., Resick, P. A., & Mueser, K. T. (2001). Sleep difficulties and alcohol use motives in female rape victims with posttraumatic stress disorder. *Journal of Traumatic Stress, 14*(3), 469–479. https://doi.org/10.1023/A:1011152405048

Nock, M. K., Hwang, I., Sampson, N. A., & Kessler, R. C. (2010). Mental disorders, comorbidity and suicidal behavior: Results from the National Comorbidity Survey Replication. *Molecular Psychiatry, 15*(8), 868–876. https://doi.org/10.1038/mp.2009.29

Noordsy, D. L., Mishra, M. K., & Mueser, K. T. (2013). Models of relationships between substance use and mental disorders. In P. Miller (Ed.), *Comprehensive addictive behaviors and disorders: Vol. 1. Principles of addiction* (pp. 489–495). Academic Press. https://doi.org/10.1016/B978-0-12-398336-7.00051-6

Norris, F. H., Tracy, M., & Galea, S. (2009). Looking for resilience: Understanding the longitudinal trajectories of responses to stress. *Social Science & Medicine, 68*(12), 2190–2198. https://doi.org/10.1016/j.socscimed.2009.03.043

North, C. S., Smith, E. M., & Spitznagel, E. L. (1997). One-year follow-up of survivors of a mass shooting. *The American Journal of Psychiatry, 154*(12), 1696–1702. https://doi.org/10.1176/ajp.154.12.1696

Nuechterlein, K. H., & Dawson, M. E. (1984). A heuristic vulnerability/stress model of schizophrenic episodes. *Schizophrenia Bulletin, 10*(2), 300–312. https://doi.org/10.1093/schbul/10.2.300

Nurius, P. S., Green, S., Logan-Greene, P., & Borja, S. (2015). Life course pathways of adverse childhood experiences toward adult psychological well-being: A stress process analysis. *Child Abuse & Neglect, 45*, 143–153. https://doi.org/10.1016/j.chiabu.2015.03.008

O'Hare, T., & Sherrer, M. (2011a). Drinking motives as mediators between PTSD symptom severity and alcohol consumption in persons with severe mental illnesses. *Addictive Behaviors, 36*(5), 465–469. https://doi.org/10.1016/j.addbeh.2011.01.006

O'Hare, T., & Sherrer, M. (2011b). Subjective distress associated with sudden loss in clients with severe mental illness. *Community Mental Health Journal, 47*(6), 646–653. https://doi.org/10.1007/s10597-011-9382-0

O'Hare, T., Sherrer, M. V., & Shen, C. (2006). Subjective distress from stressful events and high-risk behaviors as predictors of PTSD symptom severity in clients with severe mental illness. *Journal of Traumatic Stress, 19*(3), 375–386. https://doi.org/10.1002/jts.20131

OConghaile, A., & DeLisi, L. E. (2015). Distinguishing schizophrenia from post-traumatic stress disorder with psychosis. *Current Opinion in Psychiatry, 28*(3), 249–255. https://doi.org/10.1097/YCO.0000000000000158

Okkels, N., Trabjerg, B., Arendt, M., & Pedersen, C. B. (2017). Traumatic stress disorders and risk of subsequent schizophrenia spectrum disorder or bipolar disorder: A nationwide cohort study. *Schizophrenia Bulletin, 43*(1), 180–186. https://doi.org/10.1093/schbul/sbw082

Olfson, M. (2016). Building the mental health workforce capacity needed to treat adults with serious mental illnesses. *Health Affairs, 35*(6), 983–990. https://doi.org/10.1377/hlthaff.2015.1619

Pacella, M. L., Hruska, B., & Delahanty, D. L. (2013). The physical health consequences of PTSD and PTSD symptoms: A meta-analytic review. *Journal of Anxiety Disorders, 27*(1), 33–46. https://doi.org/10.1016/j.janxdis.2012.08.004

Pagura, J., Stein, M. B., Bolton, J. M., Cox, B. J., Grant, B., & Sareen, J. (2010). Comorbidity of borderline personality disorder and posttraumatic stress disorder in the U.S. population. *Journal of Psychiatric Research, 44*(16), 1190–1198. https://doi.org/10.1016/j.jpsychires.2010.04.016

Panagioti, M., Gooding, P. A., & Tarrier, N. (2012). A meta-analysis of the association between posttraumatic stress disorder and suicidality: The role of comorbid depression. *Comprehensive Psychiatry, 53*(7), 915–930. https://doi.org/10.1016/j.comppsych.2012.02.009

Parabiaghi, A., Bonetto, C., Ruggeri, M., Lasalvia, A., & Leese, M. (2006). Severe and persistent mental illness: A useful definition for prioritizing community-based mental health service interventions. *Social Psychiatry and Psychiatric Epidemiology, 41*(6), 457–463. https://doi.org/10.1007/s00127-006-0048-0

Penney, D., El-Baalbaki, G., & Lepage, M. (2023). Exploring the factor structure of the PTSD checklist for *DSM-5* in psychotic disorders. *Psychological Trauma: Theory, Research, Practice, and Policy, 15*(5), 767–771. https://doi.org/10.1037/tra0001146

Phelps, A. J., Lethbridge, R., Brennan, S., Bryant, R. A., Burns, P., Cooper, J. A., Forbes, D., Gardiner, J., Gee, G., Jones, K., Kenardy, J., Kulkarni, J., McDermott, B., McFarlane, A. C., Newman, L. R. V., Worth, C., & Silove, D. (2022). Australian guidelines for the prevention and treatment of posttraumatic stress disorder: Updates in the third edition. *Australian & New Zealand Journal of Psychiatry, 56*, 230–247. https://doi.org/10.1177/00048674211041917

Phoenix Australia Centre for Posttraumatic Mental Health. (2020). *Australian guidelines for the treatment of acute stress disorder and posttraumatic stress disorder.*

Picken, A., & Tarrier, N. (2011). Trauma and comorbid posttraumatic stress disorder in individuals with schizophrenia and substance abuse. *Comprehensive Psychiatry, 52*(5), 490–497. https://doi.org/10.1016/j.comppsych.2010.10.008

Pietrzak, R. H., Feder, A., Singh, R., Schechter, C. B., Bromet, E. J., Katz, C. L., Reissman, D. B., Ozbay, F., Sharma, V., Crane, M., Harrison, D., Herbert, R., Levin, S. M., Luft, B. J., Moline, J. M., Stellman, J. M., Udasin, I. G., Landrigan, P. J., & Southwick, S. M. (2014). Trajectories of PTSD risk and resilience in World Trade Center responders: An 8-year prospective cohort study. *Psychological Medicine, 44*(1), 205–219. https://doi.org/10.1017/S0033291713000597

Pitman, R. K., Altman, B., Greenwald, E., Longpre, R. E., Macklin, M. L., Poiré, R. E., & Steketee, G. S. (1991). Psychiatric complications during flooding therapy for posttraumatic stress disorder. *The Journal of Clinical Psychiatry, 52*(1), 17–20. https://pubmed.ncbi.nlm.nih.gov/1988412/

Pollice, R., Bianchini, V., Conti, C. M., Mazza, M., Roncone, R., & Casacchia, M. (2010). Cognitive impairment and perceived stress in schizophrenic inpatients with post-traumatic stress disorder. *European Journal of Inflammation, 8*(3), 211–219. https://doi.org/10.1177/1721727X1000800311

Polusny, M. A., & Follette, V. M. (1995). Long-term correlates of child sexual abuse: Theory and review of the empirical literature. *Applied & Preventive Psychology, 4*(3), 143–166. https://doi.org/10.1016/S0962-1849(05)80055-1

Pratt, S. I., Rosenberg, S. D., Mueser, K. T., Brancato, J., Salyers, M. P., Jankowski, M. K., & Descamps, M. (2005). Evaluation of a PTSD psychoeducational program for psychiatric inpatients. *Journal of Mental Health*, *14*(2), 121–127. https://doi.org/10.1080/09638230500066356

Prochaska, J. O., & DiClemente, C. C. (1984). *The transtheoretical approach: Crossing the traditional boundaries of therapy*. Dow-Jones; Irwin.

Ratcliffe, M. (2021). Sensed presence without sensory qualities: A phenomenological study of bereavement hallucinations. *Phenomenology and the Cognitive Sciences*, *20*(4), 601–616. https://doi.org/10.1007/s11097-020-09666-2

Read, J. (1997). Child abuse and psychosis. *Professional Psychology: Research and Practice*, *28*(5), 448–456. https://doi.org/10.1037/0735-7028.28.5.448

Read, J., Perry, B. D., Moskowitz, A., & Connolly, J. (2001). The contribution of early traumatic events to schizophrenia in some patients: A traumagenic neurodevelopmental model. *Psychiatry*, *64*(4), 319–345. https://doi.org/10.1521/psyc.64.4.319.18602

Rector, N. A., Beck, A. T., & Stolar, N. (2005). The negative symptoms of schizophrenia: A cognitive perspective. *Canadian Journal of Psychiatry*, *50*(5), 247–257. https://doi.org/10.1177/070674370505000503

Reed, G. L., & Enright, R. D. (2006). The effects of forgiveness therapy on depression, anxiety, and posttraumatic stress for women after spousal emotional abuse. *Journal of Consulting and Clinical Psychology*, *74*(5), 920–929. https://doi.org/10.1037/0022-006X.74.5.920

Resick, P. A., Bovin, M. J., Calloway, A. L., Dick, A. M., King, M. W., Mitchell, K. S., Suvak, M. K., Wells, S. Y., Stirman, S. W., & Wolf, E. J. (2012). A critical evaluation of the complex PTSD literature: Implications for *DSM-5*. *Journal of Traumatic Stress*, *25*(3), 241–251. https://doi.org/10.1002/jts.21699

Resick, P. A., Galovski, T. E., Uhlmansiek, M. O., Scher, C. D., Clum, G. A., & Young-Xu, Y. (2008). A randomized clinical trial to dismantle components of cognitive processing therapy for posttraumatic stress disorder in female victims of interpersonal violence. *Journal of Consulting and Clinical Psychology*, *76*(2), 243–258. https://doi.org/10.1037/0022-006X.76.2.243

Resick, P. A., Monson, C. M., & Chard, K. M. (2024). *Cognitive processing therapy for PTSD: A comprehensive manual* (2nd ed.). Guilford Press.

Resick, P. A., Nishith, P., Weaver, T. L., Astin, M. C., & Feuer, C. A. (2002). A comparison of cognitive-processing therapy with prolonged exposure and a waiting condition for the treatment of chronic posttraumatic stress disorder in female rape victims. *Journal of Consulting and Clinical Psychology*, *70*(4), 867–879. https://doi.org/10.1037/0022-006X.70.4.867

Resnick, S. G., Bond, G. R., & Mueser, K. T. (2003). Trauma and posttraumatic stress disorder in people with schizophrenia. *Journal of Abnormal Psychology*, *112*(3), 415–423. https://doi.org/10.1037/0021-843X.112.3.415

Roberts, N. P., Kitchiner, N. J., Lewis, C. E., Downes, A. J., & Bisson, J. I. (2021). Psychometric properties of the PTSD Checklist for *DSM-5* in a sample of trauma exposed mental health service users. *European Journal of Psychotraumatology*, *12*(1), Article 1863578. https://doi.org/10.1080/20008198.2020.1863578

Rodrigues, R., & Anderson, K. K. (2017). The traumatic experience of first-episode psychosis: A systematic review and meta-analysis. *Schizophrenia Research*, *189*, 27–36. https://doi.org/10.1016/j.schres.2017.01.045

Roe, D., & Chopra, M. (2003). Beyond coping with mental illness: Toward personal growth. *American Journal of Orthopsychiatry*, *73*(3), 334–344. https://doi.org/10.1037/0002-9432.73.3.334

Roe, D., & Davidson, L. (2005). Self and narrative in schizophrenia: Time to author a new story. *Medical Humanities, 31*(2), 89–94. https://doi.org/10.1136/jmh.2005.000214

Ronconi, J. M., Shiner, B., & Watts, B. V. (2015). A meta-analysis of depressive symptom outcomes in randomized, controlled trials for PTSD. *Journal of Nervous and Mental Disease, 203*(7), 522–529. https://doi.org/10.1097/NMD.0000000000000322

Rosen, A. J., Sussman, S., Mueser, K. T., Lyons, J. S., & Davis, J. M. (1981). Behavioral assessment of psychiatric inpatients and normal controls across different environmental contexts. *Journal of Behavioral Assessment, 3*(1), 25–36. https://doi.org/10.1007/BF01321349

Rosenberg, S. D., Lu, W., Mueser, K. T., Jankowski, M. K., & Cournos, F. (2007). Correlates of adverse childhood events among adults with schizophrenia spectrum disorders. *Psychiatric Services, 58*(2), 245–253. https://doi.org/10.1176/ps.2007.58.2.245

Rosenberg, S. D., Mueser, K. T., Jankowski, M. K., Salyers, M. P., & Acker, K. (2004). Cognitive-behavioral treatment of posttraumatic stress disorder in severe mental illness: Results of a pilot study. *American Journal of Psychiatric Rehabilitation, 7*(2), 171–186. https://doi.org/10.1080/15487760490476200

Rosenfield, P. J., Jiang, D., & Pauselli, L. (2022). Childhood adversity and psychotic disorders: Epidemiological evidence, theoretical models and clinical considerations. *Schizophrenia Research, 247*, 55–66. https://doi.org/10.1016/j.schres.2021.06.005

Roy, L., Crocker, A. G., Nicholls, T. L., Latimer, E. A., & Ayllon, A. R. (2014). Criminal behavior and victimization among homeless individuals with severe mental illness: A systematic review. *Psychiatric Services, 65*(6), 739–750. https://doi.org/10.1176/appi.ps.201200515

Russinova, Z., Bloch, P., Wewiorski, N., Shappell, H., & Rogers, E. S. (2018). Predictors of sustained employment among individuals with serious mental illness: Findings from a 5-year naturalistic longitudinal study. *Journal of Nervous and Mental Disease, 206*(9), 669–679. https://doi.org/10.1097/NMD.0000000000000876

Russinova, Z., Rogers, E. S., Ellison, M. L., & Lyass, A. (2011). Recovery-promoting professional competencies: Perspectives of mental health consumers, consumer–providers and providers. *Psychiatric Rehabilitation Journal, 34*(3), 177–185. https://doi.org/10.2975/34.3.2011.177.185

Ryder, A. L., Azcarate, P. M., & Cohen, B. E. (2018). PTSD and physical health. *Current Psychiatry Reports, 20*(12), Article 116. https://doi.org/10.1007/s11920-018-0977-9

Rygh, J. L., & Sanderson, W. C. (2004). *Treating generalized anxiety disorder: Evidence-based strategies, tools, and techniques.* Guilford Press.

Sacks, S. A., Schwartz, B., & Mueser, K. T. (2017). A pilot study of the trauma recovery group for veterans with post traumatic stress disorder and co-occurring serious mental illness. *Journal of Mental Health, 26*(3), 237–241. https://doi.org/10.1080/09638237.2016.1222057

Santayana, G. (1905). *The life of reason: Reason in common sense.* Scribners.

Sariaslan, A., Arseneault, L., Larsson, H., Lichtenstein, P., & Fazel, S. (2020). Risk of subjection to violence and perpetration of violence in persons with psychiatric disorders in Sweden. *JAMA Psychiatry, 77*(4), 359–367. https://doi.org/10.1001/jamapsychiatry.2019.4275

Sautter, F. J., Cornwell, J., Johnson, J. J., Wiley, J., & Faraone, S. V. (2002). Family history study of posttraumatic stress disorder with secondary psychotic symptoms. *The American Journal of Psychiatry, 159*(10), 1775–1777. https://doi.org/10.1176/appi.ajp.159.10.1775

Schäfer, I., Morgan, C., Demjaha, A., Morgan, K., Dazzan, P., Fearon, P., Jones, P. B., Doody, G. A., Leff, J., Murray, R. M., & Fisher, H. L. (2011). Assessment of posttraumatic symptoms in patients with first-episode psychosis. *Journal of Nervous and Mental Disease, 199*(11), 896–898. https://doi.org/10.1097/NMD.0b013e318234a037

Scheller-Gilkey, G., Moynes, K., Cooper, I., Kant, C., & Miller, A. H. (2004). Early life stress and PTSD symptoms in patients with comorbid schizophrenia and substance abuse. *Schizophrenia Research, 69*(2–3), 167–174. https://doi.org/10.1016/S0920-9964(03)00188-9

Schmidt, S. J., Schultze-Lutter, F., Bendall, S., Groth, N., Michel, C., Inderbitzin, N., Schimmelmann, B. G., Hubl, D., & Nelson, B. (2017). Mediators linking childhood adversities and trauma to suicidality in individuals at risk for psychosis. *Frontiers in Psychiatry, 8*, Article 242. https://doi.org/10.3389/fpsyt.2017.00242

Schnurr, P. P., Vielhauer, M. J., Weathers, F., & Findler, M. (1999). *The Brief Trauma Questionnaire*. National Center for PTSD.

Seedat, S., Stein, M. B., Oosthuizen, P. P., Emsley, R. A., & Stein, D. J. (2003). Linking posttraumatic stress disorder and psychosis: A look at epidemiology, phenomenology, and treatment. *Journal of Nervous and Mental Disease, 191*(10), 675–681. https://doi.org/10.1097/01.nmd.0000092177.97317.26

Segal, Z. V., Williams, J. M. G., & Teasdale, J. D. (2002). *Mindfulness-based cognitive therapy for depression*. Guilford Press.

Seow, L. S. E., Ong, C., Mahesh, M. V., Sagayadevan, V., Shafie, S., Chong, S. A., & Subramaniam, M. (2016). A systematic review on comorbid post-traumatic stress disorder in schizophrenia. *Schizophrenia Research, 176*(2–3), 441–451. https://doi.org/10.1016/j.schres.2016.05.004

Shah, R., Shah, A., & Links, P. (2012). Post-traumatic stress disorder and depression comorbidity: Severity across different populations. *Neuropsychiatry, 2*(6), 521–526. https://doi.org/10.2217/npy.12.56

Shaner, A., & Eth, S. (1989). Can schizophrenia cause posttraumatic stress disorder? *American Journal of Psychotherapy, 43*(4), 588–597. https://doi.org/10.1176/appi.psychotherapy.1989.43.4.588

Shapiro, F. (2017). *Eye movement desensitization and reprocessing: Basic principles, protocols, and procedures* (3rd ed.). Guilford Press.

Sheffield, J. M., Karcher, N. R., & Barch, D. M. (2018). Cognitive deficits in psychotic disorders: A lifespan perspective. *Neuropsychology Review, 28*(4), 509–533. https://doi.org/10.1007/s11065-018-9388-2

Sherrer, M. V. (2011). The role of cognitive appraisal in adaptation to traumatic stress in adults with serious mental illness: A critical review. *Trauma, Violence & Abuse, 12*(3), 151–167. https://doi.org/10.1177/1524838011404254

Shevlin, M., Armour, C., Murphy, J., Houston, J. E., & Adamson, G. (2011). Evidence for a psychotic posttraumatic stress disorder subtype based on the National Comorbidity Survey. *Social Psychiatry and Psychiatric Epidemiology, 46*(11), 1069–1078. https://doi.org/10.1007/s00127-010-0281-4

Sin, G. L., Abdin, E., & Lee, J. (2012). The PSS-SR as a screening tool for PTSD in first-episode psychosis patients. *Early Intervention in Psychiatry, 6*(2), 191–194. https://doi.org/10.1111/j.1751-7893.2011.00327.x

Sin, G. L., Abdin, E., Lee, J., Poon, L. Y., Verma, S., & Chong, S. A. (2010). Prevalence of post-traumatic stress disorder in first-episode psychosis. *Early Intervention in Psychiatry, 4*(4), 299–304. https://doi.org/10.1111/j.1751-7893.2010.00199.x

Sin, J., & Spain, D. (2016). Psychological interventions for trauma in individuals who have psychosis: A systematic review and meta-analysis. *Psychosis, 9*(1), 67–81. https://doi.org/10.1080/17522439.2016.1167946

Slade, M. (2009). *Personal recovery and mental illness: A guide for mental health professionals.* Cambridge University Press. https://doi.org/10.1017/CBO9780511581649

Slade, E. P., Gottlieb, J. D., Lu, W., Yanos, P. T., Rosenberg, S., Silverstein, S. M., Minsky, S. K., & Mueser, K. T. (2017). Cost-effectiveness of a PTSD intervention tailored for individuals with severe mental illness. *Psychiatric Services, 68*(12), 1225–1231. https://doi.org/10.1176/appi.ps.201600474

Slade, M., Bird, V., Clarke, E., Le Boutillier, C., McCrone, P., Macpherson, R., Pesola, F., Wallace, G., Williams, J., & Leamy, M. (2015). Supporting recovery in patients with psychosis through care by community-based adult mental health teams (REFOCUS): A multisite, cluster, randomised, controlled trial. *The Lancet Psychiatry, 2*(6), 503–514. https://doi.org/10.1016/S2215-0366(15)00086-3

Smucker, M. R., Grunert, B. K., & Weis, J. M. (2003). Posttraumatic stress disorder: A new algorithm treatment model. In R. L. Leahy (Ed.), *Roadblocks in cognitive-behavioral therapy: Transforming challenges into opportunities for change* (pp. 175–194). Guilford Press.

Sobell, M. B., & Sobell, L. C. (2000). Stepped care as a heuristic approach to the treatment of alcohol problems. *Journal of Consulting and Clinical Psychology, 68*(4), 573–579. https://doi.org/10.1037/0022-006X.68.4.573

Solomon, P., Draine, J., & Delaney, M. A. (1995). The working alliance and consumer case management. *Journal of Mental Health Administration, 22*(2), 126–134. https://doi.org/10.1007/BF02518753

Spinazzola, J., Blaustein, M., & van der Kolk, B. A. (2005). Posttraumatic stress disorder treatment outcome research: The study of unrepresentative samples? *Journal of Traumatic Stress, 18*(5), 425–436. https://doi.org/10.1002/jts.20050

Srivastava, A., Miller, A. N., Tai, M.-H., Coles, M. S., Brigham, R., Peterson, E. R., Kreida, E., Mueser, K. T., & Ng, L. C. (2022). Development of a primary care intervention for PTSD in adolescents. *Clinical Practice in Pediatric Psychology, 10*(1), 54–65. https://doi.org/10.1037/cpp0000382

Stanovich, K. E. (2019). *How to think straight about psychology* (11th ed.). Pearson.

Steel, C., Haddock, G., Tarrier, N., Picken, A., & Barrowclough, C. (2011). Auditory hallucinations and posttraumatic stress disorder within schizophrenia and substance abuse. *Journal of Nervous and Mental Disease, 199*(9), 709–711. https://doi.org/10.1097/NMD.0b013e318229d6e8

Steel, C., Hardy, A., Smith, B., Wykes, T., Rose, S., Enright, S., Hardcastle, M., Landau, S., Baksh, M. F., Gottlieb, J. D., Rose, D., & Mueser, K. T. (2017). Cognitive-behaviour therapy for post-traumatic stress in schizophrenia. A randomized controlled trial. *Psychological Medicine, 47*(1), 43–51. https://doi.org/10.1017/S0033291716002117

Stein, L. I., & Santos, A. B. (1998). *Assertive community treatment of persons with severe mental illness*. W.W. Norton.

Stein, M. B., Walker, J. R., & Forde, D. R. (2000). Gender differences in susceptibility to posttraumatic stress disorder. *Behaviour Research and Therapy, 38*(6), 619–628. https://doi.org/10.1016/S0005-7967(99)00098-4

Steinert, T., Schmid, P., & Bergbauer, G. (2006). History of trauma in people with schizophrenia predicts need for seclusion and restraint. *The Journal of Clinical Psychiatry, 67*(6), Article 995. https://doi.org/10.4088/JCP.v67n0619a

Straus, J. H., & Sarvet, B. (2014). Behavioral health care for children: The Massachusetts Child Psychiatry Access Project. *Health Affairs, 33*(12), 2153–2161. https://doi.org/10.1377/hlthaff.2014.0896

Strauss, G. P., Duke, L. A., Ross, S. A., & Allen, D. N. (2011). Posttraumatic stress disorder and negative symptoms of schizophrenia. *Schizophrenia Bulletin, 37*(3), 603–610. https://doi.org/10.1093/schbul/sbp122

Strauss, J. L., Calhoun, P. S., Marx, C. E., Stechuchak, K. M., Oddone, E. Z., Swartz, M. S., & Butterfield, M. I. (2006). Comorbid posttraumatic stress disorder is associated with suicidality in male veterans with schizophrenia or schizo-affective disorder. *Schizophrenia Research, 84*(1), 165–169. https://doi.org/10.1016/j.schres.2006.02.010

Street, A. E., Gibson, L. E., & Holohan, D. R. (2005). Impact of childhood traumatic events, trauma-related guilt, and avoidant coping strategies on PTSD symptoms in female survivors of domestic violence. *Journal of Traumatic Stress, 18*(3), 245–252. https://doi.org/10.1002/jts.20026

Suarez, R., Mills, R. C., & Stewart, D. G. (1987). *Sanity, insanity, and common sense: The groundbreaking new approach to happiness*. Fawcett Columbine.

Subica, A. M., Claypoole, K. H., & Wylie, A. M. (2011). PTSD's mediation of the relationships between trauma, depression, substance abuse, mental health, and physical health in individuals with severe mental illness: Evaluating a comprehensive model. *Schizophrenia Research, 136*(1), 104–109. https://doi.org/10.1016/j.schres.2011.10.018

Substance Abuse and Mental Health Services Administration. (2012). *SAMHSA's working definition of recovery*. Center for Mental Health Services, Substance Abuse and Mental Health Services Administration, U.S. Department of Health and Human Services. https://store.samhsa.gov/sites/default/files/pep12-recdef.pdf

Substance Abuse and Mental Health Services Administration. (2017). *Mental and substance use disorders*. https://www.samhsa.gov/disorders

Switzer, G. E., Dew, M. A., Thompson, K., Goycoolea, J. M., Derricott, T., & Mullins, S. D. (1999). Posttraumatic stress disorder and service utilization among urban mental health center clients. *Journal of Traumatic Stress, 12*(1), 25–39. https://doi.org/10.1023/A:1024738114428

Tarrier, N., Khan, S., Cater, J., & Picken, A. (2007). The subjective consequences of suffering a first episode psychosis: Trauma and suicide behaviour. *Social Psychiatry and Psychiatric Epidemiology, 42*(1), 29–35. https://doi.org/10.1007/s00127-006-0127-2

Tarrier, N., & Sommerfield, C. (2004). Treatment of chronic PTSD by cognitive therapy with exposure: 5-year follow-up. *Behavior Therapy, 35*(2), 231–246. https://doi.org/10.1016/S0005-7894(04)80037-6

Teplin, L. A., McClelland, G. M., Abram, K. M., & Weiner, D. A. (2005). Crime victimization in adults with severe mental illness: Comparison with the National

Crime Victimization Survey. *Archives of General Psychiatry, 62*(8), 911–921. https://doi.org/10.1001/archpsyc.62.8.911

Tomassi, S., Tosato, S., Mondelli, V., Faravelli, C., Lasalvia, A., Fioravanti, G., Bonetto, C., Fioritti, A., Cremonese, C., Lo Parrino, R., De Santi, K., Meneghelli, A., Torresani, S., De Girolamo, G., Semrov, E., Pratelli, M., Cristofalo, D., Ruggeri, M., & the GET UP Group. (2017). Influence of childhood trauma on diagnosis and substance use in first-episode psychosis. *The British Journal of Psychiatry, 211*(3), 151–156. https://doi.org/10.1192/bjp.bp.116.194019

van den Berg, D. P. G., de Bont, P. A. J. M., van der Vleugel, B. M., de Roos, C., de Jongh, A., van Minnen, A., & van der Gaag, M. (2015). Prolonged exposure versus eye movement desensitization and reprocessing versus waiting list for posttraumatic stress disorder in patients with a psychotic disorder. *JAMA Psychiatry, 72*(3), 259–267. https://doi.org/10.1001/jamapsychiatry.2014.2637

van den Berg, D. P. G., de Bont, P. A. J. M., van der Vleugel, B. M., de Roos, C., de Jongh, A., van Minnen, A., & van der Gaag, M. (2016). Trauma-focused treatment in PTSD patients with psychosis: Symptom exacerbation, adverse events, and revictimization. *Schizophrenia Bulletin, 42*(3), 693–702. https://doi.org/10.1093/schbul/sbv172

van den Berg, D. P. G., & van der Gaag, M. (2012). Treating trauma in psychosis with EMDR: A pilot study. *Behavior Therapy and Experimental Psychiatry, 43*(1), 664–671. https://doi.org/10.1016/j.jbtep.2011.09.011

van't Veer-Tazelaar, P. J., van Marwijk, H. W., van Oppen, P., van Hout, H. P., van der Horst, H. E., Cuijpers, P., Smit, F., & Beekman, A. T. (2009). Stepped-care prevention of anxiety and depression in late life: A randomized controlled trial. *Archives of General Psychiatry, 66*(3), 297–304. https://doi.org/10.1001/archgenpsychiatry.2008.555

van Zyl, M., Oosthuizen, P. P., & Seedat, S. (2008). Post traumatic stress disorder: Undiagnosed cases in a tertiary inpatient setting. *African Journal of Psychiatry, 11*(2), 119–122. https://doi.org/10.4314/ajpsy.v11i2.30263

Varese, F., Smeets, F., Drukker, M., Lieverse, R., Lataster, T., Viechtbauer, W., Read, J., van Os, J., & Bentall, R. P. (2012). Childhood adversities increase the risk of psychosis: A meta-analysis of patient–control, prospective- and cross-sectional cohort studies. *Schizophrenia Bulletin, 38*(4), 661–671. https://doi.org/10.1093/schbul/sbs050

Waldfogel, S., & Mueser, K. T. (1988). Another case of chronic PTSD with auditory hallucinations. *The American Journal of Psychiatry, 145*(10), 1314–1314. https://doi.org/10.1176/ajp.145.10.1314b

Wason, P. C. (1960). On the failure to eliminate hypotheses in a conceptual task. *The Quarterly Journal of Experimental Psychology, 12*(3), 129–140. https://doi.org/10.1080/17470216008416717

Watts, B. V., Schnurr, P. P., Mayo, L., Young-Xu, Y., Weeks, W. B., & Friedman, M. J. (2013). Meta-analysis of the efficacy of treatments for posttraumatic stress disorder. *The Journal of Clinical Psychiatry, 74*(6), e541–e550. https://doi.org/10.4088/JCP.12r08225

Weathers, F. W., Bovin, M. J., Lee, D. J., Sloan, D. M., Schnurr, P. P., Kaloupek, D. G., Keane, T. M., & Marx, B. P. (2018). The Clinician-Administered PTSD Scale for *DSM-5* (CAPS-5): Development and initial psychometric evaluation in military veterans. *Psychological Assessment, 30*(3), 383–395. https://doi.org/10.1037/pas0000486

Weathers, F. W., Litz, B., Keane, T. M., Marx, B. P., & Schnurr, P. (2013). *PTSD Checklist for DSM-5 (PCL-5)*. National Center for PTSD.

Weinberg, M., & Gil, S. (2016). Trauma as an objective or subjective experience: The association between types of traumatic events, personality traits, subjective experience of the event, and posttraumatic symptoms. *Journal of Loss and Trauma, 21*(2), 137–146. https://doi.org/10.1080/15325024.2015.1011986

Weinberg, M., Harel, H., Shamani, M., Or-Chen, K., Ron, P., & Gil, S. (2017). War and well-being: The association between forgiveness, social support, posttraumatic stress disorder, and well-being during and after war. *Social Work, 62*(4), 341–348. https://doi.org/10.1093/sw/swx043

Wells, A. (2009). *Metacognitive therapy for anxiety and depression*. Guilford Press.

Wells, R., Jacomb, I., Swaminathan, V., Sundram, S., Weinberg, D., Bruggemann, J., Cropley, V., Lenroot, R. K., Pereira, A. M., Zalesky, A., Bousman, C., Pantelis, C., Weickert, C. S., & Weickert, T. W. (2020). The impact of childhood adversity on cognitive development in schizophrenia. *Schizophrenia Bulletin, 46*(1), 140–153. https://doi.org/10.1093/schbul/sbz033

Wells, S. Y., Morland, L. A., Torres, E. M., Kloezeman, K., Mackintosh, M. A., & Aarons, G. A. (2019). The development of a brief version of the Posttraumatic Cognitions Inventory (PTCI-9). *Assessment, 26*(2), 193–208. https://doi.org/10.1177/1073191116685401

Wigham, S., & Emerson, E. (2015). Trauma and life events in adults with intellectual disability. *Current Developmental Disorders Reports, 2*(2), 93–99. https://doi.org/10.1007/s40474-015-0041-y

Williamson, J. B., Porges, E. C., Lamb, D. G., & Porges, S. W. (2015). Maladaptive autonomic regulation in PTSD accelerates physiological aging. *Frontiers in Psychology, 5*, Article 1571. https://doi.org/10.3389/fpsyg.2014.01571

Wilson, A. E., Calhoun, K. S., & Bernat, J. A. (1999). Risk recognition and trauma-related symptoms among sexually revictimized women. *Journal of Consulting and Clinical Psychology, 67*(5), 705–710. https://doi.org/10.1037/0022-006X.67.5.705

Wolf, E. J., Miller, M. W., Kilpatrick, D., Resnick, H. S., Badour, C. L., Marx, B. P., Keane, T. M., Rosen, R. C., Friedman, M. J., & Friedman, M. J. (2015). *ICD-11* complex PTSD in U.S. national and veteran samples: Prevalence and structural associations with PTSD. *Clinical Psychological Science, 3*(2), 215–229. https://doi.org/10.1177/2167702614545480

Wolford, G., Rosenberg, S. D., Rosenberg, H. J., Swartz, M. S., Butterfield, M. I., Swanson, J. W., & Jankowski, M. K. (2008). A clinical trial comparing interviewer and computer-assisted assessment among clients with severe mental illness. *Psychiatric Services, 59*(7), 769–775. https://doi.org/10.1176/ps.2008.59.7.769

Wong, S. E., Terranova, M. D., Bowen, L., Zarate, R., Massel, H. K., & Liberman, R. P. (1987). Providing independent recreational activities to reduce stereotypic vocalizations in chronic schizophrenics. *Journal of Applied Behavior Analysis, 20*(1), 77–81. https://doi.org/10.1901/jaba.1987.20-77

World Health Organization. (2019). *International statistical classification of diseases and related health problems* (11th ed.). https//icd.who.int

Yanchus, N. J., Periard, D., & Osatuke, K. (2017). Further examination of predictors of turnover intention among mental health professionals. *Journal of Psychiatric and Mental Health Nursing, 24*(1), 41–56. https://doi.org/10.1111/jpm.12354

Yanos, P. T., Roe, D., & Lysaker, P. H. (2011). Narrative enhancement and cognitive therapy: A new group-based treatment for internalized stigma among persons with severe mental illness. *International Journal of Group Psychotherapy, 61*(4), 577–595. https://doi.org/10.1521/ijgp.2011.61.4.576

Zammit, S., Lewis, C., Dawson, S., Colley, H., McCann, H., Piekarski, A., Rockliff, H., & Bisson, J. (2018). Undetected post-traumatic stress disorder in secondary-care mental health services: Systematic review. *The British Journal of Psychiatry, 212*(1), 11–18. https://doi.org/10.1192/bjp.2017.8

Zanarini, M. C., Athanasiadi, A., Temes, C. M., Magni, L. R., Hein, K. E., Fitzmaurice, G. M., Aguirre, B. A., & Goodman, M. (2021). Symptomatic disorders in adults and adolescents with borderline personality disorder. *Journal of Personality Disorders, 35*(Suppl. B), 48–55. https://doi.org/10.1521/pedi_2021_35_502

Zanarini, M. C., Frankenburg, F. R., Dubo, E. D., Sickel, A. E., Trikha, A., Levin, A., & Reynolds, V. (1998). Axis I comorbidity of borderline personality disorder. *The American Journal of Psychiatry, 155*(12), 1733–1739. https://doi.org/10.1176/ajp. 155.12.1733

Zatzick, D., Rivara, F., Jurkovich, G., Russo, J., Trusz, S. G., Wang, J., Wagner, A., Stephens, K., Dunn, C., Uehara, E., Petrie, M., Engel, C., Davydow, D., & Katon, W. (2011). Enhancing the population impact of collaborative care interventions: Mixed method development and implementation of stepped care targeting posttraumatic stress disorder and related comorbidities after acute trauma. *General Hospital Psychiatry, 33*(2), 123–134. https://doi.org/10.1016/j. genhosppsych.2011.01.001

Zeifman, R. J., Landy, M. S. H., Liebman, R. E., Fitzpatrick, S., & Monson, C. M. (2021). Optimizing treatment for comorbid borderline personality disorder and posttraumatic stress disorder: A systematic review of psychotherapeutic approaches and treatment efficacy. *Clinical Psychology Review, 86*, Article 102030. https://doi.org/10.1016/j.cpr.2021.102030

Zimmerman, M., & Mattia, J. I. (1999). Psychiatric diagnosis in clinical practice: Is comorbidity being missed? *Comprehensive Psychiatry, 40*(3), 182–191. https://doi.org/10.1016/S0010-440X(99)90001-9

Zlotnick, C., Johnson, D. M., Yen, S., Battle, C. L., Sanislow, C. A., Skodol, A. E., Grilo, C. M., McGlashan, T. H., Gunderson, J. G., Bender, D. S., Zanarini, M. C., & Shea, M. T. (2003). Clinical features and impairment in women with borderline personality disorder (BPD) with posttraumatic stress disorder (PTSD), BPD without PTSD, and other personality disorders with PTSD. *Journal of Nervous and Mental Disease, 191*(11), 706–713. https://doi.org/10.1097/01.nmd.0000095122. 29476.ff

Zlotnick, C., Rodriguez, B. F., Weisberg, R. B., Bruce, S. E., Spencer, M. A., Culpepper, L., & Keller, M. B. (2004). Chronicity in posttraumatic stress disorder and predictors of the course of posttraumatic stress disorder among primary care patients. *Journal of Nervous and Mental Disease, 192*(2), 153–159. https://doi.org/10. 1097/01.nmd.0000110287.16635.8e

Zubin, J., & Spring, B. (1977). Vulnerability: A new view of schizophrenia. *Journal of Abnormal Psychology, 86*(2), 103–126. https://doi.org/10.1037/0021-843X.86.2.103

Zuehlke, J. B., Kotecki, R. M., Kern, S., Sholty, G., & Hauser, P. (2016). Transformation to a recovery-oriented model of care on a veterans administration inpatient unit. *Psychiatric Rehabilitation Journal, 39*(4), 361–363. https://doi.org/10.1037/prj0000198

INDEX

NOTE: Page numbers followed by e, f, and t denote exhibits, figures, and tables, respectively. Page numbers with prefix A denote the Appendix.

ABOUT THE AUTHORS

Kim T. Mueser, PhD, is a professor in the Department of Occupational Therapy and Department of Psychological and Brain Sciences at Boston University. He has published over 400 peer-reviewed articles, 100 book chapters, and 15 books primarily on psychosocial treatments for serious mental illness and has given numerous conference presentations, workshops, and invited lectures in the United States and abroad. Dr. Mueser began adapting empirically supported treatment methods for posttraumatic stress disorder (PTSD) in the general population to the serious mental illness population in the late 1990s, which resulted in the first standardization and feasibility testing of the Cognitive Restructuring for PTSD program in the early 2000s, followed by randomized controlled trials evaluating the program.

Jennifer D. Gottlieb, PhD, is a diplomate in the Academy of Cognitive and Behavioral Therapies whose work has been dedicated to the development, evaluation, and implementation of effective psychotherapeutic interventions for persons with severe psychiatric conditions. She is a founding member and former president of the North America CBT for Psychosis Network (NACBTpN) and is affiliated with the Cambridge Health Alliance/Harvard Medical School Department of Psychiatry. In addition to numerous publications and presentations related to cognitive behavioral therapies for psychosis and other serious mental illness, Dr. Gottlieb has focused on the Cognitive Restructuring for PTSD intervention for over 18 years, as both a coinvestigator and a program development consultant. She has provided extensive workshop training, clinical supervision, and treatment fidelity evaluation to hundreds of clinicians and has worked with multiple mental health agencies, nationally and internationally, to implement and sustain this intervention (https://www.jennifergottliebphd.com).